PULMONARY EMBOLISM

LUNG BIOLOGY IN HEALTH AND DISEASE

Executive Editor

Claude Lenfant
Director, National Heart, Lung and Blood Institute
National Institutes of Health
Bethesda, Maryland

1. Immunologic and Infectious Reactions in the Lung, *edited by Charles H. Kirkpatrick and Herbert Y. Reynolds*
2. The Biochemical Basis of Pulmonary Function, *edited by Ronald G. Crystal*
3. Bioengineering Aspects of the Lung, *edited by John B. West*
4. Metabolic Functions of the Lung, *edited by Y. S. Bakhle and John R. Vane*
5. Respiratory Defense Mechanisms (in two parts), *edited by Joseph D. Brain, Donald F. Proctor, and Lynne M. Reid*
6. Development of the Lung, *edited by W. Alan Hodson*
7. Lung Water and Solute Exchange, *edited by Norman C. Staub*
8. Extrapulmonary Manifestations of Respiratory Disease, *edited by Eugene Debs Robin*
9. Chronic Obstructive Pulmonary Disease, *edited by Thomas L. Petty*
10. Pathogenesis and Therapy of Lung Cancer, *edited by Curtis C. Harris*
11. Genetic Determinants of Pulmonary Disease, *edited by Stephen D. Litwin*
12. The Lung in the Transition Between Health and Disease, *edited by Peter T. Macklem and Solbert Permutt*
13. Evolution of Respiratory Processes: A Comparative Approach, *edited by Stephen C. Wood and Claude Lenfant*
14. Pulmonary Vascular Diseases, *edited by Kenneth M. Moser*
15. Physiology and Pharmacology of the Airways, *edited by Jay A. Nadel*
16. Diagnostic Techniques in Pulmonary Disease (in two parts), *edited by Marvin A. Sackner*
17. Regulation of Breathing (in two parts), *edited by Thomas F. Hornbein*
18. Occupational Lung Diseases: Research Approaches and Methods, *edited by Hans Weill and Margaret Turner-Warwick*
19. Immunopharmacology of the Lung, *edited by Harold H. Newball*
20. Sarcoidosis and Other Granulomatous Diseases of the Lung, *edited by Barry L. Fanburg*
21. Sleep and Breathing, *edited by Nicholas A. Saunders and Colin E. Sullivan*
22. *Pneumocystis carinii* Pneumonia: Pathogenesis, Diagnosis, and Treatment, *edited by Lowell S. Young*

23. Pulmonary Nuclear Medicine: Techniques in Diagnosis of Lung Disease, *edited by Harold L. Atkins*
24. Acute Respiratory Failure, *edited by Warren M. Zapol and Konrad J. Falke*
25. Gas Mixing and Distribution in the Lung, *edited by Ludwig A. Engel and Manuel Paiva*
26. High-Frequency Ventilation in Intensive Care and During Surgery, *edited by Graziano Carlon and William S. Howland*
27. Pulmonary Development: Transition from Intrauterine to Extrauterine Life, *edited by George H. Nelson*
28. Chronic Obstructive Pulmonary Disease: Second Edition, Revised and Expanded, *edited by Thomas L. Petty*
29. The Thorax (in two parts), *edited by Charis Roussos and Peter T. Macklem*
30. The Pleura in Health and Disease, *edited by Jacques Chrétien, Jean Bignon, and Albert Hirsch*
31. Drug Therapy for Asthma: Research and Clinical Practice, *edited by John W. Jenne and Shirley Murphy*
32. Pulmonary Endothelium in Health and Disease, *edited by Una S. Ryan*
33. The Airways: Neural Control in Health and Disease, *edited by Michael A. Kaliner and Peter J. Barnes*
34. Pathophysiology and Treatment of Inhalation Injuries, *edited by Jacob Loke*
35. Respiratory Function of the Upper Airway, *edited by Oommen P. Mathew and Giuseppe Sant'Ambrogio*
36. Chronic Obstructive Pulmonary Disease: A Behavioral Perspective, *edited by A. John McSweeny and Igor Grant*
37. Biology of Lung Cancer: Diagnosis and Treatment, *edited by Steven T. Rosen, James L. Mulshine, Frank Cuttitta, and Paul G. Abrams*
38. Pulmonary Vascular Physiology and Pathophysiology, *edited by E. Kenneth Weir and John T. Reeves*
39. Comparative Pulmonary Physiology: Current Concepts, *edited by Stephen C. Wood*
40. Respiratory Physiology: An Analytical Approach, *edited by H. K. Chang and Manuel Paiva*
41. Lung Cell Biology, *edited by Donald Massaro*
42. Heart–Lung Interactions in Health and Disease, *edited by Steven M. Scharf and Sharon S. Cassidy*
43. Clinical Epidemiology of Chronic Obstructive Pulmonary Disease, *edited by Michael J. Hensley and Nicholas A. Saunders*
44. Surgical Pathology of Lung Neoplasms, *edited by Alberto M. Marchevsky*
45. The Lung in Rheumatic Diseases, *edited by Grant W. Cannon and Guy A. Zimmerman*
46. Diagnostic Imaging of the Lung, *edited by Charles E. Putman*
47. Models of Lung Disease: Microscopy and Structural Methods, *edited by Joan Gil*

48. Electron Microscopy of the Lung, *edited by Dean E. Schraufnagel*
49. Asthma: Its Pathology and Treatment, *edited by Michael A. Kaliner, Peter J. Barnes, and Carl G. A. Persson*
50. Acute Respiratory Failure: Second Edition, *edited by Warren M. Zapol and Francois Lemaire*
51. Lung Disease in the Tropics, *edited by Om P. Sharma*
52. Exercise: Pulmonary Physiology and Pathophysiology, *edited by Brian J. Whipp and Karlman Wasserman*
53. Developmental Neurobiology of Breathing, *edited by Gabriel G. Haddad and Jay P. Farber*
54. Mediators of Pulmonary Inflammation, *edited by Michael A. Bray and Wayne H. Anderson*
55. The Airway Epithelium, *edited by Stephen G. Farmer and Douglas Hay*
56. Physiological Adaptations in Vertebrates: Respiration, Circulation, and Metabolism, *edited by Stephen C. Wood, Roy E. Weber, Alan R. Hargens, and Ronald W. Millard*
57. The Bronchial Circulation, *edited by John Butler*
58. Lung Cancer Differentiation: Implications for Diagnosis and Treatment, *edited by Samuel D. Bernal and Paul J. Hesketh*
59. Pulmonary Complications of Systemic Disease, *edited by John F. Murray*
60. Lung Vascular Injury: Molecular and Cellular Response, *edited by Arnold Johnson and Thomas J. Ferro*
61. Cytokines of the Lung, *edited by Jason Kelley*
62. The Mast Cell in Health and Disease, *edited by Michael A. Kaliner and Dean D. Metcalfe*
63. Pulmonary Disease in the Elderly Patient, *edited by Donald A. Mahler*
64. Cystic Fibrosis, *edited by Pamela B. Davis*
65. Signal Transduction in Lung Cells, *edited by Jerome S. Brody, David M. Center, and Vsevolod A. Tkachuk*
66. Tuberculosis: A Comprehensive International Approach, *edited by Lee B. Reichman and Earl S. Hershfield*
67. Pharmacology of the Respiratory Tract: Experimental and Clinical Research, *edited by K. Fan Chung and Peter J. Barnes*
68. Prevention of Respiratory Diseases, *edited by Albert Hirsch, Marcel Goldberg, Jean-Pierre Martin, and Roland Masse*
69. *Pneumocystis carinii* Pneumonia: Second Edition, Revised and Expanded, *edited by Peter D. Walzer*
70. Fluid and Solute Transport in the Airspaces of the Lungs, *edited by Richard M. Effros and H. K. Chang*
71. Sleep and Breathing: Second Edition, Revised and Expanded, *edited by Nicholas A. Saunders and Colin E. Sullivan*
72. Airway Secretion: Physiological Bases for the Control of Mucous Hypersecretion, *edited by Tamotsu Takishima and Sanae Shimura*
73. Sarcoidosis and Other Granulomatous Disorders, *edited by D. Geraint James*
74. Epidemiology of Lung Cancer, *edited by Jonathan M. Samet*

75. Pulmonary Embolism, *edited by Mario Morpurgo*

ADDITIONAL VOLUMES IN PREPARATION

Sports and Exercise Medicine, *edited by Stephen C. Wood and Robert C. Roach*

Endotoxin and the Lungs, *edited by Kenneth L. Brigham*

Regulation of Breathing: Second Edition, Revised and Expanded, *edited by Jerome A. Dempsey and Allan I. Pack*

The Mesothelial Cell and Mesothelioma, *edited by Jean Bignon and Marie-Claude Jaurand*

PULMONARY EMBOLISM

Edited by

Mario Morpurgo

San Carlo Borromeo Hospital
Milan, Italy

Marcel Dekker, Inc. **New York • Basel • Hong Kong**

Pulmonary embolism / edited by Mario Morpurgo.
p. cm. -- (Lung biology in health and disease; 75)
Includes bibliographical references and index.
ISBN 0-8247-9178-9 (alk. paper)
1. Pulmonary embolism. I. Morpurgo, M. II. Series: Lung biology in health and disease; v. 75.
[DNLM: 1. Pulmonary Embolism. W1 LU62 v.75 1994 / WG 420 P9875 1994]
RC776.P85P823 1994
616.2'49--dc20
DNLM/DLC
for Library of Congress 93-46951
CIP

The publisher offers discounts on this book when ordered in bulk quantities. For more information, write to Special Sales/Professional Marketing at the address below.

This book is printed on acid-free paper.

MARCEL DEKKER, INC.
270 Madison Avenue, New York, New York 10016

Current printing (last digit):
10 9 8 7 6 5 4 3 2 1

Printed in the United States of America

INTRODUCTION

> A thrombus having formed in some part of the venous system becomes detached, and, passing through the right cavities of the heart, blocks either the trunk of the pulmonary artery or one of its main branches or a secondary branch.
>
> *Fowler and Godler, 1898*

Simple, one could say! But, not so indeed. In their introduction to this volume, Drs. Brochier, Denolin, and Morpurgo provide the history of pulmonary embolism. It appears that Galen (2nd century A.D.) made reference to this condition. Yet, today it remains one of the most puzzling diseases, feared by physician and patient alike. But, at the same time, it is so preventable!

The villain is a blood clot.

The complexity of the blood clot was best illustrated by the great pathologist Julius Cohnheim who, in his *Lectures on General Pathology*, remarked, "Now, the vessels are not merely the channels for the blood, but are still more intimately related to it by reciprocity of action." This says it all. We are facing a truly complex interplay between two systems, the blood and the blood vessel. Whenever this relationship is disrupted, "the blood passes from the fluid into the solid state, it coagulates, a thrombosis occurs." Sometimes the clot stays wherever it formed. Other times it migrates upstream until it becomes lodged in distant vessels, usually those of the lungs, and then we have pulmonary embolism.

Simple? Well, it is not, because as yet the prodromal signs of pulmonary embolism are not uniformly recognized, and then, its cardinal signs are sometimes mistaken. For these reasons, the World Health Organization convened a group of experts to discuss this disease and what should be done about it. This volume on pulmonary embolism—epidemiology to prevention—owes its existence to the leadership of Dr. Mario Morpurgo. It presents a panoramic, yet detailed and comprehensive, approach to the problem. Schools of thought from many countries are represented. The international roster of authors illustrates very well that there are no borders in medicine and science. It took foresight and wisdom to gather the best-informed authors from around the world to structure this volume.

At the end, the question "Can we prevent pulmonary embolism?" is answered even in the face of high worldwide incidence and prevalence. The answer is that both primary and secondary prevention are possible and attainable. However, it is clear that to succeed we must apply what we know. Oh, surely many research questions are still in want of an answer, but at the same time we have learned a great deal since Galen! This volume gives the reader the means, and the opportunity, to apply what is known. There is no doubt that the readership and the patients will gain from this volume.

Dr. Morpurgo and his authors must be commended for making such an important contribution. Pulmonary embolism is an old problem, indeed, but one that needs continued attention and vision. This is what Dr. Morpurgo and his colleagues have given us.

Claude Lenfant, M.D.
Bethesda, Maryland

FOREWORD

Cardiovascular diseases are a major cause of preventable morbidity and premature mortality. Moreover, the human and economic costs are extremely high. They are not diseases of the developed world alone, but are of growing concern now and in the future for developing countries, especially as the major communicable diseases come increasingly under control.

The World Health Organization's (WHO) Constitution identifies as the ultimate objective of the Organization the attainment, by all peoples, of the highest possible level of health. One of the two main functions of WHO is directing and coordinating international health work. WHO's normative function is to standardize and harmonize the diagnosis, prophylaxis, and treatment of disease.

The International Society and Federation of Cardiology (ISFC), based in Geneva, Switzerland, is a close partner of WHO's special Cardiovascular Diseases Unit, and joint WHO/ISFC projects are continuously being carried out. ISFC membership consists of national societies of cardiology and heart foundations in 69 countries, and continental members covering the regions of Asia and the Pacific, Europe, the Americas, and Africa.

Nine scientific councils, composed of experts from all over the world, carry out multinational research projects and teaching and training seminars. They are involved in all aspects of cardiology, in clinical diagnosis and treatment, and basic research and prevention.

The objectives of the ISFC are, among others: to promote the study, prevention, and relief of cardiovascular diseases; to promote, coordinate, and assist scientific programs relating to cardiovascular problems; and to cooperate with other voluntary and official agencies with related interests.

The historical background of WHO/ISFC Task Forces covers 15 years of collaboration between the two organizations. The first report of a joint meeting was published in 1978 (1) and the last one in 1992 (2). In between, a series of WHO/ISFC Task Forces have been convened at regular intervals and their reports published in scientific journals.

The need for guidelines on pulmonary embolism was raised by the medical profession because necropsy studies revealed that 40% to 60% of patients die of pulmonary embolism due to incorrect diagnosis and treatment (3). Major hemorrhagic complications occurred in 10% to 15% of patients receiving anti-coagulant drugs, showing the importance of avoiding unnecessary and potentially harmful treatment of patients with no specific diagnosis.

The importance of the problem justified the WHO/ISFC Task Force Meeting on Pulmonary Embolism held in Geneva, Switzerland, in November 1991. WHO and ISFC selected the most distinguished scientists in the field to review the present state of the art of pulmonary embolism, including epidemiology, prevention, and clinical and research aspects of the problem, and also to provide recommendations for the medical profession on prevention, diagnosis and management of pulmonary embolism, and further research.

The participants of the meeting presented background papers which formed the basis for the discussion during the meeting, the report (2), and this monograph.

This monograph is an excellent scientific and practical basis for their everyday needs, but WHO and ISFC still owe health professionals guidelines on how to deal with the serious problem of pulmonary embolism at different health care levels and in various sociocultural and economic settings.

W. Rutishauser
Past-President
International Society and Federation of Cardiology
Geneva, Switzerland

Ivan Gyarfas
Chief, Cardiovascular Diseases Unit
World Health Organization
Geneva, Switzerland

References

1. WHO/ISFC Task Force on Cardiac Arrhythmias. Definition of terms related to cardiac rhythm. Amer Heart Journal 1978; 95:796–806.
2. WHO/ISFC Task Force on Pulmonary Embolism. Diagnosis, treatment and prevention of pulmonary embolism. JAMA 1992; 268:1727–1733.
3. Goldhaber SZ, et al. Factors associated with correct antemortem diagnosis of major pulmonary embolism. Amer Journ Med 1982; 73:822–826.

PREFACE

In recent years, pulmonary embolism and venous thrombosis were given ample discussion in scientific periodicals and textbooks. Notwithstanding, as tersely put by Moser and Fedullo (Chest 1983; 83:117), ". . . clinicians dealing with venous thromboembolism do not work *in the literature*—they work with specific patients, in specific facilities, with specific colleagues." Facilities, to begin with, are distressingly apt to vary from one place to another according to what we might call "local reality"—to which our Chapters 3 and 4 bear witness—or, in fact, reveal some unexpected situations. Besides, we must make a fundamental distinction between the physical presence of specific facilities and their actual utilization. In many places, indeed, the diagnostic (hence therapeutic) approach to a patient with possible pulmonary embolism may differ according to whether the patient is being admitted during a weekend, with only a skeleton staff on duty, or on a fully operative weekday. Curiously, also, many diagnostic algorithms so far proposed for pulmonary embolism begin with ventilation–perfusion scintigraphy, as if its equipment and skills were available everywhere, while even the simpler echocardiography, whose diagnostic usefulness in massive pulmonary embolism is documented in our Chapter 13, is not so readily feasible.

An unduly rigid mental frame and operational attitude may be at least partly responsible for impeded progress in terms of diagnostic indices over the last four decades, as explored in the recent study by Anderson and his associates (JAMA 1989; 261:1610). This appears all the more important if we consider that aging of patient populations, the increasing incidence of tumoral pathology, and other factors discussed in our Chapter 2 will confront tomorrow's physicians not only with greater numbers of venous thrombosis and pulmonary embolism candidates, but indeed with a heavier proportion of diagnostically difficult cases; hence the urgent need for broader, systematic preventive action, to which our book devotes three chapters.

Also in the field of pulmonary embolism, more markedly in some institutions and among younger physicians, clinical work seems to be dominated by increasingly complex technology. Of course, clinical observation alone does not afford foolproof diagnosis; hence the rational use of therapeutic measures, not always free of risk, is sometimes necessary. Yet, used intelligently, clinical observation goes a long way toward solving problems of differential diagnosis and referring patients promptly for scintiscanning (Chapter 12) or pulmonary angiography (Chapter 14). Such an attitude not only saves time and taxpayer's money but spares the patient needless risk and discomfort. So the respective authors aptly emphasize the often neglected value of clinical examination (Chapter 6), ECG (Chapter 7), and conventional roentgenography (Chapter 12).

The sections dealing with medical and surgical treatment cover not only the acute episode of pulmonary embolism but its subsequent time course all the way to the chronic phase of thromboembolic pulmonary hypertension, including such poorly defined territories as its anatomical substrates (Chapter 5) and modes of onset (Chapter 10).

As stated by Bosken and Lenfant, "There will undoubtedly be many exciting advances in our ability to diagnose and treat pulmonary embolism in the years ahead. However, none of that information will benefit patients unless it is widely disseminated throughout the medical community" (Meeting of the WHO/ISFC Task Force on Pulmonary Embolism, Geneva, 1991). I feel that in view of the multidisciplinary spread of the subject matter, this book will prove of value to physicians of different specialties, including surgeons, obstetricians and gynecologists, orthopedic surgeons, urologists, anaesthesiologists, internists, cardiologists, pneumologists, geriatricians, and, of course, general practitioners.

And now, also on behalf of my colleagues in the Steering Committee of the WHO/ISFC Task Force on Pulmonary Embolism, I take pleasure in extending special thanks to Dr. S. Z. Goldhaber, who first thought of assembling this book; to Dr. I. Gyarfas, Chief of WHO's Cardiovascular Branch, and Mrs. M. de Figueiredo, Secretary of the International Society and Federation of Cardiology, for their most valuable help in organization; and to the staff of Marcel Dekker, Inc., for their unstinting patience and dedication.

Mario Morpurgo

CONTRIBUTORS

William R. Auger, M.D. Assistant Professor of Medicine, Pulmonary and Critical Care Division, School of Medicine, University of California, San Diego, and UCSD Medical Center, San Diego, California

Henri Bounameaux, M.D. Chief, Division of Angiology and Hemostasis, Department of Medicine, University Hospital of Geneva, Geneva, Switzerland

Mireille L. Brochier, M.D., F.E.S.C., F.A.S.C. Emeritus Professor of Cardiology, Department of Cardiovascular Medicine, University of Tours, Tours, France

Richard N. Channick, M.D. Assistant Professor of Medicine, Pulmonary and Critical Care Division, School of Medicine, University of California, San Diego, and UCSD Medical Center, San Diego, California

Xian-Sheng Cheng, M.D. Professor of Cardiology and Chief, Cardiopulmonary Division, Fu Wai Hospital, Chinese Academy of Medical Sciences, Beijing, China

James E. Dalen, M.D. Vice Provost for Health Sciences, and Dean, College of Medicine, University of Arizona, Tucson, Arizona

Henri Denolin, M.D., F.E.S.C. Honorary Professor, Department of Cardiology, Hôpital Universitaire Saint-Pierre, Brussels, Belgium

Peter F. Fedullo, M.D. Associate Clinical Professor of Medicine, Pulmonary and Critical Care Division, School of Medicine, University of California, San Diego, and UCSD Medical Center, San Diego, California

François Feihl, M.D. Privat-Dozent, Agrégé, Institute of Pathophysiology, University Hospital (CHUV), Lausanne, Switzerland

Carlo Giuntini, M.D. Professor of Pulmonary Medicine, Respiratory Pathophysiology Unit, 2nd Medical Clinic, University of Pisa, Pisa, Italy

Samuel Z. Goldhaber, M.D. Associate Professor of Medicine, Harvard Medical School, and Cardiovascular Division, Brigham and Women's Hospital, Boston, Massachusetts

Stewart W. Jamieson, M.B., F.R.C.S. Professor and Head, Division of Cardiothoracic Surgery, School of Medicine, University of California, San Diego, and UCSD Medical Center, San Diego, California

V. V. Kakkar, M.B., B.S., F.R.C.S., F.R.C.S.E. Professor of Surgical Science, and Honorary Consultant Vascular Surgeon, National Heart and Lung Institute, Royal Brompton Hospital, Thrombosis Research Institute, London, England

Maurizio Marzegalli, M.D. Department of Cardiology, San Carlo Borromeo Hospital, Milan, Italy

Mario Morpurgo, M.D., F.E.S.C. Head, Department of Cardiology, San Carlo Borromeo Hospital, Milan, Italy

Kenneth M. Moser, M.D. Professor and Director, Pulmonary and Critical Care Division, School of Medicine, University of California, San Diego, and UCSD Medical Center, San Diego, California

Walinjom F. T. Muna, M.D., Ph.D. The University Center for Health Sciences and The General Hospital of Yaoundé, Yaoundé, Cameroon

Antonio Palla, M.D. Assistant Professor of Pulmonary Medicine, Respiratory Pathophysiology Unit, 2nd Medical Clinic, University of Pisa, Pisa, Italy

Claude H. Perret, M.D., F.C.C.M., F.C.C.P. Professor of Pathophysiology and Head of the Medical Intensive Care Service, Institute of Pathophysiology, University Hospital (CHUV), Lausanne, Switzerland

Robert C. Schlant, M.D. Professor of Medicine, Division of Cardiology, Emory University School of Medicine, Atlanta, Georgia

R. Sergysels Clinique de Pneumologie, Hôpital Universitaire Saint-Pierre, Brussels, Belgium

Adam Torbicki, M.D. Department of Hypertension and Angiology, Medical Academy, Warsaw, Poland

Makis J. Tsapogas, M.D., D.Sc., M.Ch., F.A.C.S., Ph.D.(Hon.), D.M.(Hon.) Professor of Vascular Diseases, State University of New York at Stony Brook, Stony Brook, Professor, Albany Medical College, Albany, New York, Hunterian Professor, Royal College of Surgeons of England, London, Honorary Professor, King's College School of Medicine and University of London, London, England, and Corresponding Member, Academy of Athens, Athens, Greece

Marc Verstraete, M.D., Ph.D., F.R.C.P.(Edin.), F.A.C.P.(Hon.) Professor of Medicine, Center for Molecular and Vascular Biology, University of Leuven, Leuven, Belgium

C. A. Wagenvoort, M.D. Emeritus Professor of Pathology and Honorary Consultant Pathologist, Department of Pathology, Erasmus University, Rotterdam, The Netherlands

Qi Wang, M.D. Professor and Chief of Cardiology, Wu Jing General Hospital, Beijing, China

Jiří Widimský, M.D. Department of Cardiology, Postgraduate Medical Institute, Prague, Czech Republic

CONTENTS

1

Introduction

MIREILLE L. BROCHIER

University of Tours
Tours, France

HENRI DENOLIN

Hôpital Universitaire Saint-Pierre
Brussels, Belgium

MARIO MORPURGO

San Carlo Borromeo Hospital
Milan, Italy

An indirect reference to the disorders this book will deal with may be found in Galen (second century A.D.): "In asthmatic patients when the amount of inspired air does not match the size of the rib cage, an infarct of the pulmonary vessels is very likely . . . " (quoted by Luzzatto [1]). However, the first direct reference to pulmonary embolism and infarction probably is in the work by Laennec (2), "De l'auscultation médiate ou Traité du diagnostic des maladies des poumons et du coeur," where he deals with "pulmonary apoplexy." "The disease I call by this name," wrote Laennec in 1819, "is very common, but nevertheless its features are almost unknown. On the contrary, its main symptom—serious and abundant hemoptysis—is very well known."

The first description of a case of pulmonary embolism is usually attributed to Helie (3), who in 1837 published a paper under the title, "Inflammation de l'artère pulmonaire, mort subite." The frequent coexistence of obstruction of the pulmonary artery and diseased peripheral veins was found—among others—by James Paget from London, who in 1844 published a paper "On obstructions of the pulmonary arteries" (quoted in Luzzatto [1]).

However, we owe the discovery of the connection between venous thrombi and the obstruction of the pulmonary artery to the intuition of von Virchow (4): "These stoppers originated in a part of the cardiovascular system upstream of the lungs, namely the veins and the right heart. They are then carried to the pulmonary artery by the bloodstream." The famous Berlin pathologist was also the first to use the word *embolism* (from the Greek term *emballein*, "to throw into"). Nine years later Rokitansky(5) promoted the concept of the embolic or thrombotic origin of pulmonary infarcts, but von Virchow's theory was not accepted without reservations, because Ruault de Lalande (quoted by Luzzatto)[1]) in 1861 defined embolism as "a creation of German imagination."

However, a series of publications confirmed and completed von Virchow's ideas. Of note is the volume Beniamino Luzzatto (1) published 1880 in Milan, entitled "Embolism of the Pulmonary Artery" (Fig. 1). In 526 pages he described no fewer than 160 cases, stressing the predilection for the right lung and the lower lobes, aside from the prevalence of valvular heart disease in the underlying pathology. Futhermore, he described pulmonary stasis as a predisposing factor for pulmonary infarction, analyzed the clinical manifestations in relation to the site of embolization, and recognized the prognostic role of preexisting cardiopulmonary disease.

In 1884, Picot (6), professor of Clinical Medicine in Bordeaux, published his "Leçons de Clinique Médicale" (Fig. 2). He wrote, "Venous thrombosis is always a severe disease and is often fatal, because fragments of the thrombi may detach and occlude branches of the pulmonary artery." Even more impressive is the statement that "the occlusion of the main branches of the pulmonary artery causes a striking rise of the blood pressure in these vessels. This rise—which the right heart might fight in order to ensure circulation—may sometimes lead to cardiac arrest."

The earliest recorded report of the changes in the chest X-ray associated with acute pulmonary embolism and infarct is that of Wharton and Pierson (7) from the Johns Hopkins Hospital.

As to the treatment of embolism, Trendelenburg (8) was the first to ligate successfully the inferior vena cava, but his most important contribution to surgery was the method for pulmonary embolectomy. This operation, which also bears his name, was presented to the German Surgical Congress in 1908 (8). He illustrated the operative technique on a corpse and discussed the fact that complete occlusion of the pulmonary artery could be tolerated from 45 s to 2 min or partial occlusion for a longer period, enough to make the intraarterial maneuver feasible for a surgeon as deft as he must have been. In addition, he reported two operations performed in Leipzig in which the patients became pulseless during the operation but recovered after removal of pieces of embolus up to 34 cm in length (9).

Among further remarkable contributions on pulmonary embolism and deep-vein thrombosis are those by P. Bardin (10), R. Lériche (11), H. Neuhof (12), and P. Chiche (13). More recent contributions include, among others, the books of Hume et al. (14), Goldhaber (15), Hirsh (16), and the very recent work edited by Leclerc (17).

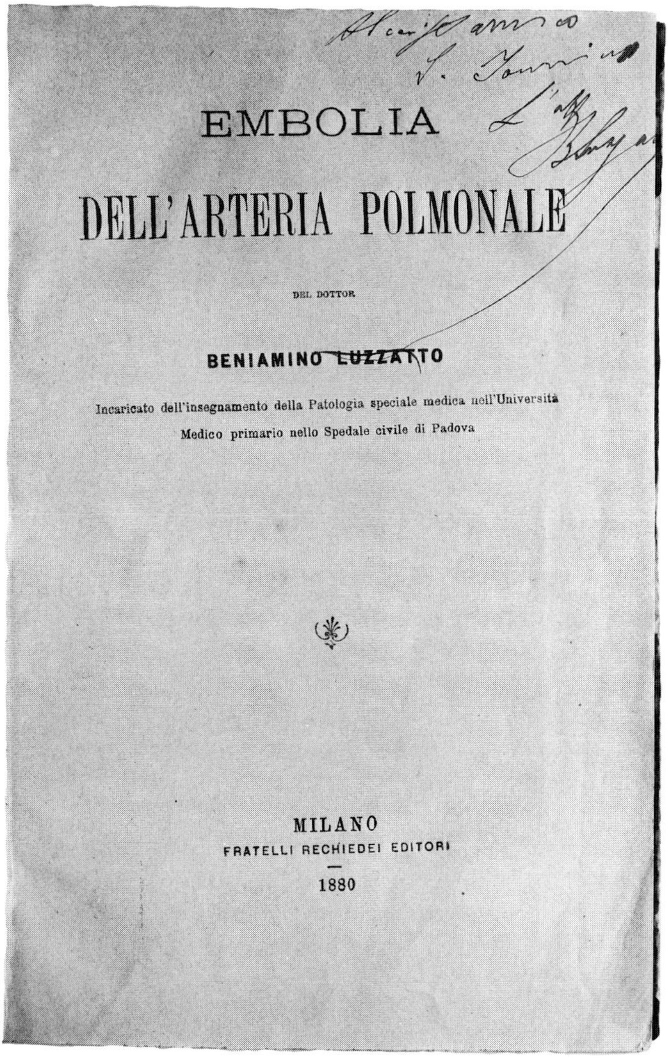

EMBOLIA

DELL'ARTERIA POLMONALE

DEL DOTTOR

BENIAMINO LUZZATTO

Incaricato dell'insegnamento della Patologia speciale medica nell'Università
Medico primario nello Spedale civile di Padova

MILANO
FRATELLI RECHIEDEI EDITORI
—
1880

Figure 1 Title page of a book devoted to pulmonary artery embolization, edited in 1880 by B. Luzzatto, Professor of Medical Pathology, University of Padua. In 526 pages the book describes 160 cases of pulmonary embolism, for the most part with autopsy findings.

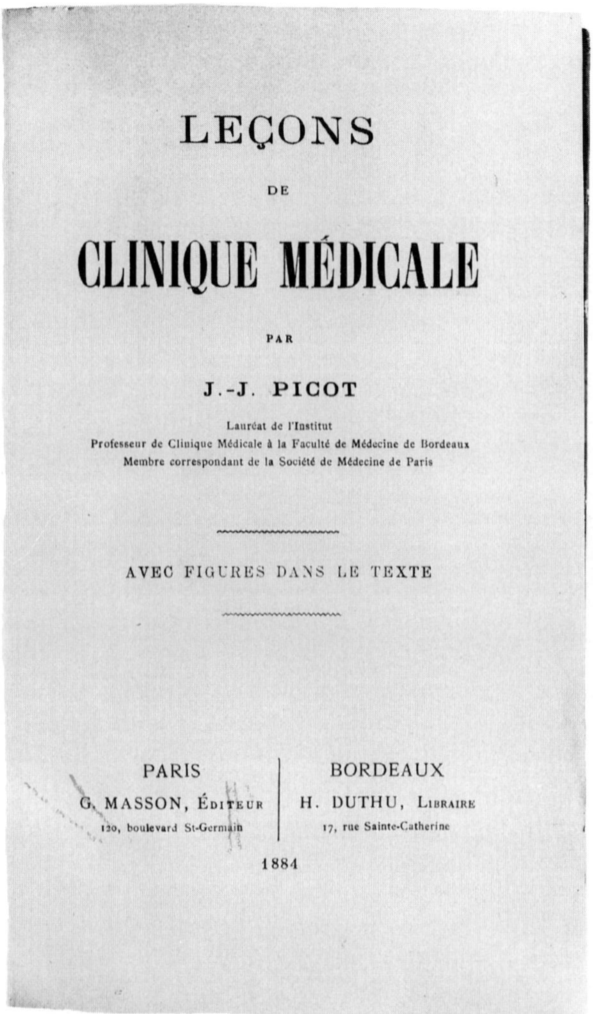

LEÇONS

DE

CLINIQUE MÉDICALE

PAR

J.-J. PICOT

Lauréat de l'Institut
Professeur de Clinique Médicale à la Faculté de Médecine de Bordeaux
Membre correspondant de la Société de Médecine de Paris

AVEC FIGURES DANS LE TEXTE

PARIS
G. MASSON, ÉDITEUR
120, boulevard St-Germain

BORDEAUX
H. DUTHU, LIBRAIRE
17, rue Sainte-Catherine

1884

Figure 2 Title page of the book "Leçons de Clinique Médicale," edited in 1884 by J. J. Picot, Professor of Clinical Medicine, University of Bordeaux. This book deals for the first time with the relationships between occlusion of main pulmonary arteries, increase in pulmonary artery pressure, right ventricular overload, and cardiac arrest.

Pulmonary embolism is still a tough diagnostic problem. In 1940, Géry et al. (18) collected 222 autopsy cases of massive pulmonary embolism; among surgical and obstetrical patients, false negatives amounted to 23% as opposed to 66% among "medical" cases. In Italy, the autopsy data of Passarino et al. (19) were even more discouraging. Out of 546 cases of pulmonary embolism in nonsurgical patients, the correct diagnosis had been made antemortem in only 8.4% of cases. In a recent experience (20) out of 92 postmortem cases of pulmonary embolism studied a posteriori from 1986 to 1989, only 28% had been diagnosed before death. It should be noted that the 66 false negatives had been hospitalized for more than 24 h. At least one chest radiograph and one electrocardiogram had been performed in all cases, which had a pulmonary embolism or a pulmonary infarction involving at least one pulmonary segment or its equivalent at autopsy.

In a large study carried out in Norway and totaling over 1900 cases of pulmonary embolism (21), it has been found that a correct clinical diagnosis had been more frequently made in the period from 1960 to 1969 than in the years from 1980 to 1984! Anderson et al. (22) noted that there had been no apparent improvement in diagnostic indices during the nearly four decades encompassed by previous studies and concluded that "clinical diagnosis in persons dying of pulmonary embolism leaves considerable room for improvement." The results of a population-based assessment of death caused by pulmonary embolism in New Mexico were published in 1990 (23). Among 812 autopsy-documented cases of pulmonary embolism, only 34.5% were correctly diagnosed before death, compared with 15,436 autopsy-negative cases, in which individuals (2.5%) had been misdiagnosed clinically as having died from pulmonary embolism. These results point out the problem of false positives, such as pulmonary embolism diagnosed clinically but not confirmed at autopsy.

In agreement with Sperry's (23) data and in contrast with the findings of Modan et al. (24), who recorded a percentage of false positives (62%) almost as high as that of false negatives (66%), Morpurgo's (20) recent study showed that false positives account for only 3% of cases. This observation causes us to agree with Lériche's (11) statement, "Silent or anomalous massive embolisms are much more numerous than false embolic syndromes."

References

1. Luzzatto B. Embolia dell'arteria polmonale. Milan: Fratelli Richiedei ed., 1880.
2. Laennec RHT. De l'auscultation médiate ou Traité du diagnostic des maladies des poumons et du coeur. Vol. I. Paris: Brosson et Chaudé, 1819.
3. Helie J. Inflammation de l'artère pulmonaire, mort subite. Bull Soc Anat Paris 1837; 8:254–7.

4. Virchow R von. Weitere Untersuchungen ueber die Verstopfung der Lungenarterien und ihre Folge. Traube's Beitraege exp Path u Physiol, Berlin 1846; 2:21–31.
5. Rokitansky J von. Handbuch der speziellen pathologischen Anatomie, Wien 1855.
6. Picot JJ. Leçons de Clinique Médicale. Paris; Masson, 1884.
7. Wharton LR, Pierson JW. Minor forms of pulmonary embolism after abdominal operations. JAMA 1922; 79:1904–10.
8. Trendelenburg F. Ueber die operative Behandlung der Embolie der Lungenarterie. Verh Dtsch Ges Chir 1908; 37:89.
9. Hume M. Pulmonary embolism. Historical aspects. Arch Surg 1963; 87:709–14.
10. Bardin P. L'embolie pulmonaire. Paris; Masson, 1937.
11. Lériche R. Les embolies de l'artère pulmonaire et des artères des membres. Paris: Masson, 1947.
12. Neuhof H. Venous thrombosis and pulmonary embolism. New York: Grune & Stratton, 1948.
13. Chiche P: La maladie thrombo-embolique pulmonaire. Paris: L'Expansion Scientifique Française, 1969.
14. Hume M, Sevitt S, Thomas DP. Venous thrombosis and pulmonary embolism. Cambridge: Harvard University Press, 1970.
15. Goldhaber SZ. Pulmonary embolism and deep venous thrombosis. Philadelphia: Saunders, 1985.
16. Hirsh J. Venous thrombosis and pulmonary embolism: diagnostic methods. Edinburgh: Churchill Livingstone, 1987.
17. Leclerc JR. Venous thromboembolic disorders. Philadelphia: Lea Febiger, 1991.
18. Géry L, Fontaine R, Blume E. Quelques reflexions à propos d'une statistique de 222 cas d'embolies pulmonaires mortelles. Presse Méd 1940; 35:390–5.
19. Passarino G, Nobili A, Colombo A, Comino A, Mollo F. La tromboembolia polmonare nelle corsie mediche: osservazioni su 546 casi. G It Cardiol 1982; 12:11–16.
20. Morpurgo M. Embolia polmonare: le dimensioni del problema. In Caturelli G, ed. Cura Intensiva Cardiologica. Milano Librex 1989: 125–9.
21. Karwinsky B, Svendsen E. Comparison of clinical and postmortem diagnosis of pulmonary embolism. J Clin Pathol 1989; 42:135–9.
22. Anderson RE, Hill RB, Key CR. The sensitivity and specificity of clinical diagnostics during five decades: toward an understanding of necessary fallibility. JAMA 1989; 261:1610–7.
23. Sperry KL, Key CR, Anderson RE. Toward a population-based assessment of death due to pulmonary embolism in New Mexico. Hum Pathol 1990; 21:159–65.
24. Modan B, Sharon E, Jelin N. Factors contributing to the incorrect diagnosis of pulmonary embolic disease. Chest 1972; 62:388–93.

Part One

FUNDAMENTALS

2

Epidemiology of Pulmonary Embolism

SAMUEL Z. GOLDHABER

Harvard Medical School
and Brigham and Women's Hospital
Boston, Massachusetts

I. Introduction

Venous thrombosis has been described only for the past few centuries and is, therefore, an illness of modern society (1). Pulmonary embolism (PE) and deep venous thrombosis (DVT) now account for approximately 300,000 hospitalizations per year in the United States (2) and constitute the third most common cardiovascular disease, after acute ischemic syndromes and stroke. About two thirds of cases are first-time episodes; the remaining third arise in patients with recurrent venous thromboembolism (Fig. 1) (3).

Unfortunately, PE causes as many as 50,000 deaths per year in the United States, and, in the past two decades, there has been no decline in the PE death rate (Fig. 2) (4). The death rate from PE is higher in men than in women and in nonwhites than whites. In Canada, the PE death rate is slightly lower than in the United States (5). However, in Canada as in the United States, more men than women die of PE, and there has been no decline in the death rate for the past 25 years. In both the United States and in Canada, death from PE occurs more frequently with increasing age (4,5).

Venous thromboembolism occurs much less often in Asian (6) and African (7) populations compared with Western communities. The lower rates in other

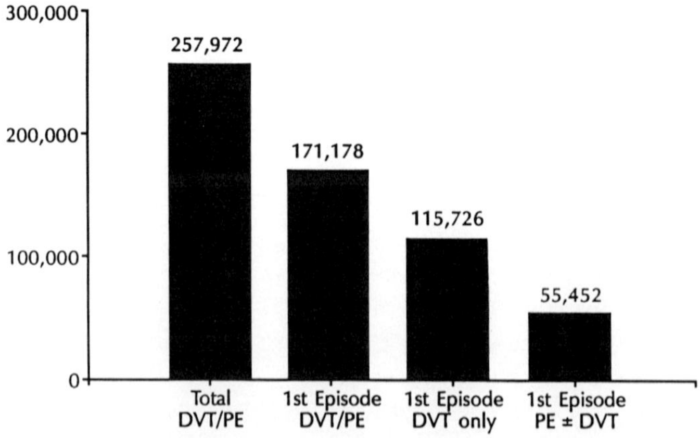

Figure 1 Estimated number of cases of venous thromboembolism in the United States in 1986, based on a 15-hospital survey in the Worcester, MA area. (Adapted from data in Anderson FA et al., 1991.)

parts of the world may provide clues to etiologic factors in the West. For example, differences in diet, exercise, and bowel habits may contribute to the lower rates of PE and DVT in non-Western societies.

Contemporary autopsy studies reveal that PE continues to be underdiagnosed among hospitalized patients, despite the availability of lung scanning and pulmonary angiography (8,9). Several studies have found that PE contrib-

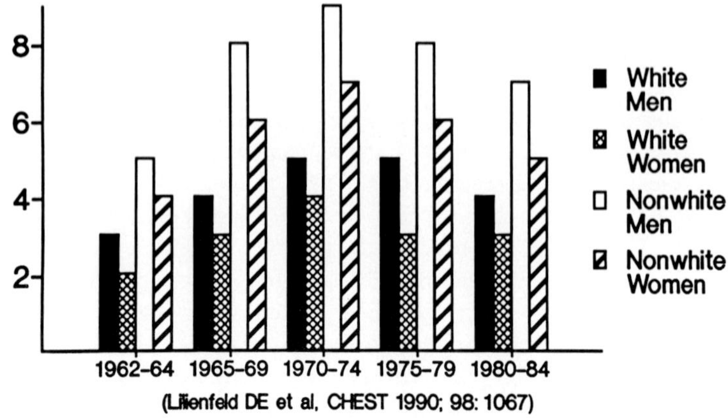

Figure 2 Death rate from pulmonary embolism in the United States from 1962–1984, based on data from the National Hospital Discharge Survey. (Adapted from data in Lilienfeld DE et al., 1990.)

uting to patient death is diagnosed antemortem only in one of approximately every three cases (8,9). Autopsy studies have shown that PE is especially difficult to diagnose antemortem among elderly institutionalized patients (10,11).

II. Acquired Conditions Associated with PE (Table 1)

Certain types of surgery, such as orthopedic surgery of the lower extremity, gynecologic cancer surgery, or major abdominal surgery, confer a particularly high risk for postoperative PE, which may occur as late as a month after hospital discharge. Less well appreciated is that venous thrombosis occurs with high frequency after coronary artery bypass grafting (12), renal transplantation (13), and splenectomy (14). Patients immobilized because of trauma or because of medical illness are also at special risk for developing PE (15).

Occult cancer may be present among patients with PE (16) or DVT (17). The most frequently associated malignancies are adenocarcinomas of the lung, gastrointestinal tract, breast, and uterus. Among patients with DVT younger than 50 years, the relative risk of occult cancer in one study (17) was 19.0, but the confidence intervals were very wide (95% CI 2.2, 168.0). For patients with established cancer, the chemotherapy itself appears to contribute to the risk of venous thrombosis (18). Another problem for cancer patients is that they are prone to tumor as well as thrombotic PE. Tumor PE, which has a clinical presentation similar to thrombotic PE, is more difficult to diagnose than thrombotic PE among cancer patients (19).

Pulmonary embolism is also associated with use of oral contraceptives and with pregnancy (20), particularly among women confined to bed because of preeclampsia, eclampsia, or cesarean section. The risk of PE is much greater

Table 1 Acquired Conditions Associated with PE

Surgery
Orthopedic
Gynecological cancer
Major abdominal
Coronary artery bypass grafting
Renal transplantation
Splenectomy
Trauma
Immobilized medical patients
Cancer
Pregnancy/oral contraceptives
Obesity
Air travel

during the first 6 weeks postpartum than during the pregnancy itself. One study demonstrated that PE is the leading medical cause of maternal mortality: four times more common among obstetrical patients than death from hemorrhage or an anesthetic accident and twice as common as death from an ectopic pregnancy or infection (21).

Data from the Framingham Heart Study have indicated that obesity among women is a long-term risk factor for PE (22). Among hospitalized patients, obesity may also increase the likelihood of PE.

In otherwise apparently healthy individuals, PE can be associated with long air flights (23). The mechanism is presumed to be an increase in venous stasis in the legs caused by immobility and dehydration.

III. Hypercoagulable States (Table 2)

It is not cost-effective to screen all PE patients for hypercoagulable states. Instead, tests for these conditions should be undertaken selectively, particularly among young patients without obvious risk factors for PE. In an unselected population study of patients with DVT, deficiencies of antithrombin III, protein C, and protein S were the most commonly identified hypercoagulable disorders and accounted for 8% of the patients (24). In a study of 141 venous thrombosis patients less than 45 years of age, 9% had protein C or S deficiency, 3% had antithrombin III deficiency, 2% had a plasminogen abnormality, and 1% had a fibrinogen abnormality (25). In another study of 88 patients with venous thrombosis, 19% had increased levels of plasminogen activator inhibitor (26).

"Lupus anticoagulant," an antibody that interferes with phospholipid-dependent coagulation reactions, is often present in patients without lupus. It usually prolongs the activated partial thromboplastin time (PTT) but, despite its name and its effect on the PTT, is a procoagulant rather than an anticoagulant. Patients with lupus anticoagulant often have elevated titers of anticardiolipin antibodies, which are assayed with the negatively charged phospholipid, cardiolipin, as the antigen. The presence of lupus anticoagulant and elevated anticardiolipin antibodies may be especially ominous in pregnant women. These markers of a

Table 2 Hypercoagulable States

Antithrombin III deficiency
Protein C deficiency
Protein S deficiency
Excessive plasminogen activator inhibitor
Lupus anticoagulant
Anticardiolipin antibodies

Table 3 The PE–DVT Relationship: Frequent Sources of PE

Proximal leg DVT
Isolated calf vein thrombosis
Pelvic thrombosis
Renal vein/inferior vena caval thombosis
Upper extremity thrombosis
Central venous catheters

hypercoagulable state are associated with recurrent venous thrombosis during pregnancy as well as recurrent first- or second-trimester miscarriages.

IV. The PE–DVT Relationship (Table 3)

Silent PE frequently accompanies clinically apparent DVT of the legs. Approximately half of patients with DVT proximal to the calf have asymptomatic PE (27). It is often not appreciated that as many as one in three patients with isolated calf vein thrombosis also has asymptomatic PE (28). Symptomatic patients with isolated calf vein thrombosis who do not receive anticoagulation had, in one randomized controlled trial, a 29% likelihood of recurrent proximal leg DVT or PE (29).

Upper extremity venous thrombosis is occurring with greater frequency because of increasing intravenous drug abuse, especially cocaine-related arm thrombosis (30), and because of more frequently inserted indwelling central venous catheters for hyperalimentation or for cancer chemotherapy (31,32). One group of investigators obtained lung scans prospectively in 20 patients with central venous catheter related thrombosis. They found that 5 of the 20 patients had high-probability scans for PE (33).

V. Future Perspectives (Table 4)

During the next decade, the frequency of upper-extremity thrombosis will continue to rise because of increased use of long-term, in-dwelling central venous

Table 4 Future Perspectives

Increased frequency of upper extremity thrombosis
Increased recognition of isolated calf thrombosis
Increased diagnosis of PE after hospital discharge
Increased identification of PE among the institutionalized elderly population
Increased emphasis on prevention of PE

catheters. As compression ultrasound becomes more widespread and as technology in noninvasive diagnosis improves, not only upper extremity thrombosis but also isolated calf vein thrombosis (34) will be recognized more often.

In the future, there will also be an increased appreciation for the surprisingly large proportion of PE that occurs after patients are discharged from hospital (35,36). Improved home health care services will have to be developed because many patients are less mobile at home than in the hospital and, therefore, more susceptible to PE.

As the population ages, an increasing number of elderly individuals will be institutionalized. Their risk of PE will need to be addressed more thoroughly.

In the 1990s, research in PE prophylaxis will intensify as more sophisticated risk assessment methodology is developed and as more widespread implementation of PE prevention protocols is encouraged. By utilizing knowledge gained from PE epidemiology, the World Health Organization can devise effective preventive strategies that will conserve financial resources and yet minimize the frequency of this common cardiovascular disease.

References

1. Dexter L. The chair and venous thrombosis. Transactions of the American Clinical and Climatological Association 1973; 84:1–15.
2. Gillum RF. Pulmonary embolism and thrombophlebitis in the United States, 1970–1985. Am Heart J 1987; 114:1262–4.
3. Anderson FA Jr, Wheeler HB, Goldberg RJ, Hosmer DW, Patwardhan NA, Jovanovic B, Forcier A, Dalen JE: A population-based perspective of the hospital incidence and case-fatality rates of venous thrombosis and pulmonary embolism: The Worcester DVT Study. Arch Intern Med 1991; 151:933–8.
4. Lilienfeld DE, Chan E, Ehland J, Godbold JH, Landrigan PJ, Marsh G: Mortality from pulmonary embolism in the United States: 1962 to 1984. Chest 1990; 98:1067–72.
5. Soskolne CL, Wong AW, Lilienfeld DE: Trends in pulmonary embolism death rates for Canada and the United States, 1962–87. Can Med Assoc J 1990; 142:321–4.
6. Woo KS, Tse LKK, Tse CY, Metreweli C, Vallance-Owen J. The prevalence and pattern of pulmonary thromboembolism in the Chinese in Hong Kong. Int J Cardiol 1988; 20:373–80.
7. Thomas WA, Davies JNP, O'Neal RM, Dimakulangan AA. Incidence of myocardial infarction correlated with venous and pulmonary thrombosis and embolism. A geographic study based on autopsies in Uganda, East Africa and St. Louis, U.S.A. Am J Cardiol 1960; 5:41–7.
8. Goldhaber SZ, Hennekens CH, Evans DA, Newton EC, Godleski JJ. Factors associated with correct antemortem diagnosis of major pulmonary embolism. Am J Med 1982; 73:822–6.

9. Rubinstein I, Murray D, Hoffstein V. Fatal pulmonary emboli in hospitalized patients. An autopsy study. Arch Intern Med 1988; 148:1425–6.
10. Taubman LB, Silverstone FA. Autopsy proven pulmonary embolism among the institutionalized elderly. J Am Geriatr Soc 1986; 34:752–6.
11. Gross JS, Neufeld RR, Libow LS, Gerber I, Rodstein M. Autopsy study of the elderly institutionalized patient. Review of 234 autopsies. Arch Intern Med 1988; 148:173–6.
12. Josa M, Siouffi SY, Silverman AB, Barsamian EM, Khuri SF, Sharma GVRK. Pulmonary embolism after cardiac surgery. J Am Coll Cardiol 1993; 21:990–6.
13. Allen RDM, Michie CA, Murie JA, Morris PJ. Deep venous thrombosis after renal transplantation. Surg Gynecol Obstet 1987; 164:137–42.
14. Pimpl W, Dapunt O, Kaindl H, Thalhamer J. Incidence of septic and thromboembolic-related deaths after splenectomy in adults. Br J Surg 1989; 76:517–21.
15. Gardlund B. Fatal pulmonary embolism in hospitalized non-surgical patients. Acta Med Scand 1985; 218:417–21.
16. Gore JM, Appelbaum JS, Greene HL, Dexter L, Dalen JE: Occult cancer in patients with acute pulmonary embolism. Ann Intern Med 1982; 96:556–60.
17. Goldberg RJ, Seneff M, Gore JM, Anderson PA, Jr, Greene HL, Wheeler HB, Dalen JE: Occult malignancy in patients with deep venous thrombosis. Arch Intern Med 1987; 147:251–3.
18. Levine MN, Gent M, Hirsh J, Arnold A, Goodyear MD, Hryniuk W, De Pauw S. The thrombogenic effect of anticancer drug therapy in women with stage II breast cancer. N Engl J Med 1988; 318:404–7.
19. Goldhaber SZ, Dricker E, Buring JE, Eberlein K, Godleski JJ, Mayer RJ, Hennekens CH: Clinical suspicion of autopsy-proven thrombotic and tumor pulmonary embolism in cancer patients. Am Heart J 1987; 114:1432–5.
20. Dixon JE. Pregnancies complicated by previous thromboembolic disease. Br J Hosp Med 1987; 37:449–52.
21. Sachs BP, Brown DAJ, Driscoll SG, Schulman E, Acker D, Ransil BJ, Jewett JF. Maternal mortality in Massachusetts. Trends and prevention. N Engl J Med 1987; 316:667–72.
22. Goldhaber SZ, Savage DD, Garrison RJ, Castelli WP, Kannel WB, McNamara PM, Gherardi G, Feinleib M. Risk factors for pulmonary embolism. The Framingham Study. Am J Med 1983; 74: 1023–8.
23. Cruickshank JM, Gorlin R, Jennett B. Air travel and thrombotic episodes: The economy class syndrome. Lancet 1988; 2:497–8.
24. Heijboer H, Brandjes DP, Büller HR, Sturk A, ten Cate JW: Deficiencies of coagulation-inhibiting and fibrinolytic proteins in outpatients with deep-vein thrombosis: N Engl J Med 1990; 323:1512–6.
25. Gladson CL, Scharrer I, Hach V, Beck KH, Griffin JH: The frequency of type I heterozygous protein S and protein C deficiency in 141 unrelated young patients with venous thrombosis. Thromb Haemost 1988; 59:18–22.
26. Tabernero MD, Estellés A, Vicente V, Alberca I, Aznar J: Incidence of increased plasminogen activator inhibitor in patients with deep venous thrombosis and/or pulmonary embolism. Thromb Res 1989; 56:565–70.
27. Huisman MV, Buller HR, ten Cate JW, van Royen EA, Vreeken J, Kersten M-J,

Bakx R. Unexpected high prevalence of silent pulmonary embolism in patients with deep venous thrombosis. Chest 1989; 95:498–502.

28. Doyle DJ, Turpie AGG, Hirsh J, Best C, Kinch D, Levine MN, Gent M. Adjusted subcutaneous heparin or continuous intravenous heparin in patients with acute deep vein thrombosis: A randomized trial. Ann Intern Med 1987; 107:441–5.
29. Lagerstedt CI, Olsson C-G, Fagher BO, Öqvist BW, Albrechtsson U: Need for long-term anticoagulant treatment in symptomatic calf-vein thrombosis. Lancet 1985; 2:515–8.
30. Lisse JR, Davis CP, Thurmond-Anderle ME: Upper extremity deep venous thrombosis: Increased prevalence due to cocaine abuse. Am J Med 1989; 87:457–8.
31. Anderson AJ, Krasnow SH, Boyer MW, Raucheisen ML, Grant CE, Gasper OR, Hoffmann JK, Cohen MH: Hickman catheter clots: a common occurrence despite daily heparin flushing. Cancer Treat Rep 1987; 71:651–3.
32. Anderson AJ, Krasnow SH, Boyer MW, Cutler DJ, Jones BD, Citron ML, Ortega LG, Cohen MH: Thrombosis: The major Hickman catheter complication in patients with solid tumor. Chest 1989; 95:71–5.
33. Monreal M, Lafoz E, Ruiz J, Valls R, Alastrue A. Upper-extremity deep venous thrombosis and pulmonary embolism. A prospective study. Chest 1991; 99:280–3.
34. Yucel EK, Fisher JS, Egglin TK, Geller SC, Waltman AC. Isolated calf venous thrombosis: diagnosis with compression US. Radiology 1991; 179:443–6.
35. Scurr JH, Coleridge-Smith PD, Hasty JH. Deep vein thrombosis: a continuing problem. Br Med J 1988; 297:28.
36. Huber O, Bounameaux H, Borst F, Rohner A. Postoperative pulmonary embolism after hospital discharge. An underestimated risk. Arch Surg 1992; 127:310–3.

3

Experience with Pulmonary Embolism in a Developing Country

WALINJOM F. T. MUNA

The University Center for Health Sciences
and The General Hospital of Yaoundé
Yaoundé, Cameroon

I. Introduction

The frequency of deep-vein thrombosis (DVT), pulmonary embolism (PE), and thromboembolic disease (TED) in general appears to vary within and between ethnic or population groups and when different geographic areas are taken into consideration (1). Although the reasons for this apparent variation in the frequency of these conditions are incompletely understood, it must be emphasized that clinical criteria frequently used in suspecting the existence or making the diagnosis of these conditions are notoriously unreliable (2–6). Consequently, some of the published frequencies based on these criteria must be considered speculative or at best a crude estimate of trends. Possibly, they may be useful for comparisons when study protocols are similar or consistent. Unfortunately, these clinical criteria are frequently the only diagnostic tools available to most of the developing countries of Asia and Africa where these conditions are reportedly rare (7,8). The relative paucity of publications or knowledge about TED in developing countries can be partially explained by their so-called low-technology environments that lack the minimal or adequate diagnostic facilities and appropriately trained human resources or health professionals. It is important to emphasize the point that the usage of the concept of a "developed" or "developing" country may involve some generalizations (about socioeconomic and environmental variables not taken into consideration in either the original definition or classification). Consequently, "developing" countries may have a somewhat heterogeneous environment with some urban centers that are either equally or more developed than some centers in the "developed" countries. The discussion of the potential effect of this observation on certain findings and their subsequent implications on interpretations and/or analyses, however critical or important, is beyond the scope of the intended discussion here.

The evidence for DVT, PE, and TED in developing countries will be briefly reviewed here. An illustrative example (Cameroon) of an experience with PE in a developing country will also be presented. Finally, some of the reasons for the observed trends for DVT, PE, and TED in developing countries will be either explained where possible or at least evoked.

II. Frequency of DVT, PE, and TED in Developing Countries

Most of the relatively few reports, based either on clinical experience or studies, undoubtedly leave one with the impression that DVT, PE, or TED are rare and occur with a considerably lower frequency in developing countries. This is especially true when the reported frequencies for these conditions in Europe and the United States are compared with those obtained from developing African and Asian countries (1). In Asia, DVT has been reported to be an uncommon event among the Thai (9,10). In fact, in a more recent study evaluating postoperative DVT (documentation by phlebography) in group of Thai patients undergoing hip surgery (no anticoagulant therapy), the reported incidence was 4%, a figure considerably lower than the 40%–70% for most studies concerned with Western population groups (10). Asian populations of Chinese origin also have comparatively lower frequencies of TED (11,12). A recent autopsy-based study (13) of pulmonary thromboembolism in Hong Kong Chinese, however, showed a dramatic rise in the incidence from 0.58% to 2.08% over a recent 5-year period. Although this suggests either a change in pattern or a rapidly rising trend, these frequencies are still considerably less than those from similar autopsy-based studies, 12.8% in Europe (14) and 3.8%–9.3% in the United States (15).

There are relatively fewer published data available on the frequencies of DVT, PE, and TED in developing African countries. Furthermore, differences in study protocols or designs and our current understanding of the heterogeneous nature of most African population groups makes any meaningful comparisons a difficult task at best, if not impossible. Earlier studies had suggested that venous diseases were generally rare in black Africans. In one such study (16), 2 cases of phlebitis were observed in the course of 1000 surgical interventions in Dakar (West Africa). This notion was further strengthened by reports of low frequencies of postoperative TED in Morocco, North Africa (17); in Natal province, South Africa (17); and in Madagascar (17), which is an island off the southeast African coastline with a mixed African-Asian population. A comparative and autopsy-based study in Uganda (East Africa) suggested a frequency of 2% for TED in a population of adults aged 40 years and over (8). Another study of 13 cases of pulmonary thromboembolic disease in Côte-D'Ivoire (West Africa) suggested that this condition may be more common (frequency estimated at 2%) than previously thought (18). This impression was confirmed in a more recent publication (using diagnostic techniques that included Doppler examination, phlebography, and, where indicated, pulmonary angiography) from Côte-D'Ivoire showing a frequency of about 2.5% among hospitalized patients (17). This study looked at both African and European patients living in Côte-D'Ivoire. The prevalence for the Africans was 9.5 per 100,000, and this was considerably much lower than the prevalence of 88 per 100,000 reported for the Europeans. On the contrary, a controlled study of postoperative patients in South Africa showed no significant differences in the prevalence of venous thrombosis in the European, Bantu, "colored," and Indian patients (19).

III. Pulmonary Embolism in a Developing Country: The Experience in Cameroon

Cameroon is a central African country with a population currently estimated at 12 million inhabitants, a gross national product (GNP) of $970 (US), a percentage of school-age secondary school enrollment of 25–30, and an estimated life expectancy of about 53 years. It has a physician to population ratio of about 1 to 12,000 inhabitants. Most of these physicians (over 75%) are general practitioners. Over 70% of its population is either rural or semiurban. It has two major urban centers (the capital city of Yaoundé and Douala, its major port and the center of most of its economic activities) where most of the locally available diagnostic capabilities are concentrated. Laboratory capabilities for determining basic clinical parameters for coagulation such as clotting time, platelet count, fibrinogen level, prothrombin time, partial thromboplastin time, and others are available. Sonography (including Doppler capabilities with vascular applications), phlebography, and possibilities for performing pulmonary angiography and determining blood gases are available at two medical centers. Scintigraphy (and other isotope-based techniques), plethysmography, and other recently developed immunological and biological techniques for detecting TED are not available.

In a review of randomly selected medical records of 4500 patients admitted over a period extending from 1981 to 1991, PEs were clinically suspected in 415 (0.9%) patients. The most common symptoms that led to this suspicion included the sudden onset of shortness of breath (80%) and/or chest pain (67%), unexplained or unusual restlessness and/or anxiety (45%) in an appropriate clinical setting (e.g., postoperatively, obesity, trauma, prolonged bed rest, severe heart failure, etc.). Of these 415 patients with clinical suspicion of PE, 150 (29%) had phlebography done because of either persistent symptoms in the face of a deteriorating clinical state or prominent and highly suggestive clinical signs. Sixty-six of 150 (44%) were positive, 15 (10%) were either inconclusive or uninterpretable, and 69 (46 percent) were negative. Thirty-three of 150 (22%) pulmonary angiograms were performed, and the usual indications were a rapidly deteriorating clinical state (15 patients), shock and hypotension (4 patients), inability to advance a central pulmonary catheter (1 patient), a previous history of gastrointestinal bleeding (7 patients), and recent surgery (6 patients). Twenty (61%) of 33 pulmonary angiograms were positive, 8 (24%) were either uninterpretable or inconclusive, and 5 (15%) were considered negative.

Of the 415 patients initially suspected of having pulmonary emboli on clinical grounds, 260 (62%) were empirically placed on low-dose heparin for variable periods. In the 150 patients whose clinical state suggested the performance of phlebography, full heparinisation was initiated in 85 patients (57%) prior to the procedure. In the 66 patients in whom the phlebography was subsequently positive, full heparinization was continued and generally stopped in individuals with a negative study. Full heparinization was discontinued in all patients with negative pulmonary angiograms. Patients with positive pulmonary angiograms were generally discharged on oral anticoagulants to be taken for periods that varied between 6 months and 1 year.

Over the past 5 years, phlebography has been systematically performed (in one of the hospitals with such a capability) on outpatients and inpatients with clinical signs and symptoms suggestive of DVT. This initiative was begun by the radiologist and some clinicians who were interested in the frequency of this condition in a population that went beyond, either hospitalized or postoperative cases. Of the 46 patients (age ranged from 26 to 61 years, with a mean age of 32 years) who underwent phlebography, 26 (54%) had positive studies, and it was concluded that this condition was not as uncommon as previously thought. However, it was unclear if the classic risk groups were equally applicable to the patients in the environment of developing countries.

IV. General Comments

The Cameroonian experience described earlier is typical of most developing countries in general, but more specific for sub-Saharan African countries (17). Several generalizations can be made, based on this experience and similar reports in the literature: DVT, PE, and TED are much less of a clinical concern in hospitalized patients in developing countries. It is rare to find any group of patients (that are usually classified in the usual high-risk group in developed countries) on pharmacological or nonpharmacological prophylaxis to prevent DVT, PE, or TED. Although this attitude is based on the extensive clinical experience in several regions, it is becoming apparent that as clinical competence, awareness, and diagnostic possibilities become available to these countries, these conditions may not be as rare as such past experience may have suggested. This may partially explain the rising frequency over time, noted in the Hong Kong Chinese (13) and West Africans (17), as mentioned earlier, although changes in disease patterns and life-styles must also constitute important considerations (13).

Finally (where clinical competence and awareness are available), it is evident that as technological capabilities permit a higher diagnostic certainty, therapeutic and preventive applications will ultimately be limited by cost. Eventually, other elements related to the system of health-care financing and delivery that may be specific for each country (including socioeconomic and cultural factors) will be equally important in determining the efficacy of each therapeutic and/or preventive measure applied and subsequent clinical outcomes. Cultural attitudes toward procedures, such as autopsies, will continue to delay our understanding of some aspects of the current extent of the problem.

Are some population groups "naturally" protected against DVT, PE, and TED? What is the relationship of "the development process" (including changes in culture, life-style, diet, other disease patterns and risk factors for these conditions) to the apparent difference in frequencies for DVT, PE, and TED between "developing" and "developed" countries? There is no doubt that the most critical element that may increase our chances of understanding these differences will depend on the systematic collection of clinical data as well as the undertaking of basic studies. Changes in diet, obesity, level of physical activity, and the patterns of several disease entities and aging have been incriminated by several authors (1,12,13,17,20). Populations in developing countries are, in general, much younger, and age is a well-known risk factor for DVT, PE, and TED. However, TED occurs in children (1,21–23), and there are increasing case reports from some developing countries (24). Consumption of fish by some African populations has been suggested as possibly playing a protective role (17,25). However, there is no adequate explanation for the different frequencies for TED observed in different parts of some regions of Europe (26). Genetic or biological factors have been incriminated by several observations. Higher levels of fibrinolytic activity in the Thais are thought to, at least partially, explain the lower frequencies of DVT, PE, and TED (27). Some African populations have been shown to have lower platelet counts (25), lower platelet aggregability (25,28), a more precocious and a higher fibrinolytic activity (25,28,29), lower fibrinogen level (25), consistently lower prothrombin activity and maybe other factors related to vascular reactivity and integrity (25).

These changes have been evoked as a possible explanation for this "natural" protection and relatively lower frequencies for TED observed in these population groups.

In conclusion, there is some evidence to suggest that DVT, PE, and TED are much less frequent in developing countries, although there is a strong tendency toward an increase. More reliable studies will have to be performed to define further the frequencies of these conditions and either the etiologies or major risk factors involved. Changing patterns for chronic diseases and noncommunicable diseases in general and cardiovascular disorders in particular have been observed in most developing countries, and consequently the trends observed for DVT, PE, and TED are consistent with this phenomenon (30,31). The significant morbidity and mortality associated with DVT, PE, and TED may require that some of these developing countries (especially the "rapidly" developing ones) reconsider their health priorities. However, it is evident that, for rational preventive, diagnostic, and therapeutic strategies to be developed and eventually applied in the overall schema of health-care planning and delivery, the extent and reasons for these disease trends must be identified and understood. Given the limited health-care resources and research capabilities of most of these countries, the significant investments required in human resource training and infrastructure development will remain a major challenge for the future. Consequently, these countries will require significant international support and collaboration in the understanding and management of DVT, TED, and PE in particular, if we all share the emerging concept of health as, ultimately, a global issue requiring a matching approach.

References

1. Coon WW. Venous thromboembolism. Prevalence, risk factors, and prevention. Clin Chest Med 1984; *5*:391–400.
2. Alderson PO, Martin EC. Pulmonary embolism: diagnosis with multiple imaging modalities. Radiology 1987; *164*:297–312.
3. Kipper SM, Moser KM, Kortman KE, Ashburn WL. Longterm follow-up of patients with suspected pulmonary embolism and a normal lung scan. Chest 1982; *82*:411–25.
4. The PIOPED Investigators. Value of the ventilation/perfusion scan in acute pulmonary embolism. Results of the prospective investigation of pulmonary embolism diagnosis (PIOPED). JAMA 1990; *263*:2753–9.
5. Dalen JE, Alpert JS. Natural history of pulmonary embolism. Prog Cardiovasc Dis 1975; *17*:259–70.
6. Karwinski B, Svendsen E. Comparison of clinical and postmortem diagnosis of pulmonary embolism. J Clin Pathol 1989; *42*:135–9.
7. Burkitt DP. Varicose veins, deep vein thrombosis and haemorrhoids: Epidemiology and suggested aetiology. Br Med J 1972; *2*:556–61.

8. Thomas WA, Davies JNP, O'Neal RM, et al. Incidence of myocardial infarction correlated with venous and pulmonary thrombosis and embolism: a geographic study based on autopsies in Uganda, East Africa and St. Louis, U.S.A. Am J Cardiol 1960; *5*:41–7.
9. Talakak P. Thromboembolism in Thailand: incidence, coagulogram and its significance in therapeutic implications and prognosis. J Med Assoc Thai 1976; *59*:6–11.
10. Atichartakarn V, Pathepcjotiwong K, Keorochana S, Eurvilaichit C. Deep vein thrombosis after hip surgery among Thai. Arch Intern Med 1988; *148*:1349–53.
11. Hwang WS. The rarity of pulmonary thrombo-embolism in Asians. Singapore Med J 1968; *9*:269–79.
12. Woo KS, Tse LKK, Tse CY, Metreweli C, Vallance-Owen J. Int J Cardiol 1988; *20*:373–80.
13. Chau KY, Yuen ST, Ng THK, Ng WF. An autopsy study of pulmonary thromboembolism in Hong Kong Chinese. Pathology 1991; *23*:181–4.
14. Bergqvist D, Lindblad B. A 30 year survey of pulmonary embolism verified at autopsy: an analysis of 1274 surgical patients. Br J Surg 1985; *72*:105.
15. Bismuke SE, Wagner EH. Pulmonary embolism as a cause of death. JAMA 1986; *255*:2039.
16. Vorvor M. De la rareté de la pathologie veineuse en Afrique Noire. These, 1956, Montpellier.
17. Adoh A, Moncany G, Bogui-Ferron A, N'dori R, Bertrand Ed. Etude de 115 cas de maladies thrombo-emboliques veino-pulmonaires chez le Noir African a Abidjan. Aspects épidémiologiques, étiologiques, radiologiques et évolutifs. Cardiologie Tropicale 1989; *15*:91–6.
18. Touze JE, Moncany G, Amonkou A, Cailleau G, Monnier A, Kacou M, Bertrand Ed. La Maladie Thrombo-embolique Pulmonaire en Côte D'Ivoire: A propos de 13 cas. Med Trop 1985; *45*:43–6.
19. Joffe SN. Racial incidence of postoperative deep vein thrombosis in South Africa. Br J Surg 1974; *61*:982–3.
20. Gans H, Mori K, Quinlan R, et al. The intestine as a source of plasminogen activator activity. Ann Surg 1971; *174*:826.
21. Byard RW, Cutz E. Sudden and unexpected death in infancy and childhood due to pulmonary thromboembolism. An autopsy study. Arch Pathol Lab Med 1990; *114*:142–4.
22. Buck JR, Connors RH, Coon WW, Weintraub WH, Wesley JR, Coran AG. Pulmonary embolism in children. J Pediatr Surg 1981; *16*:385–91.
23. Bernstein D, Coupey S, Schonberg SK. Pulmonary embolism in adolescents. AJDC 1986; *140*:667–71.
24. Tetanye E, Bonnin-Bernard AC, N'Koulou H. Un cas de thrombophlébite poplitée chez un garçon de 15 ans. Ann Univ Sci Sante 1985; *2*:91–7.
25. Bertrand E, Cloitre B, Ticolat R, Darracq R, Rain SF. Activité plaquettaire, fibrinolyse et facteurs d'environement comparés chez 50 africains et 50 européens. Rôle de la consommation de poisson. Nouv Rev Fr Hematol 1987; *29*:237–45.
26. Kagan A. Information on thrombosis as a cause of death from studies promoted

by the World Health Organisation. In Sherry S, ed. Thrombosis. Washington, DC: National Academy of Sciences, 1969.
27. Visudhiphan S, Poolsuppasit S, Piboonnukarintr O, et al. The relationship between high fibrinolytic activity and daily capsicum ingestion in the Thais. Am J Clin Nutri 1982; *35*:1452–58.
28. Buchanan GR, Holtkamp CA, Levy EN. Racial differences in Ristocetin induced platelet aggregation. Br J Haematol 1981; *49*:455.
29. Howell M. Comparison of fibrinolysis and coagulation in Nigerian and European men. J Atheroscl Res 1965; *5*:80.
30. Feachem RG, Jamison DT, Bos ER. Changing patterns of disease and mortality in Sub-Saharan Africa. In Feachem RG and Jamison DT (eds.). Disease and Mortality in Sub-Saharan Africa. New York: Oxford University Press; 1991.
31. Ghali JK. Should cardiovascular diseases be a health priority for developing countries? A brief overview of mortality data. Ethnicity Dis 1991; *1*:295–9.

4

Experience of Pulmonary Embolism in China

XIAN-SHENG CHENG

Fu Wai Hospital
Chinese Academy of Medical Sciences
Beijing, China

QI WANG

Wu Jing General Hospital
Beijing, China

I. Introduction

China is a developing country in the east of Asia with a population of 1158 million (1991), about 80% of whom live in rural areas. Pulmonary embolism (PE) is considered to be an uncommon disease in China, and little attention has been paid to it, and the understanding of the disease is accordingly much less and incomplete.

II. The Epidemiology of PE

No exact and systematic epidemiological data of PE in China are as yet available, and only a few investigations were made on the peripheral vascular diseases and PE. From November 1, 1990, to October 31, 1991, an analysis of 75,140 visits in out-patient departments (OPDs) of peripheral vascular diseases was conducted in 35 medical centers. The results showed that deep phlebitis and varicosity amounted to 11.6% and 9.6%, respectively (Table 1). Another group of 4395 visits in an OPD of a special clinic for peripheral vascular diseases was found to have deep phlebitis in 859 cases (19.6%) and superficial phlebitis in 514 cases

Table 1 Disease Distribution of 75,140 Outpatients with Peripheral Vascular Diseases

Diseases	n	Percent
Arteriosclerosis obliterans	11,609	15.45
Thromboangiitis obliterans	21,263	28.30
Takayasu's disease	1091	1.45
Raynaud's disease	1939	2.58
Deep phlebitis	8714	11.60
Superficial phlebitis	9566	12.73
Venous varicosity	6905	9.19
Ecthyma	13,835	18.41
Miscellaneous	218	0.29

(11.7%) with a lower percentage of associated PE as compared with that in the Western countries (about 50%)(1). The incidence of PE in general hospitals is still unclear, whereas in a cardiovascular hospital, the incidence of autopsy proved PE larger than one segment was 11% (Table 2), of which 76% were confirmed to have pulmonary infarction with an antemortem diagnosis of only 13% (2).

Every year there are about 650,000 cases of PE in the United States (3); compared with China, the U.S. population is much less but the incidence of PE in the United States is much more. The causes of the difference may be: (1) Blood lipids: the data furnished by the USA-PRC collaborative study on cardiovascular and cardiopulmonary epidemiology showed that there was a

Table 2 Analysis of 100 Patients with Pulmonary Embolism (PE) Associated with Cardiovascular Diseases

		PE	
Diseases	Cases autopsied	n	Percent
Rheumatic heart disease	155	45	29.03
Cardiomyopathy	46	12	26.09
Cor pulmonale	84	16	19.05
Congenital heart disease	250	10	4.00
Coronary heart disease	175	7	4.00
Hypertension	100	2	2.00
Aortitis	5	3	
Cardiac tumor	8	2	
Others		3	

significant difference in serum lipids between the Chinese and the American. The concentration of serum total cholesterol and triglyceride of the Chinese were lower than those of the American, and the level of serum HDL-C of the Chinese was higher than that in the American (4). Hyperlipemia might induce thrombosis because of the increase in coagulability and the decrease in fibrinolytic activity. (2) Genetic background: Sukumaran et al. (5) analyzed 190 patients with autopsy proved PE. They include 21 Chinese descendants and 169 Americans in metropolitan New York city. No statistical difference in the detection rate of PE was found between the two groups. This indicates that the racial difference might not be concerned in the development of PE. (3) Diagnostic techniques: the difference in diagnostic technique between China and the western developed countries might affect the diagnostic rate of PE, e.g., in our hospital no diagnosis of PE was made in patients without associated heart diseases or lung diseases until the application of lung scan in 1973. Since then the number of cases of PE had been found to increase gradually, and the relative incidence of PE in hospitalized patients went up to 29.40% of pulmonary vascular diseases in 1981 (6). This suggests that the lower incidence of PE in China is related not only to the absolute small number of patients with PE but also to the lack of advanced diagnostic techniques. Thus, it is important to carry out a joint program of oriental and occidental countries, so as to clarify whether there is really any difference in the incidence, to explore the etiology and to provide new strategies of the prevention and treatment of PE.

III. The Clinical Aspects of PE

A. The Diagnosis of PE

Deep Venous Thrombosis in the Lower Extremities

In 82 patients with PE, 72 (87.8%) had lower-extremity venous disorders including 54 cases (75.0%) of thrombophlebitis and 18 of venous thrombosis (7). The results of radionuclide venography-documented 94 cases of deep venous thrombosis in the lower extremities were divided into four patterns: (1) normal venous flow in 15 cases, (2) complete obstruction in 51 cases with 2 subtypes: (a) complete obstruction with collateral vessels in 5 cases, (b) complete obstruction with no collateral vessels in 46 cases, (3) incomplete obstruction in 14 cases, and (4) venous insufficiency in 14 cases (8).

Pulmonary Embolism

Because PE used to be regarded as an uncommon disease, some physicians were not much aware of this disorder. As a result, patients with PE were often misdiagnosed. Sixty-three cases (76.83%) of 82 cases of PE were misdiagnosed as follows: pneumonia in 52 cases (82.54%); pleuritis in 9 (14.29%), myocardial infarction in 2 (3.17%) (7). About 50% of the patients with Takayasu's disease have the lung vessels involved, which accounted to 3.73% of 241 cases of pulmonary vascular diseases in Fu Wai Hospital (9). Takayasu's disease often shows defects in lung scan and pulmonary angiography, so it may be confused with PE. Therefore, the differentiation between the two is important, because their treatment is quite different.

Because the diagnosis of some patients with PE was not made promptly, the successful treatment was difficult in such cases, and recurrent PE would induce chronic thromboembolic pulmonary hypertension, which became even more difficult to diagnose. The misdiagnostic rate of 43 patients with chronic thromboembolic pulmonary hypertension was as high as 79.1% (34 cases); the misdiagnostic analysis of them is shown in Table 3.

The hemodynamics of 46 inpatients with chronic thromboembolic pulmonary hypertension is illustrated in Table 4. Most of the patients admitted to the hospital had severe pulmonary hypertension.

The causes of the higher incidence of thromboembolic pulmonary hypertension in China are unknown; it might be related to recurrent emboli, especially infectious emboli, which are resistant to lysis, or to acute PE without treatment. We analyzed the relationship between the number of segments of radionuclide lung perfusion defects and the level of pulmonary arterial pressure, and found that mean pulmonary arterial pressure of 6 cases with 5 segments or less was 25 ± 6.0 mm Hg (M ± SD), while mean pulmonary arterial pressure of 27 cases

Table 3 Misdiagnostic Analysis of 34 Patients with Thromboembolic Pulmonary Hypertension

Misdiagnosed diseases	*n*	Percent
Cardiomyopathy	16	37.21
Coronary heart disease	8	18.61
Myocarditis	3	7.00
Mitral disease	6	13.96
Pulmonic stenosis	1	2.33
Aortic stenosis	1	2.33
Atrial septal defect	5	11.63
Ventricular septal defect	3	7.08
Trilogy of Fallot	1	2.33
Other congenital heart diseases	2	4.65
Pulmonary tuberculosis	2	4.65
Pneumonia	2	4.65
Pleuritis	1	2.33
Lung cancer	1	2.33

Table 4 Hemodynamics of 46 Patients with Thromboembolic Pulmonary Hypertension

Parameters	*n*	X ± SD	Parameters	*n*	X ± SD
HR (bpm)	46	81.4 ± 1.7	PAPm (mm Hg)	46	48.7 ± 1.9
SAPs (mm Hg)	46	115.7 ± 1.8	CI (L/min/m^2)	44	1.85 ± 0.08
SAPd (mm Hg)	46	77.9 ± 1.9	TPRI (U/m^2)	40	27.9 ± 1.7
RAP (mm Hg)	41	8.7 ± 0.8	SaO_2 (%)	39	91.0 ± 0.9
PAPs (mm Hg)	46	89.7 ± 3.1	SvO_2 (%)	39	55.2 ± 1.6
PAPd (mm Hg)	46	30.7 ± 1.7			

with more than 5 segments was 51 ± 11 mm Hg, which was statistically a significant difference between the two groups ($P < 0.01$). Meanwhile, the number of defects in lung scan was much less than the level of pulmonary hypertension, which might be due to the occluded vessels being too small to be detected in perfusion scan or certain humoral mediators being involved in the pathogenesis of thromboembolic pulmonary hypertension (10). The radionuclide lung scans of 32 patients with unexplained pulmonary hypertension were studied with the method developed by D'Alonzo and colleagues (11). The results revealed normal or scattered defects of lung perfusion scan imaging in 12 patients (37.50%) in accordance with the diagnosis of the plexogenic pulmonary arteriopathy and the irregular perfusion defects (nonsegmental distribution) in 20 cases (62.50%) with recurrent pulmonary embolism (12). A comparative study of the concentration of serum cyclic GMP between the chronic thromboembolic pulmonary hypertension and the unexplained pulmonary hypertension showed that the level of serum cyclic GMP was significantly higher in the former than that in the latter. The serum cyclic GMP may be used to differentiate the chronic thromboembolic pulmonary hypertension from the unexplained pulmonary hypertension (13). A Bayes probability model was established in a study of 71 cases of primary pulmonary hypertension and 55 cases of chronic thromboembolic pulmonary hypertension with the diagnosis conducted by clinical history (particularly deep venous thrombosis of the lower extremities), cardiac catheterization, radionuclide lung scans, or pulmonary angiography. By means of this model, it was found that the correct diagnostic rate of both disorders was 86.51% (14).

B. The Treatment of PE

Acute pulmonary embolism in China is usually treated with anticoagulants (heparin or warfarin), thrombolytic agents (urokinase), snake venom, and traditional Chinese medicine as well as general care. Eighteen patients with deep venous thrombosis of the lower extremities were treated with small daily doses of 50 mg heparin, among whom 11 cases (61.11%) were improved after 2-week

Table 5 Hemodynamic Response of the Patients with Thromboembolic Pulmonary Hypertension to Pure Oxygen Inhalation

		Inhalation		
Parameters	*n*	Before	After	*P*
PAPs (mm Hg)	28	94.5 ± 21.7	86.3 ± 19.6	<0.001
PAPd (mm Hg)	27	33.4 ± 11.4	30.5 ± 11.8	NS
PAPm (mm Hg)	28	51.9 ± 12.5	47.1 ± 12.0	<0.01
CI (L/min/m^2)	28	1.99 ± 0.48	2.55 ± 0.43	<0.05
TPRI (U/m^2)	21	27.8 ± 10.3	21.6 ± 7.2	<0.01

treatment, while the others did not. The effect of some drugs was studied because humoral factors are probably involved in the development of thromboembolic pulmonary hypertension besides mechanical occlusion of the lung vessels. The hemodynamic response to pure oxygen inhalation of 28 patients with thromboembolic pulmonary hypertension was observed. The average reduction of mean pulmonary arterial pressure was 4.8 ± 0.5 mm Hg; however, the paradoxical rise in the mean pulmonary arterial pressure was 5.9 ± 5.6 mm Hg in five cases (Table 5). The hemodynamic changes after a single dose of 20 mg sublingual nifedipine in 10 patients with chronic thromboembolic pulmonary hypertension showed an increase in the cardiac index, a decrease in the total pulmonary resistance index, but no significant decrease in the mean pulmonary arterial pressure (Table 6).

The patients with chronic thromboembolic pulmonary hypertension were treated mainly with anticoagulants, vasodilators, antiplatelet agents, and traditional Chinese medicine. A long-term follow-up (average 4.2 years) in 13 patients with chronic thromboembolic pulmonary hypertension revealed a remarkable

Table 6 Hemodynamic Changes After Sublingual Nifedipine (20 mg) in 10 Patients with Thromboembolic Pulmonary Hypertension

	Nifedipine		
Parameters	Before	After	*P*
HR (bpm)	79.3 ± 14.1	87.9 ± 8.8	<0.05
SAPm (mm Hg)	92.0 ± 11.8	84.4 ± 11.3	<0.01
PAPm (mm Hg)	51.9 ± 14.7	51.0 ± 16.2	NS
RAP (mm Hg)	8.4 ± 5.9	9.1 ± 4.6	NS
CI (L/min/m^2)	2.37 ± 0.76	2.66 ± 0.84	NS
TPRI (U/m^2)	24.8 ± 13.4	22.0 ± 9.9	NS
PAPm/SAPm (%)	56.6 ± 13.5	61.6 ± 15.9	<0.05

improvement in 8 cases, some improvement in 2, no change in 1, and deterioration in 2 (15). Patients who had anticoagulant therapy for 4 years had to go on with it because of deterioration in the withdrawing of the anticoagulant. The longest period of therapy at present was 5 years.

In China PE is not as uncommon as conventionally expected, and it shows a rising trend professionally and has been given more and more attention. However, the characteristic features of PE in China and occidental countries remain to be studied.

Acknowledgment

We thank Professor Chen Su-Chang, Department of Peripheral Vascular Disease, Dong Zhi Men Hospital, Beijing Traditional Chinese Medicine College, for her invaluable data in Table 1.

References

1. Huisman MV, Biiller HR, Cate JW, Royen EA, Vreeken J, Kersten MJ, Baks R. Unexpected high prevalence of silent pulmonary embolism in patients with deep venous thrombosis. Chest 1989; 95:498–502.
2. Ruan Ying-mao, Cheng Xian-sheng, Shi Wen-xue, Zhang Lian-zhuang, Liang Feng-ling. A clinico-pathological analysis of 100 autopsy cases of massive or submassive pulmonary thrombo-obstruction in cardiovascular and pulmonary disease. Chinese J Tuber Resp Dis 1991; 14:5–6.
3. Bell WR, Simon TL. Current status of pulmonary thromboembolic disease: pathophysiology, diagnosis, prevention and treatment. Am Heart J 1982; 103:239–62.
4. Data preview from the People's Republic of China. Data from USA-PRC collaborative study of cardiovascular and cardiopulmonary epidemiology: baseline serum lipids, 1990.
5. Sukumaran M, AbuNasser S, Savajiyani B, Flynn JT. The incidence of pulmonary thromboembolism in the Chinese population: a comparative study. The New York Infirmary-Beekman Downtown Hospital, 1984.
6. Wang Qi, Cheng Xian-sheng. Clinical investigation in 143 cases of pulmonary vascular disease. Chinese J Tuber Resp Dis 1983; 6:39–41.
7. Ruan Cun-liang, Li Qui-lin, Zhong Cheng-zhu. Treatment observation of 82 patients with pulmonary embolism. Chinese J Tuber Resp Dis 1990; 13:88–90.
8. Xu Jin-yin, Zao Qian, Long Ming-qing. Radionuclide venography for detecting deep vein thrombosis and evaluating heparin treatment. Chinese J Nuclear Med 1991; 11:71–3.
9. Cheng Xiang-sheng, Zhao Yi-ju. Classification of pulmonary vascular disease. Chinese Circulation J 1991; 6:158–160.
10. Malik AB, Johnson A. Role of humoral mediators in the pulmonary vascular

response to pulmonary embolism. In: Weir EN, Reeves JT, eds, Pulmonary vascular physiology and pathophysiology. New York, Marcel Dekker, 1989:445–67.

11. D'Alonzo DO, Bower JS, Dantzker DR. Differentiation of patients with primary and thromboembolic pulmonary hypertension. Chest 1984; 85:457–61.
12. Chen Bai-ping, Liu Yun-he, Cheng Xian-sheng. Lung perfusion scan in unexplained pulmonary hypertension. Chinese J Intern Med 1992; 31:335–7.
13. Zu Guang-Jin, Xu Shu-huai, Zhou Chao-feng, Xue Quan-fu, Ma Xiu-e, Cheng Xian-sheng. Preliminary study of differential diagnostic significance of serum cGMP level for thromboembolic pulmonary hypertension. Physiol Sci 1988; 8:398.
14. Zhao Yi-ju, Cai Ru-sheng, Cheng Xian-sheng. Discrimination between primary pulmonary hypertension and pulmonary hypertension secondary to thromboembolism. Chinese Circulation J 1990; 5:423–6.
15. Cheng Xian-sheng, Ma Xiu-e, Zhang Hai-ying. Analysis of natural history and long-term follow-up of 59 patients with obliterative pulmonary hypertension. Acta Academicae Medicine Sinicae 1992; 14:295–300.

5

Pathomorphology of Pulmonary Thromboembolism

C. A. WAGENVOORT

Erasmus University
Rotterdam, The Netherlands

I. Introduction

An embolus is an intravascular corpuscle or mass that is carried by the blood stream, subsequently to become impacted in a vessel. These particles or masses may consist of cells; pieces of tissue, fat, air, or foreign material; but they are most often thrombi. For all emboli, the lungs are the most common target organs, because they receive the total cardiac output. Moreover, prospective emboli are most often formed in or are introduced into the systemic veins so that eventually they are sieved out in the pulmonary arterial tree.

Although pulmonary thromboembolism is undoubtedly common, its incidence is unknown. Not only is the clinical diagnosis very difficult so that reliable statistical data are lacking, but also the contribution of autopsy investigation is limited for two reasons. First, pulmonary emboli may completely disappear as a result of thrombolysis, so that there is no longer postmortem evidence of embolism. Second, there is no morphological difference between the lesions resulting from embolism and from primary thrombosis.

These thrombotic lesions are exceedingly common. Depending on the number of blocks of lung tissue studied microscopically, the autopsy incidence of pulmonary embolism in consecutive adult hospital patients may be as high as

51.7% (1), 64% (2), or higher (3). However, what percentage of these lesions have an embolic origin remains questionable (4).

Grossly recognized clots are likely to be thromboemboli. Even so, the postmortem incidence of gross thromboembolism, mentioned in various reports, shows a considerable variation in the range of 5%–30% (3). This clearly depends on factors such as definition of gross or massive embolism, the extent to which peripheral pulmonary arteries are opened, and accuracy of investigation.

Pulmonary thromboembolism has a very wide spectrum not only of its clinical manifestations but also of its morphology. With time, thrombi entrapped in the lung vessels may undergo various, striking alterations. The variation is also related to the size of the thromboemboli and consequently to the caliber of the pulmonary arteries and arterioles obstructed by them.

In massive pulmonary thromboembolism, the source of the emboli is usually formed by the deep leg veins, particularly iliac, femoral, and calf veins. However, in recent times upper-extremity venous thrombosis has increased as a result of invasive diagnostic and therapeutic procedures and of intravenous drug abuse. Other sources of the embolism include the pelvic veins, responsible for many of the smaller thromboemboli; the right atrium, particularly patients with atrial fibrillation; and the right ventricle in some patients with myocardial infarction involving the ventricular septum.

II. Massive Thromboembolism

In massive pulmonary thromboembolism causing sudden death, the pulmonary trunk and/or main pulmonary arteries are blocked by a mass of thromboemboli (Fig. 1). In some cases this mass extends well into the right ventricle. Obstruction of a single main artery may be fatal when previous bouts of embolism have occluded multiple pulmonary arterial branches.

In shape and size, thromboemboli conform to their veins of origin, of which they are the casts. Sometimes they are V- or Y-shaped when the source was confluent veins. The ends of thromboemboli are usually blunt, and they may show the impressions of venous valves, which are often the sites of thrombus formation (5). Thromboemboli are generally fresh without or with no more than early organization, already present at the site of origin. They are dry and brittle and dark red in color. On their cut surface pale, gray lines, the “lines of Zahn,” represent platelets and leucocytes that separate the dark red masses of erythrocytes.

In massive pulmonary embolism, the emboli are usually large but not always occlusive. One reason is that they may be V-shaped or folded, allowing a residual blood flow. Moreover, thromboemboli are often arrested at the bifurcation of the pulmonary trunk or at more distal points of ramification. Often

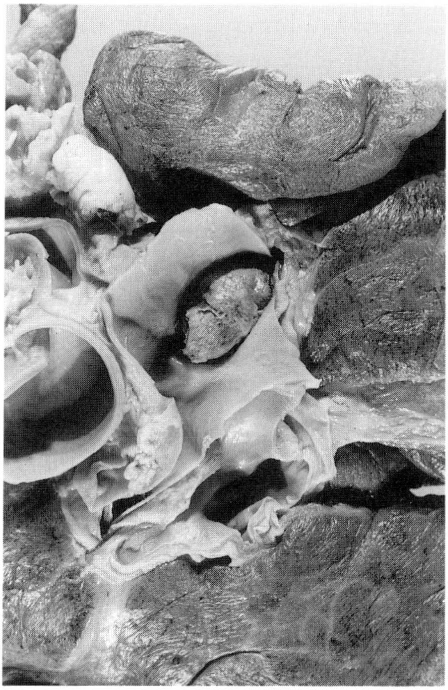

Figure 1 Left main pulmonary artery blocked by a large thromboembolus.

by riding on a bifurcation, such a "saddle embolus" is prevented from completely occluding the vessels involved. These circumstances may contribute to prevent sudden death.

If the patient survives, his or her fate may be coupled to that of the emboli. Many clots will be removed by lysis. It is believed that approximately 60% of thromboemboli disappear within weeks or months as a result of thrombolysis. The remaining thromboemboli become adherent to the arterial wall, undergo organization, and are converted into fibrous masses, which may occupy much of the lumina of the main pulmonary arteries and its branches. Gradually, retraction of the mass results in some luminal widening. Almost simultaneously recanalization occurs, which further contributes to restoration of blood flow. The recanalization channels developing within the thrombus tend to become very wide, so that the remnants of the thromboembolus stand out as fibrous septa or networks, the so-called bands and webs (Fig. 2).

These various processes explain that chronic thromboembolic pulmonary hypertension as a result of occlusion of large vessels is uncommon. It may be treated surgically (6,7) (see Chap. 17).

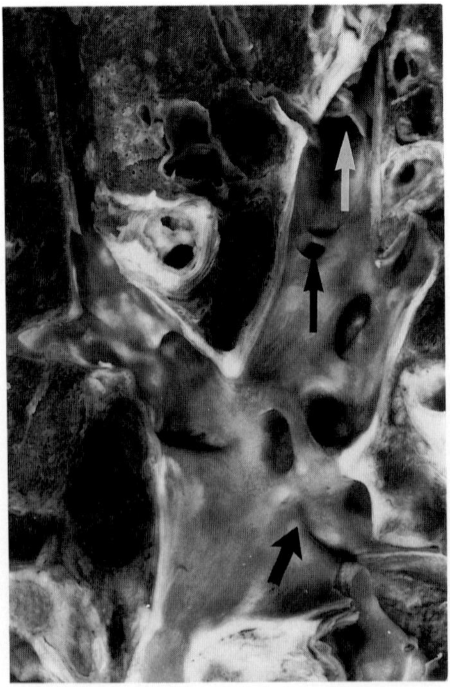

Figure 2 A band (small arrows) and a weblike structure (large arrow) resulting from organization and recanalization of thromboembolus within major elastic pulmonary artery.

III. Emboli in Intrapulmonary Elastic Arteries: Infarction

Thrombi found in elastic pulmonary arteries are often multiple; they are considered to be embolic in nature, as long as there is no inflammation or injury to the arterial wall or other reasons to suspect primary thrombosis. Thromboemboli occur more often in the right than in the left lung, which corresponds with the pulmonary flow distribution.

The morphology of thromboemboli in intrapulmonary elastic arteries is essentially the same as in pulmonary trunk and both main pulmonary arteries. There is usually complete occlusion by one or more emboli (Fig. 3), and this is followed by organization and recanalization, eventually leading to formation of fibrous plaques or to weblike or colanderlike structures. Occasionally obliteration with shrinkage occurs in an elastic artery, resulting in a fibrous strand.

The effect of thromboembolic occlusion of an elastic pulmonary artery is generally limited. No damage to the lung tissue that was supplied by the

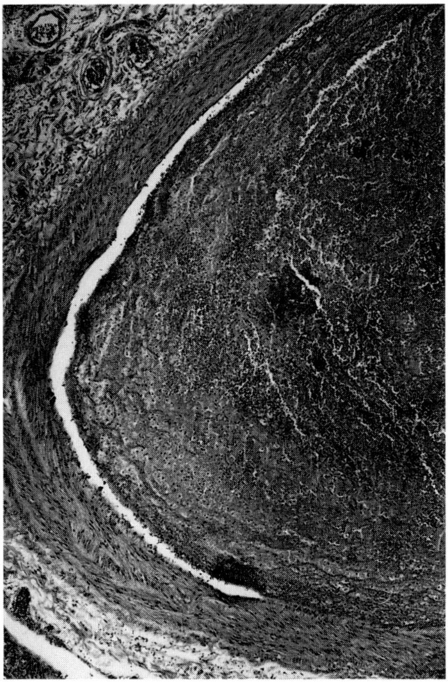

Figure 3 Major elastic pulmonary artery occluded by fresh thromboembolus.

obstructed artery will ensue as long as the bronchial circulation is adequate. Anastomosing capillary networks provide a scant but usually sufficient collateral blood supply from adjacent pulmonary arteries and particularly from the bronchial circulation. Only when a major pulmonary artery is blocked, so that a large area of lung tissue is affected, this collateral circulation may not suffice. Infarction of lung tissue, however, is more likely to occur when in addition to arterial obstruction, the bronchial circulation is insufficient. This may result from congestion of the lungs or when the cardiac output is decreased.

In an ischemic area of the lung, hemorrhage may be the first sign, because damage of endothelium leads to increased permeability. Small arterioles and venules and capillaries dilate, and there is extensive leakage of fluid and erythrocytes, but there is no destruction of lung tissue (Fig. 4). If the bronchial circulation can cope with this situation, pulmonary hemorrhage is reversible and eventually may disappear with no other remnants than deposition of iron pigment. If, however, tissue necrosis sets in, capillaries are destroyed, and an infarction develops. Because blood from the bronchial circulation seeps into the area, a pulmonary infarction is almost always hemorrhagic.

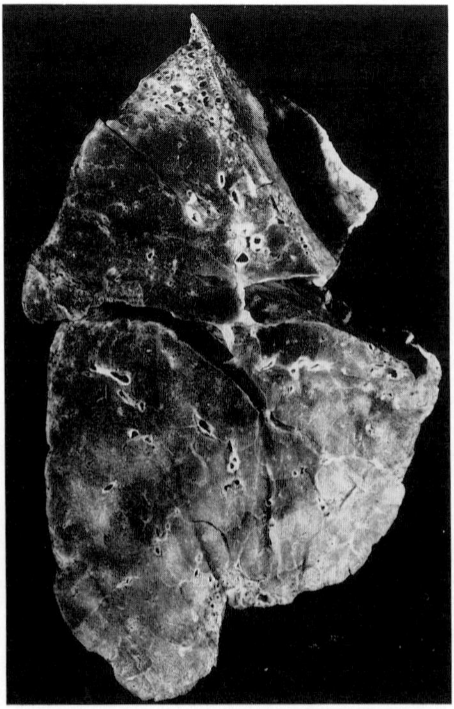

Figure 4 Cut section of lung with multiple large areas of pulmonary hemorrhage following thromboembolic obstruction of main pulmonary artery. Within these areas, the structure of lung tissue is still recognizable.

Hemorrhagic pulmonary infarctions are often multiple and, like the thromboemboli, are observed somewhat more often in the lower than in the upper lobes. They are wedge-shaped on cross section, bordering the pleura with the apex close to the thromboembolus. Infarctions are dark red with a sharp delimitation; on cut section they are soft and friable, and the various structures in the lung tissue such as bronchi, vessels, and septa are no longer recognizable (Fig. 5). In the long run, organization occurs so that gradually a scar develops, which may be difficult to detect on gross inspection unless the lung is expanded by inflation.

Microscopically, the infarcted tissue is engorged with blood, and capillary walls, bronchioles, and vessels are recognized as ghostlike structures or are hardly

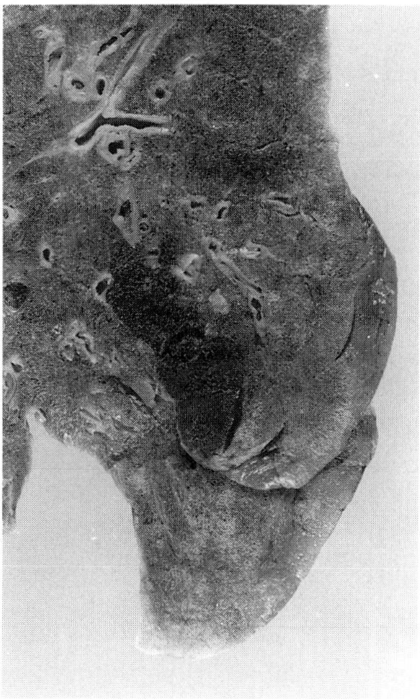

Figure 5 Cut section of lung with hemorrhagic pulmonary infarction; the structure of the lung tissue in this area is no longer recognizable.

identifiable (Fig. 6). In the margins necrosis may not have occurred, so that here the lung tissue can be still viable.

When the embolus initiating the infarction was infected, or when there was pneumonia or sepsis, the hemorrhagic infarction may become septic; it usually is then grayish-white in color. A pulmonary abscess may develop in this area.

IV. Emboli in Muscular Arteries: Thrombotic Arteriopathy

While clots in intact elastic pulmonary arteries are likely to be embolic in origin, this is questionable when it concerns thrombi within muscular pulmonary arteries, i.e., arterial branches of less than 1 mm in diameter. Just as with larger clots, the morphology does not allow one to distinguish between small thrombi of embolic and of primary origin, and the same is true for their sequelae: the

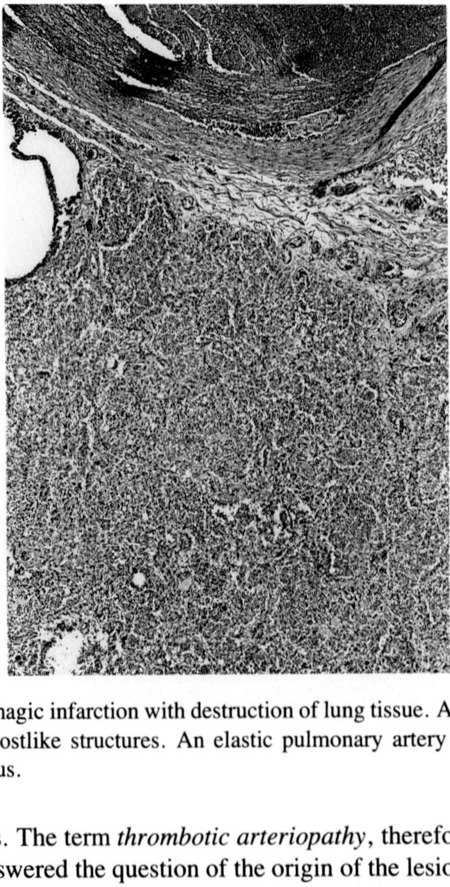

Figure 6 Hemorrhagic infarction with destruction of lung tissue. Alveolar walls can still be recognized as ghostlike structures. An elastic pulmonary artery (top) is occluded by fresh thromboembolus.

thrombotic lesions. The term *thrombotic arteriopathy*, therefore, is a descriptive one, leaving unanswered the question of the origin of the lesions (3). Obviously, arteriopathy implies a disease, and, thus, this term should only be used when there is widespread involvement of the arterial tree. While thrombotic arteriopathy is not common, isolated lesions occur in a great variety of conditions as complicating lesions. They are particularly numerous in older age groups and in the presence of pulmonary hypertension by whatever cause (8). In fact, occasional lesions are often seen in otherwise normal individuals.

There is little doubt that in some cases, thrombotic arteriopathy results from thromboembolism, while in other cases, primary thrombosis is responsible. Thromboemboli, small enough to become impacted in muscular pulmonary arteries, may be released from systemic venous plexuses, but in part they will represent pieces of larger emboli. Fragmentation of thombi may occur during their passage through the right heart and the larger pulmonary arteries. Thrombolysis may well play an important part, because it leads to gradual disintegration of the thrombus (4).

In many cases of unmistakable thromboembolism, there is, in addition to embolic occlusion of major pulmonary arteries, also a thrombotic arteriopathy involving the muscular pulmonary arteries. This suggests that, rather than dealing with two different, unrelated processes as embolism and primary thrombosis, both are embolic in nature.

On the other hand, there are also cases in which exclusively small arteries and arterioles are blocked in such numbers that this is almost certainly due to primary thrombosis. Also, in conditions with increased tendency to thrombosis, e.g., in tetralogy of Fallot, the thrombotic lesions in the lung vessels are primary rather than embolic.

The ratio between embolic and primary thrombotic arteriopathy is unknown. Embolic lesions tend to be more numerous in the lower lobes and lesions based upon primary thrombosis more in the upper lobes (Wagenvoort, unpublished data). This also applies to the so-called age changes, plaques of the intimal fibrosis that increase in number with age. These lesions, which probably are thrombotic in origin, appear to be more common in the upper parts of the lungs (9). Such a dual distribution of lesions is not surprising. The pulmonary flow, particularly at rest, is much larger through the lower than through the upper lobes. Consequently, as we have seen, emboli will favor the lower parts of the lungs, but the tendency to in situ thrombosis will be greater in the upper parts, where the flow is slow or even stagnant. In practice, however, for distinguishing the lesions, the consequences of this distribution are limited in view of the very time-consuming assessment involved.

As discussed earlier, thrombotic lesions can be found in a very large percentage of routine autopsies but uncommonly in such large numbers that we are dealing with thrombotic arteriopathy. Even more rare are patients with sustained pulmonary hypertension on the basis of this arterial disease. In these patients, the mechanism of the increased pulmonary arterial pressure is believed to be mechanical rather than vasoconstrictive (10–12). This is also suggested by the morphology of the pulmonary arteries. In most cases of patients with severe pulmonary hypertension caused by thrombotic arteriopathy, the media of the pulmonary arteries is not or only mildly thickened. If vasoconstriction should play the major part, medial hypertrophy would be expected. In a minority of such patients, however, there is indeed prominent medial hypertrophy, and it is certainly possible that in these instances microemboli elicited vasoconstriction contributing to an elevated pulmonary vascular resistance.

When there is chronic pulmonary hypertension, segmental and/or muscular pulmonary arteries are obstructed. Most of these thrombi, also when they have an embolic origin, are asymptomatic, and the signs and symptoms of pulmonary hypertension may be the first indication that thromboembolism is involved. This "silent embolic pulmonary hypertension" is uncommon and very difficult to diagnose clinically (12,13). In these instances of unexplained pulmonary hypertension, an open-lung biopsy may be the only way to establish a diagnosis (14).

In thrombotic arteriopathy, recent thrombi are almost always scarce. Even in patients with severe thromboembolic pulmonary hypertension, clots that are fresh or with no more than early organization are few or absent. The reason is the rapid turnover of the clots into organized plaques. At the site of a thrombus, the artery remains wide, while, as a result of collapse and fixation shrinkage, the adjacent parts of the vessel will narrow (Fig. 7).

The process of organization can be easily demonstrated in muscular pulmonary arteries. Following a stage of adherence to the arterial wall, endothelial cells form a thin lining over the surface of the thrombus, while myofibroblasts grow from the media through the internal elastic lamina into the clot. Gradually the thrombus is replaced by these cells (Fig. 7). Thereafter, increasing amounts of collagen and elastic fibers are formed. In this way the thrombus is incorporated into the arterial wall as a patch of intimal fibrosis (Fig.

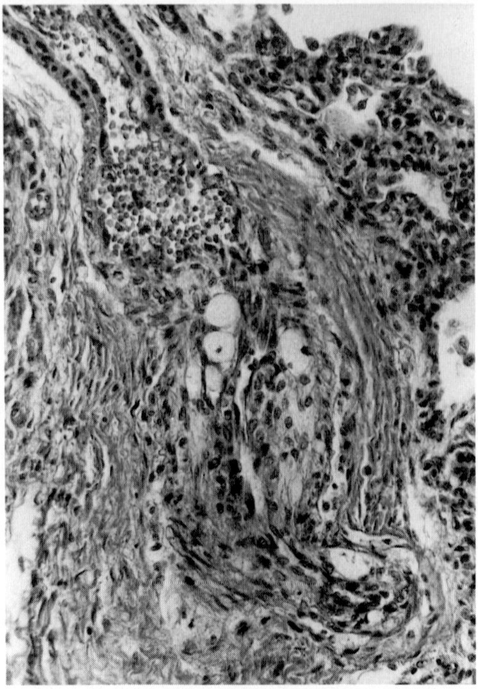

Figure 7 Early organization of thrombus in muscular pulmonary artery. The clot is replaced by proliferating cells. In this area, the artery is much wider than in the adjacent parts, which are collapsed and shrunken.

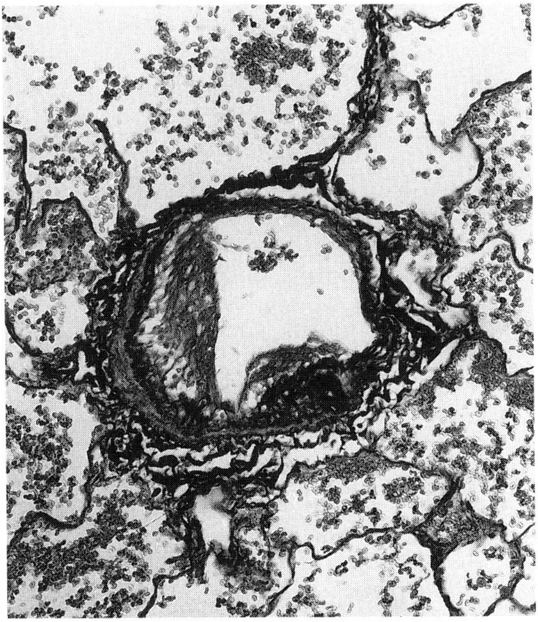

Figure 8 Irregular patch of intimal fibrosis resulting from organization of a thrombus in muscular pulmonary artery.

8). This patch is usually eccentric and irregular but, even when it is circumferential or occlusive, it does not have the concentric-laminar or "onionskin" appearance that is characteristic of plexogenic arteriopathy.

Postthrombotic intimal fibrosis often obliterates the arterial lumen completely (Fig. 9), although it usually extends only over short distances within the arteries. As a consequence, the significance of these intimal lesions is sometimes underestimated when too few histological sections are available for the pathologist. The few lesions caught in a single random slide are seemingly in contrast to the pulmonary hypertension attributed to them (15). In most cases of thrombotic pulmonary hypertension, however, this problem does not occur because the lesions are usually numerous.

Simultaneously with, or soon after, the myofibroblasts, capillaries grow into the clot, particularly when this is occlusive (Fig. 10). These capillaries communicate with each other and with the arterial lumen on either side of the thrombus, forming networks. Some of these anastomosing vessels widen at the cost of others so that a limited number of channels remain (Fig. 11). This recanalization may allow some blood flow through the obstructing thrombotic

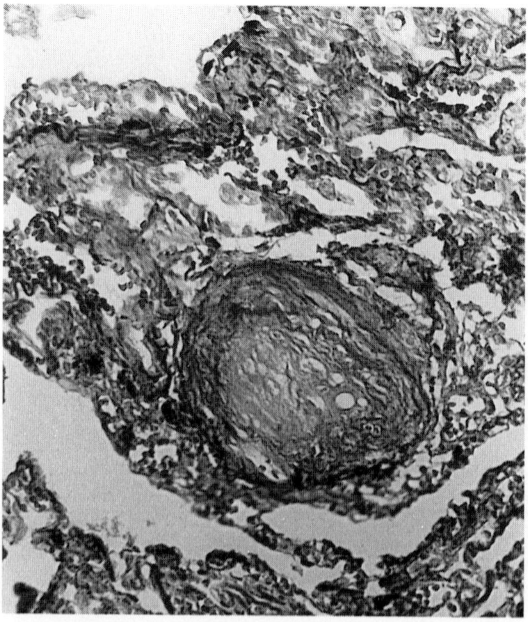

Figure 9 Complete obliteration of muscular pulmonary artery by organizing thrombus, retraction of which has caused partial thickening of the media.

lesions. In a number of instances, the channels become so wide that the remnants of the original thrombus stand out as fibrous septa separating the channels (Fig. 12). These intravascular septa are equivalents of the "band and webs" in the elastic arteries, and pathognomonic for organized thrombotic lesions.

Some features, although not exclusively occurring in thrombotic changes, are commonly observed in these lesions so that they may help in the diagnosis of thrombotic arteriopathy. One of these is proliferation of longitudinal smooth muscle cells within the patch of intimal fibrosis (Fig. 13). These cells may lie in dense bundles or layers, or widely apart in the fibrous tissue (3). In hypoxic pulmonary hypertension and in some patients with plexogenic arteriopathy, longitudinal smooth muscle is found in pulmonary arterioles. In contrast, in thrombotic arteriopathy it occurs in muscular arteries, even of fairly large caliber. This feature may also be observed in patients with pulmonary venous hypertension, and then in intimal fibrosis that is probably not of thrombotic origin.

Smooth muscle cells within thrombotic lesions sometimes form a circular layer around the remaining or newly formed lumen. This layer may even be bounded on either side by an elastic lamina so that a complete new muscular

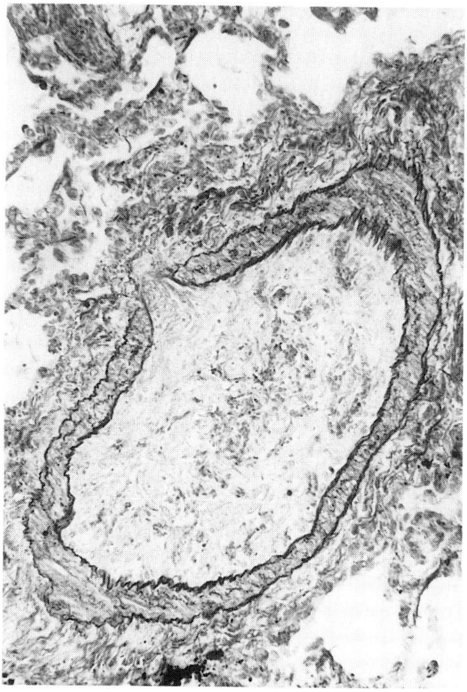

Figure 10 Muscular pulmonary artery obliterated by organized thrombus. There is early recanalization by multiple capillaries.

coat is formed (Fig. 14). Pulmonary arteries with such a "double media" are regularly found in cases of thrombotic arteriopathy but also in some forms of lung fibrosis, particularly in systemic sclerosis.

Calcification of organized thrombi is uncommon (Fig. 15). It may be impossible to decide whether it occurred in the lung, or whether a phlebolith embolized to the lung. Deposition of iron pigment is more common but usually in small amounts either within macrophages or extracellular.

Reversibility of organized thrombotic lesions is rather limited. To some extent, retraction of an organized clot may result in widening of the remaining lumen. Recanalization also contributes to reestablishing some pulmonary flow, but the effect is probably moderate at best. Complete obliteration of pulmonary arteries is an irreversible change. Therefore, when pulmonary hypertension as a result of thromboembolism has been established, reversibility is very limited, and treatment should be directed particularly to preventing further embolic episodes.

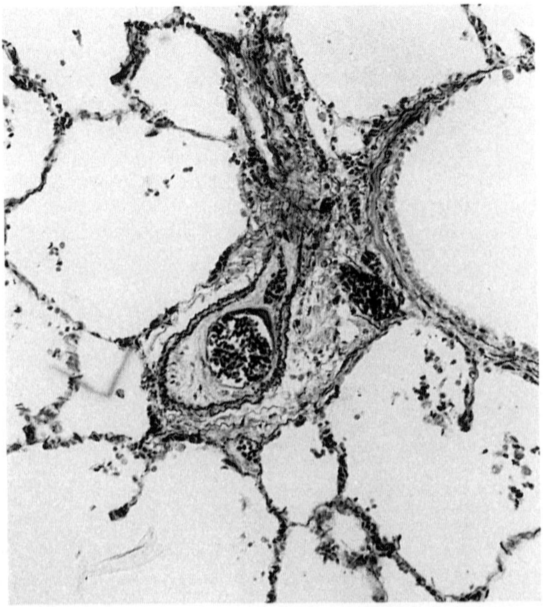

Figure 11 Muscular pulmonary artery with two fairly wide recanalization channels within organized thrombus.

In the morphological evaluation of thrombotic arteriopathy, there are a few sources of error to be taken into account (14). Incipient plexiform lesions have been confused with intravascular septa. Other characteristics of the plexiform lesion such as destruction of the media and dilatation of peripheral branches should be looked for to avoid this. Thrombotic intimal fibrosis occasionally may mimic an onionskin arrangement, indicative of plexogenic arteriopathy, in some vessels, but as a rule recanalization channels will reveal the true nature of this alteration. Concentric-laminar intimal fibrosis may also be suggested by the development of a "double media," particularly when this occurs in small arteries.

Finally, the warning must be repeated that obstructive thrombotic lesions may extend over a very short distance within an artery, so that it can be missed in a random histological section. The erroneous conclusion that the pulmonary vasculature is normal, or that at least its changes do not match the elevation of the pulmonary arterial pressure, can be avoided if more blocks or more sections are studied. When open-lung biopsies are concerned, multiple sections at different levels are necessary; this is important in any form of pulmonary vascular disease but particularly in patients with thrombosis or thromboembolism.

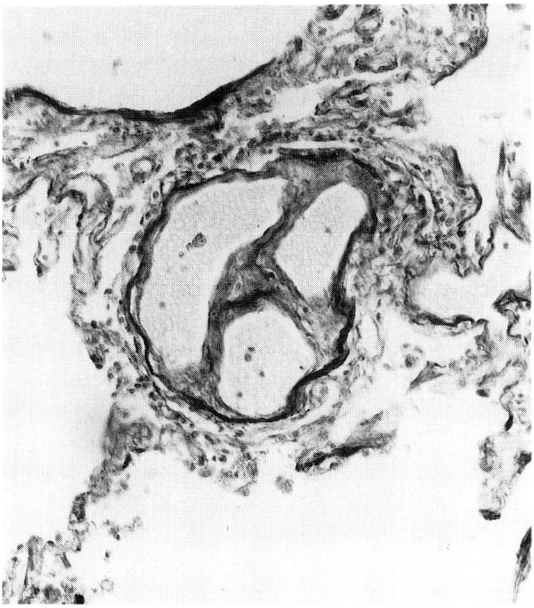

Figure 12 Coarse intravascular fibrous septa in muscular pulmonary artery resulting from recanalization of organized thrombus.

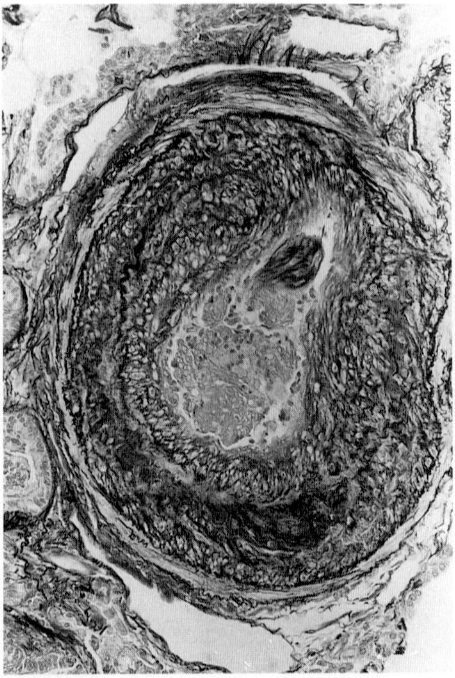

Figure 13 Muscular pulmonary artery with extensive postthrombotic intimal thickening with numerous longitudinal smooth muscle cells in cross section. The remaining lumen contains a cross section of a band and a recent thrombus.

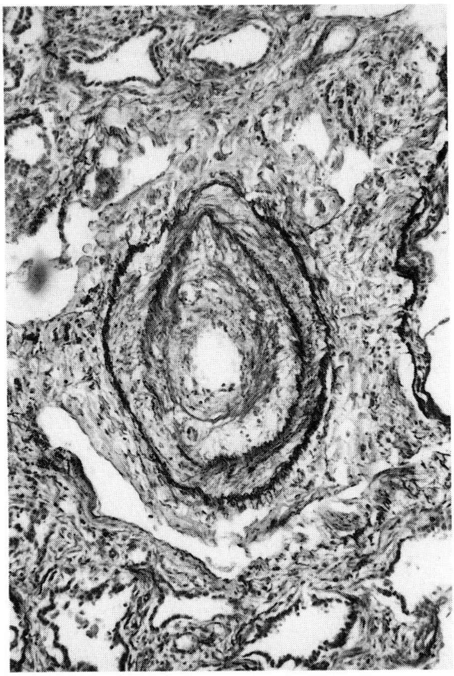

Figure 14 Muscular pulmonary artery with postthrombotic intimal fibrosis. Around the remaining lumen, a new layer of circular smooth muscle cells has developed. There is beginning formation of elastic laminae on either side of this layer so that a "double media" is formed.

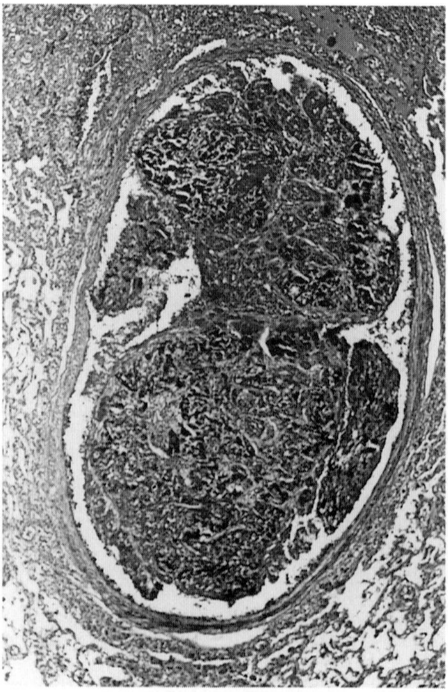

Figure 15 Elastic pulmonary artery with largely calcified organized thromboembolus.

References

1. Morrell MT, Dunnill MS. The postmortem incidence of pulmonary embolism in a hospital population. Br J Surg 1968, 55:347–52.
2. Freiman DG, Suyemoto J, Wessler S. Frequency of pulmonary thromboembolism in man. N Engl J Med 1965, 272:1278–80.
3. Wagenvoort CA, Mooi WJ. Biopsy Pathology of the Pulmonary Vasculature. London: Chapman & Hall, 1989.
4. Wagenvoort CA, Mooi WJ. Vascular diseases. In: Dail DH, Hammer SP, eds. Pulmonary Pathology. 2nd ed. New York: Springer Verlag, 1993.
5. Beckering RE, Titus JL. Femoral-popliteal venous thrombosis and pulmonary embolism. Am J Clin Pathol 1969, 52:530–7.
6. Moser KM, Olson LK, Schlusselberg M, Daily PO, Dembitsky WP. Chronic thromboembolic occlusion in the adult can mimic pulmonary artery agenesis. Chest 1989, 95:503–8.
7. Moser KM, Auger WR, Fedullo PF, Jamieson SW. Chronic thromboembolic pulmonary hypertension: clinical picture and surgical treatment. Eur Respir J 1992, 5:334–42.

8. Wagenvoort CA, Mulder PGH. Thrombotic lesions in primary plexogenic arteriopathy. Similar pathogenesis or complication? Chest 1993; 103:844–9.
9. Wagenvoort CA, Wagenvoort N. Age changes in muscular pulmonary arteries. Arch Pathol 1965, 79:524–8.
10. Knisely WH, Wallace JM, Mahaley MS, Satterwhite WM. Evidence, including in vivo observation, suggesting mechanical blockage rather than reflex vasospam as the cause of death in pulmonary embolization. Am Heart J 1957, 54:483–97.
11. Rosenow EC, Osmundson PJ, Brown ML. Pulmonary embolism. Mayo Clinic Proc 1981, 56:161–78.
12. Messer JV. Thromboembolic pulmonary hypertension. In: Weir EK, Reeves JT, eds. Pulmonary Hypertension. Mount Kisco, NY: Futura Publishing Company, 1984: 169–249.
13. Wilhelmsen L, Selander S, Söderholm B, Paulin S, Varnauskas E, Werkö L. Recurrent pulmonary embolism. Medicine 1963, 42:335–55.
14. Wagenvoort CA, Lung biopsies in the differential diagnosis of thromboembolic versus primary pulmonary hypertension. Progr Respir Res 1980, 13:16–21.
15. Wagenvoort CA, Mooi WJ. Controversies and potential errors in the histological evaluation of pulmonary vascular disease. In: Wagenvoort CA, Denolin H, eds. Pulmonary Circulation. Advances and Controversies. Amsterdam, Elsevier, 1989: 7–26.

Part Two

CLINICAL DIAGNOSIS AND COURSE OF PE

6

Clinical Diagnosis of Acute Pulmonary Embolism

JAMES E. DALEN

College of Medicine
University of Arizona
Tucson, Arizona

I. Introduction

Acute pulmonary embolism is rarely silent, and with appropriate therapy the mortality is decreased from approximately 30% to less than 10% (1). Yet, pulmonary embolism causes 100,000–200,000 deaths per year in the United States, and it is the third most common cause of death (2). The explanation for this apparent paradox is that most patients who die of pulmonary embolism have not had therapy because the diagnosis of pulmonary embolism was not made. Less than 10% of patients dying of pulmonary embolism in the United States had therapy prior to death (2).

A recent Norwegian study illustrates the failure of clinicians to recognize pulmonary embolism prior to death. Karwinski and Svendsen (3) reported the results of 21,529 autopsies performed from 1960 to 1984. The autopsy rate at their hospital was 75%–80% during the years of the study. The total incidence of pulmonary embolism at postmortem was 9%. In 75% of the cases, pulmonary embolism was the immediate cause of death; it contributed to death in the remaining 25%. Pulmonary embolism had been recognized prior to death in only 18% in those patients in whom pulmonary embolism was the immediate cause of death and 10% in those in whom pulmonary embolism contributed to death.

Furthermore, the percent of cases of pulmonary embolism recognized prior to death actually decreased from 1960 to 1984 (3)!

The clinical accuracy of the diagnosis of pulmonary embolism is very low. In the Prospective Investigation of Pulmonary Embolism Diagnosis (PIOPED) Study, 755 patients had V/Q lung scans and pulmonary angiograms because of suspected pulmonary embolism within 24 h of study (4). Only 33% of these patients were found to have angiographic evidence of pulmonary embolism. The rate of false positive clinical diagnosis was 67%.

Prior to lung scan and angiography, the PIOPED investigators estimated the probability of pulmonary embolism based upon the clinical findings, chest X-ray, EKG, and arterial blood gas analysis. As shown in Table 1, the clinical accuracy was quite good when the probability of pulmonary embolism was judged to be 80% or greater; 68% of these patients had angiographic evidence of pulmonary embolism. When the clinical estimate of pulmonary embolism was less than 20%, only 9% had pulmonary embolism. However, the clinical estimate of pulmonary embolism was high in only 10% of the patients and very low in only 26%. In the majority (64%) of the cases, the clinical estimate of pulmonary embolism was uncertain (19%–79%). The incidence of pulmonary embolism in patients with an uncertain clinical probability was 30%. Of the 251 patients with documented pulmonary embolism, the clinical estimate of pulmonary embolism had been uncertain in the vast majority (67%) (4).

The results of the PIOPED Study (4) and other studies (5) make it very clear that the clinical diagnosis of acute pulmonary embolism is highly inaccurate. V/Q lung scans and/or pulmonary angiography are required to confirm or exclude the diagnosis of acute pulmonary embolism. The task of the clinician is to determine what combination of clinical findings is sufficiently suggestive of pulmonary embolism to justify ordering a V/Q lung scan.

The two most frequent symptoms in patients with acute pulmonary embolism are dyspnea and pleuritic chest pain. One or both of these symptoms are present in the vast majority of patients as shown in Table 2 (4,6,7). The obvious problem facing the clinician is that neither of these two symptoms is

Table 1 Accuracy of the Clinical Diagnosis of Pulmonary Embolism in the PIOPED Study[a]

Clinical probability[b]	Number of patients	Percent	Percent having pulmonary embolism
80%–100%	90	10	68
19%–79%	569	64	30
0%–19%	228	26	9

[a]From PIOPED Study, JAMA (May 23/30, 1990).
[b]Without scan results.

Table 2 Incidence of Pleuritic Pain and Dyspnea in Patients with Angiographically Documented Pulmonary Embolism

Study	Number of patients	Percent with pleuritic pain	Percent with dyspnea
Bell et al. (6)	327	74	84
Dalen (7)	124	57	77
PIOPED Study[a] (4)	117	66	73

[a]Stein et al., Chest (September 1991).

specific for pulmonary embolism. Dyspnea and pleuritic chest pain are present in a wide variety of cardiac and pulmonary diseases (8). These two symptoms are most suggestive of acute pulmonary embolism when they have associated signs, symptoms, and laboratory findings suggesting one of three syndromes of acute pulmonary embolism (9). In addition, the suspicion of acute pulmonary embolism should rise markedly when these symptoms occur in patients who have evidence of, or have conditions predisposing to, venous thromboembolism.

II. Associated Venous Thrombosis

Postmortem studies have shown that venous thrombosis in the legs is present in the vast majority of patients with pulmonary embolism (10). Indeed, as first shown by Virchow (11) in 1858, pulmonary embolism is a complication of venous thrombosis in the lower extremities that occurs when clots in the lower extremities are dislodged and enter the venous circulation. Pulmonary embolism is the most frequent manifestation of venous thromboembolism.

Despite the near universal presence of deep venous thrombosis in patients dying of pulmonary embolism, recognition of deep venous thrombosis depends upon the technique used for diagnosis. As shown in Table 3, only 11% of 251 patients with documented pulmonary embolism in the PIOPED Study had

Table 3 Evidence of Deep Venous Thrombosis in Patients with Pulmonary Embolism Diagnosed by Pulmonary Angiography

	Percent	Reference
Physical exam	11	(4)
IPG	43	(12)
Venogram	70–80	(13)
Postmortem exam	100	(10)

physical findings suggesting deep venous thrombosis (4). Deep venous thrombosis in most patients is clinically silent or associated with nonspecific findings. The most reliable clinical finding of deep venous thrombosis is unilateral leg swelling. Although this finding is quite specific, it lacks sensitivity because it occurs in only a small percentage of patients with deep venous thrombosis.

The diagnosis of deep venous thrombosis in patients with acute pulmonary embolism increases to 57% when an IPG is performed (12) and to 70–80% with venography (13).

III. Predisposing Factors to Venous Thromboembolism

Venous thromboembolism rarely occurs de novo in healthy ambulatory patients; in the urokinase pulmonary embolism trial, 94% of the 167 patients with pulmonary embolism had at least one major coexisting disease (6). Rather, it occurs in patients with one or more risk factors for venous thromboembolism. These risk factors include past history of venous thromboembolism, cancer (including occult cancer), trauma, surgery, pregnancy/oral contraceptive agents, immobility, advanced age, obesity, and congestive heart failure (see Chap. 2). In the PIOPED Study (4), 82% of the patients with pulmonary embolism had one or more risk factors. Most patients with pulmonary embolism have multiple risk factors for venous thromboembolism. Table 4 demonstrates the relationship between the number of risk factors for venous thromboembolism and the probability of an IPG-demonstrated proximal deep venous thrombosis (14).

The presence of evidence of, or predisposing factors for, deep venous thrombosis greatly increases the probability of pulmonary embolism in patients with dyspnea or pleuritic pain.

Table 4 Relationship of Risk Factors to the Probability of a Positive IPG in 1074 Patients Suspected of Pulmonary Embolism[a]

Number of risk factors for venous thromboembolism	Percent positive IPG
0	11
1	24
2	36
3	50
4 or more	100

[a]From Wheeler HB, Anderson FA, Cardullo PA, et al., Arch Surg (September 1982) (14).

IV. Syndromes of Acute Pulmonary Embolism

A given episode of acute pulmonary embolism may cause one of three different syndromes: pulmonary infarction/pulmonary hemorrhage, acute cor pulmonale or acute dyspnea (9). In the PIOPED Study (4), 95% of patients with documented pulmonary embolism had clinical findings consistent with one of these three syndromes. The pathophysiology of each of these three syndromes is quite different. Therefore, they cause different signs and symptoms, and different laboratory findings.

V. Pulmonary Infarction/Pulmonary Hemorrhage

Pleuritic pain, secondary to pulmonary infarction, is the most frequent symptom that leads the clinician to suspect pulmonary embolism. Virchow (15) was the first to demonstrate that necrosis of the lung may occur in areas distal to pulmonary embolic obstruction.

The pathophysiology of pulmonary infarction was the focus of pioneering postmortem studies by Hampton and Castleman (16) in 1940. In reviewing the clinical findings in patients who were found to have pulmonary infarction at postmortem exam, they found that the most frequent clinical finding was pleuritic chest pain. Utilizing postmortem as well as premortem chest X-rays, they found that an infiltrate was nearly always present in the affected lobe. Their finding that pulmonary infarction is rare in patients without associated cardiac or pulmonary disease was confirmed by other postmortem studies (17,18).

Clinical studies utilizing pulmonary angiography rather than postmortem exam to diagnose pulmonary embolism present a different view of pulmonary infarction. Pleuritic pain and a lung infiltrate by chest X-ray are common findings in patients with pulmonary embolism diagnosed by pulmonary angiography. Furthermore, these findings are very common in patients with pulmonary embolism who do not have coexistent cardiac or pulmonary disease (7).

In a study of 124 patients with pulmonary embolism documented by pulmonary angiography, we found that pleuritic pain and a lung infiltrate are frequent findings in patients with submassive pulmonary embolism (7). These patients usually have complete obstruction of a distal branch of the pulmonary circulation. We believe that the clinical findings of pleuritic pain, hemoptysis, and a lung infiltrate are due to the sudden influx of bronchial arterial blood (at systemic pressure) into the obstructed segment. We found that in patients without associated heart or lung disease, the infiltrate by chest X-ray resolved in days or weeks. We believe that in those patients, pleuritic pain and the infiltrate are due to pulmonary hemorrhage, which resolves without leading to true pulmonary infarction. In patients with associated heart disease with left ventricular failure, the infiltrate persisted as a "scar" on the chest X-ray. In these patients, increased pulmonary venous pressure impedes resolution of pulmonary hemorrhage, and true pulmonary infarction occurs (7). Because patients with submassive pulmonary embolism who do not have associated heart disease are less likely to die, the pathologist is far more likely to examine patients with pulmonary infarction who have associated heart disease.

VI. Clinical Findings in Patients with Pulmonary Infarction

In addition to pleuritic pain, patients with pulmonary infarction usually are dyspneic and may have hemoptysis and cough. On physical examination, in addition to tachypnea (Respirations >20/min), the lungs may have rales, wheezes, or evidence of a pleural effusion (7). There usually are no signs of right ventricular failure because pulmonary embolism is nearly always submassive in patients with pulmonary infarction.

The most useful laboratory test is the chest X-ray, which will usually demonstrate an infiltrate, elevated hemi-diaphragm (caused by splinting), or a pleural effusion that is usually small and may or may not be bloody (19) (see Chap. 12).

The EKG is usually normal. Arterial blood gases (breathing room air) are not diagnostic. The PCO_2 is usually decreased, and mild alkalosis is present because of hyperventilation. However, the PO_2 is often normal or near normal because a small percentage of the pulmonary circulation is obstructed.

VII. Differential Diagnosis of Pulmonary Infarction

The most comprehensive study of pleuritic chest as a sign of pulmonary embolism was performed by Hull et al. (20). They performed an IPG and V/Q lung scan in 173 consecutive patients presenting to the emergency room with pleuritic chest pain. Venography was performed in those having positive IPGs, and pulmonary angiography was performed in those having abnormal perfusion scans. The diagnosis of pulmonary embolism was confirmed by pulmonary angiography or postmortem exam in 21% of the patients. The diagnosis of pulmonary embolism was excluded by a normal perfusion scan or normal pulmonary angiogram in 79% of the patients. The diagnoses of those without pulmonary embolism are shown in Table 5. Viral or idiopathic pleurisy was the most common final diagnosis occuring in 46% of the 173 patients with pleuritic pain.

The symptoms and clinical findings in these patients with pleuritic pain were nearly the same in those patients with and without pulmonary embolism. The diagnosis of pulmonary embolism as the cause of pleuritic pain could not be established on clinical grounds. Of the patients with documented pulmonary

Table 5 Final Diagnosis Utilizing V/Q Scan, IPG, and Pulmonary Angiogram in 173 Consecutive Patients with Pleuritic Chest Pain[a]

	Number	Percent
Pulmonary embolism	36	21
Viral or idiopathic pleurisy	80	46
Pneumonia	14	8
All other diagnoses[b]	43	25

[a]From Hull et al., Arch Int Med (April 1988) (20).
[b]Trauma, cancer, SLE, TB, etc.

embolism, 76% had predisposing factors for deep venous thrombosis, or evidence of deep venous thrombosis by IPG. However, 41% of the patients without pulmonary embolism had predisposing factors for deep venous thrombosis and/or evidence of deep venous thrombosis. Thus, the presence of predisposing factors or evidence of deep venous thrombosis is sensitive for the presence of pulmonary embolism but is not specific.

This study indicates that the incidence of pulmonary embolism is sufficiently high in patients with pleuritic pain (21%) to warrant IPG and V/Q scans; especially in patients with predisposition to, or evidence of, deep venous thrombosis.

VIII. Massive Pulmonary Embolism with Acute Cor Pulmonale

Acute cor pulmonale, the most dramatic presentation of acute pulmonary embolism, occurs in about 20% of patients in whom pulmonary embolism is diagnosed. Acute pulmonary embolism causes an increase in right ventricular and pulmonary artery systolic pressure (21,22) (see Chap. 7). When the degree of obstruction of the pulmonary circulation approaches 65%–75%, the right ventricular systolic pressure reaches 60–70 mm Hg. At this point, the previously normal right ventricle dilates and fails. Right ventricular systolic and pulmonary artery systolic pressure decrease, stroke volume and cardiac output decrease, and systemic blood pressure may fall. As the right ventricle dilates and fails, right ventricular diastolic pressure and mean right atrial pressure increase (23). The increase in right atrial pressure causes distention of the neck veins, a classic finding in acute cor pulmonale. Other signs of acute right ventricular failure include a right-sided S3 gallop and at times a parasternal lift.

The drop in cardiac output may lead to hypotension, syncope (24), or cardiac arrest often caused by electromechanical dissociation (see Chap. 11).

The classical EKG sign of acute cor pulmonale, the S1 Q3 T3 pattern, was first described by McGinn and White (25) in 1935. In addition to the S1 Q3 T3 pattern, acute cor pulmonale may be evidenced by a new incomplete right bundle branch block (19) (see Chap. 7). These two EKG findings are infrequent in the overall population of patients with pulmonary embolism (26,27), but they are very frequent in patients with acute cor pulmonale caused by massive pulmonary embolism (24).

The chest X-ray is usually normal in patients with acute cor pulmonale. However, arterial blood gases (breathing room air) demonstrate significant hypoxemia and hypocapnia (24). The key clinical findings in patients with acute cor pulmonale are signs of right ventricular failure, distended neck veins, S3 gallop, and decreased cardiac output. The most important laboratory findings are the EKG findings of a new S1 Q3 T3 pattern, new incomplete right bundle branch block, negative T wave in V1 to V3, and significant hypoxemia.

IX. Acute Unexplained Dyspnea

In patients with submassive pulmonary embolism (<60% obstruction of the pulmonary circulation), acute cor pulmonale does not occur. If pulmonary infarction does not occur, the signs and symptoms of pulmonary embolism are minimal.

The principal clinical symptom is dyspnea and the principal physical finding is tachypnea. The lungs are usually clear on physical exam and by chest X-ray. The EKG is normal.

The principal clues to the presence of pulmonary embolism as the cause of dyspnea are its occurrence in patients with predisposition to, or evidence of, deep venous thrombosis and the absence of an explanation for dyspnea.

In the absence of physical findings other than tachypnea, and with a normal EKG and chest X-ray, the clinician may consider anxiety and/or the "hyperventilation syndrome" as the cause of dyspnea. It is in this setting that measurement of arterial blood gases is critical (see Chap. 9). If the patient's dyspnea is due to pulmonary embolism, one should expect to find significant hypoxemia and hypocapnia.

X. Evaluation of Patients Once Pulmonary Embolism Has Been Suspected

The critical step in the clinical diagnosis of pulmonary embolism is to recognize that the patient has signs and symptoms suggesting one of these three syndromes.

Some (28) have suggested that once pulmonary embolism is suspected, pulmonary angiography should be performed. This is a very impractical approach, given the fact the pulmonary angiography is an expensive invasive procedure that is not available at all hospitals (see Chap. 14). There is abundant

Table 6 Results of Pulmonary Angiography in 731 Patients with V/Q Scan[a]

Scan result	Percent with pulmonary embolism
High probability	88
Intermediate probability	33
Low probability	16
Near normal/normal	9

[a]From PIOPED Study, JAMA (May 23/30, 1990) (4).

evidence that V/Q lung scans and tests for the presence of deep venous thrombosis can be very helpful and reduce the need for the pulmonary angiography.

V/Q perfusion scans are extremely useful (see Chap. 12). A normal perfusion scan essentially excludes the diagnosis of acute pulmonary embolism. At the other extreme, a lung scan that demonstrates multiple segmental or lobar perfusion defects that ventilate normally is highly consistent with pulmonary embolism, with an accuracy rate of about 90% (Table 6). Therefore, in the absence of a contraindication to therapy, a high-probability lung scan is sufficient evidence to begin therapy for pulmonary embolism.

Unfortunately, the lung scan findings in patients suspected of pulmonary embolism rarely fall at the two extremes, normal or high probability. In the PIOPED Study, of 931 patients suspected of pulmonary embolism, 86% of the perfusion scans were abnormal, but only 13% were high probability. The majority (73%) were intermediate probability or low probability.

Furthermore, a minority of patients with angiographically documented pulmonary embolism have high-probability lung scans, as shown in Table 7. In 251 patients with angiographically documented pulmonary embolism, 40% had high-probability scans, while 58% had intermediate or low-probability scans,

Table 7 Results of V/Q Scan in 251 Patients with Pulmonary Embolism Documented by Pulmonary Angiography[a]

	Percent
High probability	40
Intermediate probability	42
Low probability	16
Near normal/normal	2

[a]From PIOPED Study, JAMA (May 23/30, 1990).

and 2% were "normal" or "near normal." As shown in Table 6, the specificity of a high-probability lung scan is 88%. However, the incidence of pulmonary embolism in patients with an intermediate probability scan was 33% and it was 16% in those with a low-probability scan. These data indicate that an intermediate or low-probability scan does not exclude pulmonary embolism (29). When the lung scan results are intermediate or low probability, assessment of the lower extremities for deep venous thrombosis becomes very important.

If the IPG (12) or Doppler ultrasonogram (30) are positive in a patient with an intermediate or low-probability lung scan, the probability of proximal deep venous thrombosis is sufficiently high to begin heparin therapy. Because the treatment of proximal deep venous thrombosis is essentially the same as for acute pulmonary embolism, pulmonary angiography is not necessary unless there are contraindications to heparin therapy.

If there is no evidence of deep venous thrombosis by Doppler ultrasonogram or IPG in the patient with intermediate or low-probability lung scan results, pulmonary angiography may be indicated. Selective angiography of the segments that are abnormal by perfusion scan will determine if pulmonary embolism is present (31). When performed by experienced angiographers, the mortality and morbidity of pulmonary angiography is quite low (5). However, given the invasive nature of pulmonary angiography, it is not indicated in all patients suspected to have acute pulmonary embolism. The use of lung scans and IPG or Doppler Sonography in patients with suspected pulmonary embolism reduces the need for pulmonary angiography (12).

References

1. Alpert JS, Smith R, Carlson CJ, Ockene IS, Dexter L, Dalen JE. Mortality in patients treated for pulmonary embolism. JAMA 1976; 236:1477–80.
2. Dalen JE, Alpert JS. Natural history of pulmonary embolism. Prog Cardiovasc Dis 1975; 17:259–70.
3. Karwinski B, Svendsen E. Comparison of clinical and postmortem diagnosis of pulmonary embolism. J Clin Pathol 1989; 42:135–9.
4. PIOPED Investigators. Value of the ventilation/perfusion scan in acute pulmonary embolism: results of the prospective investigation of pulmonary embolism diagnosis (PIOPED). JAMA 1990; 263:2753–96.
5. Dalen JE, Brooks HL, Johnson LW, Meister SG, Szucs M Jr, Dexter L. Pulmonary angiography in acute pulmonary embolism. Am Heart J 1971; 81:175–85.
6. Bell WR, Simon TL, DeMets DL. The clinical features of submassive and massive pulmonary emboli. Am J Med 1977; 62:355–60.
7. Dalen JE, Haffajee CI, Alpert JS, Howe JP, Ockens IS, Paraskos JA. Pulmonary embolism, pulmonary hemorrhage, pulmonary infarction. N Engl J Med 1977; 296:1431–5.

8. Hirsh J, Hull RD, Raskob GE. Diagnosis of pulmonary embolism. JACC 1986; 8:128B–136B.
9. Dalen JE, Dexter L. Pulmonary embolism. JAMA 1969; 207:1505–7.
10. Sevitt S, Gallagher N. Venous thrombosis and pulmonary embolism: a clinico-pathological study in injured and burned patients. Br J Surg 1961; 48:475–89.
11. Virchow RLK. Cellular pathology as based upon physiological and pathohistology. 7th ed. (trans. Chance F, De Witt, RM). New York, 1860: 236.
12. Hull RD, Hirsh J, Carter CJ, Jay RM, et al. Pulmonary angiography, ventilation lung scanning, and venography for clinically suspected pulmonary embolism with abnormal perfusion lung scan. Ann Int Med 1983; 98:891–9.
13. Hirsh J. Diagnosis of venous thrombosis and pulmonary embolism. Am J Cardiol 1990; 65:45C–49C.
14. Wheeler HB, Anderson FA, Cardullo PA, et al. Suspected Deep Vein Thrombosis: Management by Impedance Plethysmography. Arch Surg 1982; 117:1206–9.
15. Virchow RLK. Gesammelte Abhandlungen zur wissenschaftlichen Medizin. Frankfurt: Meidinger Sohn u Comp, 1856; 285, 294–6.
16. Hampton AO, Castleman B. Correlation of postmortem chest teleroentgenograms with autopsy findings: with special reference to pulmonary embolism and infarction. Am J Roentgenol 1940; 43:305–26.
17. Boyd W. A Textbook of Pathology: Structure and function in disease. 8th ed. Philadelphia: Lea & Febiger, 1970: 204.
18. Robbins SLR. Pathology. 3rd ed. Philadelphia: Saunders, 1967: 705.
19. Szucs M Jr, Brooks HL, Grossman W, Banas J Jr, Meister SG, Dexter L, Dalen JE. Diagnostic sensitivity of laboratory findings in acute pulmonary embolism. Ann Int Med 1971; 74:161–6.
20. Hull RD, Raskob GE, Carter CJ, et al. Pulmonary embolism in outpatients with pleuritic chest pain. Arch Intern Med 1988; 148:838–44.
21. Dalen JE, Haynes FW, Hoppin FG Jr, Evans GL, Bhardwaji P, Dexter L. Cardiovascular responses to experimental pulmonary embolism. Am J Cardiol 1967; 20:3–9.
22. Alpert JS, Godtfredsen J, Ockene IS, Anas J, Dalen JE. Pulmonary hypertension secondary to minor pulmonary embolism. Chest 1978; 73:795–7.
23. Dalen JE, Banas J Jr, Brooks H, Evans G, Paraskos J, Dexter L. Resolution rate of acute pulmonary embolism in man. N Engl J Med. 1969; 280:1194–9.
24. Thames MD, Alpert JS, Dalen JE. Syncope in patients with pulmonary embolism. JAMA 1977; 238:2509–11.
25. McGinn S, White PD. Acute cor pulmonale resulting from pulmonary embolism. JAMA 1935; 104:1473–80.
26. Panos RJ, Barish RA, DePriest WW Jr, Groleau G. The electrocardiographic manifestations of pulmonary embolism. J Emerg Med 1988; 6:301–7.
27. Petruzzelli S, Palla A, Pieraccini F, et al. Routine electrocardiology in screening for pulmonary embolism. Respiration. 1986; 50:233–43.
28. Robin ED. Overdiagnosis and overtreatment of pulmonary embolism: the emperor may have no clothes. Ann Intern Med 1977; 87:775–81.
29. Hull RD, Raskob GE. Low-probability lung scan findings: a need for change. 1991; 114:142–3.

30. Polak JF. Doppler ultrasound of the deep leg veins: a revolution in the diagnosis of deep vein thrombosis and monitoring of thrombolysis. Chest 1991; 99:165S–172S.
31. Meister SG, Brooks HL, Szucs MM, Banas JS Jr, Dexter L, Dalen JE. Pulmonary cineangiography in acute pulmonary embolism. Am Heart J 1972; 84:33–7.

7

Cardiac Manifestations of Pulmonary Embolism

ROBERT C. SCHLANT

Emory University School of Medicine
Atlanta, Georgia

The major cardiac manifestations of pulmonary embolism include the following: an increased resistance to pulmonary blood flow that is associated with an increase in pulmonary artery and right systolic ventricular pressures, remodeling of the right ventricle, an altered left ventricular performance, a decrease in cardiac output and systemic blood pressure and tachycardia, alterations in coronary blood flow, and death. The minor cardiac manifestations of pulmonary embolism include the following: tricuspid regurgitation; opening of the foramen ovale; altered pulmonary, cerebral, renal, hepatic, and gastrointestinal tract function; and disturbances of cardiac rhythm or conduction.

A. Major Cardiac Manifestations

Increase in Resistance to Pulmonary Blood Flow

The increase in pulmonary resistance to blood flow associated with pulmonary embolism is multifactorial. The major cause is mechanical blockage of the pulmonary vasculature produced by the embolic material (1–6). This blockage and the resultant pulmonary and right ventricular hypertension may resolve as the pulmonary emboli resolve (7). There is still controversy regarding the occurrence in human beings of pulmonary arteriolar vasospasm resulting from neural reflexes from occluded small arteries and arterioles (3,5,8–20). Reflex vasoconstriction of the pulmonary arterioles is most apparent in experiments in which small arteriolar emboli occur (13). Other possible mechanisms of pulmonary vasoconstriction include the release of a wide variety of humoral factors. These may originate from platelets (serotonin, adenosine diphosphate [ADP], platelet-derived growth factor [PDGF], arachidonic acid metabolites [TXA_2 and PGH_2], or platelet-activating factor [PAF]); from neutrophils (PAF, thromboxane [TXA_2], peptidoleukotrienes [LTC_4, LTD_4, and LTE_4], oxygen-derived free radicals); from plasma (thrombin, vasoactive peptides [C3a and C5a, fragment D]); from endothelium (endothelin or a decreased release of endothelium-derived relaxing factor [EDRF] or of PGI_2) from nonsympathetic-parasympathetic nerves (substance P); or from tissue (histamine) (14,15,21–25). Systemic arterial hypoxemia may also produce pulmonary arteriolar vasoconstriction (26).

In general, the mean pulmonary arterial pressure is not elevated until either the scan or the angiogram demonstrates 25%–30% involvement (27–29). In general, the resistance and pulmonary artery pressure increase exponentially when the cross-sectional area of the pulmonary circulation is obstructed by more than about 50%–60% (5,26,30–34). As a consequence of the increase in resistance to pulmonary artery flow, the systolic pressures in the pulmonary artery and right ventricle may be markedly increased (19,35). In patients who do not have underlying cardiopulmonary disease, the mean pulmonary artery pressure is usually not elevated above 50 mm Hg, whereas in patients with preexisting disease, the mean pressure can reach systemic levels (19,27,28,36,37). Right atrial and peripheral venous pressures may be secondarily increased.

Clinically, the pulmonary hypertension and right ventricular hypertension may be evident by a sternal and left parasternal heave, an accentuation of the loudness of the pulmonary component of the second heart sound, a right ventricular S_3 or S_4 gallop, and a prominent "a" wave in the jugular venous pulse (38,39).

Remodeling of the Right Ventricle

As the result of the acute increase in resistance to blood flow through the lungs and the increase in systolic pressure in "acute cor pulmonale," the right ventricle often becomes acutely dilated with an increase in right ventricular end-diastolic pressure and dimensions (38–42) and, in some patients, alteration in the shape and function of the ventricular septum (43,44) (see Chap. 13). The increase in right ventricular end-diastolic volume and diastolic pressure produce an increase in right atrial mean pressure and in the strength of the right atrial "a" wave.

Patients with chronic pulmonary hypertension may also have left ventricular dysfunction (45–49).

Left Ventricular Performance

Left ventricular pumping performance may also be altered significantly in patients with a pulmonary embolism. In some patients with relatively small pulmonary emboli, cardiac output may actually be increased, possibly related to hypoxemia (19). In other patients, left ventricular output is decreased because the right ventricle is unable to pump blood through the severely obstructed pulmonary vasculature to the left ventricle; in addition, the blood that does reach the left atrium is less well oxygenated than normal because of an abnormal ventilation:perfusion ratio with nonhomogeneity of ventilation and perfusion, and pulmonary arteriovenous shunting (35,50–54) (see Chap. 9).

The left ventricular performance is also significantly altered because of the phenomena of ventricular interdependence and pericardial restraint (43,55–66). Thus, an acute dilatation of the right ventricle is responsible for a decrease in left ventricular distensibility or an increase in the diastolic pressure in the left ventricle, particularly when both are contained within an intact pericardium (42,62,64,67–69). This mechanism might be referred to as a type of acute "reversed Bernheim syndrome" (71,72). If the patient has preexisting left ventricular dysfunction with a mild or modest elevation of the left ventricular filling pressure, the additional elevation may be sufficient to raise the left ventricular filling pressure and the left atrial and pulmonary venous and pulmonary capillary pressures to levels that produce pulmonary edema. The development of pulmonary edema in acute pulmonary embolism is also facilitated by an increase in lung vascular permeability (73) and by endothelial injury from a variety of mechanisms, including mechanical factors (systolic pulmonary arterial pressure greater than 55 mm Hg), reflex release of histamine (74), macrophage or neutrophil activation, reperfusion injury, or endothelial-derived mediators of endothelial injury (neutrophils chemo-attractants, interleukin-1, oxygen radicals, or leukotrienes) (25). Experimentally, obstruction of pulmonary arteries with various microemboli or balloons causes increased fluid filtration and protein flux in the open microvascular bed with increased lymph drainage, possibly because of high vascular pressure and high linear blood flow velocity, although the release of substances that affect endothelial permeability may also occur (6).

Decrease in Cardiac Output and Systemic Arterial Blood Pressure with Reflex Tachycardia

The marked increase in resistance to blood flow through the lungs can result in a significant decrease in cardiac output, which can produce cardiogenic shock, despite compensatory reflex systemic vasoconstriction, and tachycardia (75). Some patients may have systemic vasodilation of uncertain origin contributing to the cardiogenic shock (76,77). Schwiegk (78) described a fall in aortic pressure after an acute elevation of pulmonary arterial pressure and postulated the existence of a depressor baroreflex. Subsequent studies, however, have not documented the presence of a Schwiegk reflex (79).

Alterations in Coronary Blood Flow

The increase in right ventricular end-diastolic dimensions, systolic pressure, and in heart rate increases the myocardial oxygen requirements, which normally should result in an increase in coronary blood flow (CBF) to the right ventricle. Experimental studies in animals have indicated that both right and left ventricular CBF may be increased following pulmonary emboli sufficient to produce moderate pulmonary hypertension (81,82). Possible factors that might produce a decrease in CBF and myocardial ischemia include the following: severe systemic hypotension, significant increase in right atrial and coronary sinus pressure, increase in myocardial angiotensin 2, or marked tachycardia. Pulmonary embolism frequently results in clinical evidence of myocardial ischemia (chest pain or electrocardiographic changes) that is presumably due predominantly to the marked increase in right ventricular myocardial oxygen requirements and a decrease in coronary flow if systemic hypotension is present. An inadequate right coronary flow may be an important factor in limiting the response of the right ventricle to an acute obstruction in the pulmonary vascular tree (82–84).

Death

Pulmonary embolism may produce death when the embolism is massive and produces a major obstruction to blood flow. Less commonly, death may be related to an acute arrhythmia (see Chap. 11).

B. Minor Cardiac Manifestations

Tricuspid regurgitation may occur secondary to the acute increase in right ventricular pressure and right ventricular dilatation. The regurgitation is due to both dilatation of the tricuspid annulus and incompetence of the tricuspid valve mechanism caused by failure of the anchoring of the tricuspid valve leaflets by the chordae tendineae and papillary muscles.

Opening of the Foramen Ovale

An acute increase in right ventricular pressure and in right atrial pressure may produce remodeling and dilatation of the right atrium with a reversal or lessening of the normal right-sided convexity of the atrial septum. In addition, the increase in right atrial pressure and size may be associated with transient opening of the foramen ovale. This may produce an acute right-to-left shunt and may also permit a paradoxic embolism to the systemic circulation.

Altered Pulmonary, Cerebral, Renal, Hepatic, and Gastrointestinal Function

Pulmonary embolus may result in bronchospasm and moderate ventilation-perfusion inequality (50–54). As a result, there may be arterial hypoxemia and an increase in airway resistance. The opening of arteriovenous communications in the embolized lungs may also contribute to the hypoxemia (10). Reflex tachypnea is also characteristic (24,85–89). Clinically, patients with saddle or massive pulmonary emboli characteristically have slow, very deep respirations, whereas patients with very small emboli have rapid, shallow respirations. Bronchial blood flow increases markedly after experimental pulmonary embolization (24). Many of the pulmonary responses that occur after microembolism appear to be mediated by humoral substances activated or released as a result of obstruction, intravascular coagulation, and leukocyte and platelet activation (24).

A decrease in cerebral blood flow and an increase in serum norepinephrine and epinephrine may contribute to the subjective feelings of apprehension, anxiety, weakness, and near-syncope. Syncope, which may occur in patients with pulmonary embolism, particularly when massive, has been explained by acute cor pulmonale with acute right ventricular failure, severe depression of the cardiac output, systemic hypotension, and a fall in cerebral blood flow. These may resolve following fragmentation and remodeling of emboli in the pulmonary vascular bed (90). Alterations in renal, hepatic, and gastrointestinal tract function may occur secondarily to an increase in systemic venous pressure or to decreased arterial blood flow or both.

Electrocardiography

Electrocardiography (ECG) is not very sensitive or specific for detecting pulmonary embolism (PE); however, it is readily available, and the findings in certain patterns and in the proper clinical setting, should alert the clinician to the diagnoses of PE (91,92). An ECG is often particularly useful in differentiating between acute myocardial infarction and acute massive PE (93).

The ECG abnormalities may be fleeting and disappear within minutes or hours, and the evaluation may be difficult in the absence of earlier tracings for comparison. In addition, the ECG is influenced by preexisting cardiopulmonary disease as well as the severity of pulmonary embolism.

In patients *without* prior cardiac or pulmonary disease, the most frequent finding is T-wave inversion in the right precordial leads and/or in limb lead III and aVF (25%–89% of cases in the studies by Lenégre et al. [94] and by Stein

Table 1 Electrocardiographic Manifestations[a]: Patients with Pulmonary Embolism Without Prior Cardiac or Pulmonary Disease[b]

	Percent		
	50 patients, massive pulmonary embolism[c]	40 patients, submassive pulmonary embolism	90 patients massive or submassive pulmonary embolism
Electrocardiogram			
Normal electrocardiogram	6	23	13
Rhythm disturbances			
Premature atrial beats	2	3	2
Premature ventricular beats	4	3	3
Atrio-ventricular conduction disturbances			
First degree A-V block	0	3	1
P pulmonale	6	5	6
QRS abnormalities			
Right axis deviation	8	5	7
Left axis deviation	4	10	7
Clockwise rotation (V_5)	10	3	7
Incomplete right bundle branch block	8	3	6
Complete right bundle branch block	8	10	9
Right ventricular hypertrophy	6	5	6
$S_1S_2S_3$ Pattern	6	8	7
$S_1Q_3T_3$ Pattern	18	5	12
Pseudoinfarction	16	5	11
Low voltage (frontal plane)	8	3	6
Primary RST segment and T wave abnormalities			
RST segment depression (not reciprocal)	28	23	26
RST segment elevation (not reciprocal)	18	13	16
T-wave inversion	46	38	42

[a]Some patients had more than one abnormality.
[b]Source: Stein PD, Dalen JE, McIntyre KM, et al. The electrocardiogram in acute pulmonary embolism. Prog Cardiovasc Dis 1975; 17:247.
[c]The prevalence of none of the various electrocardiographic abnormalities differed significantly between patients with massive or submassive pulmonary embolism (chi square greater than 0.05).

et al. [95]). A nonreciprocal S-T depression was present in 56% of cases in Lenégre's series (94) and in 26% of the cases reported by Stein et al. (95).

In patients *with* preexisting cardiac or respiratory disease, T-wave inversion in V_1–V_3 was present in 30% of Lenégre's patients (96) and in 8% of a series of 63 autopsy cases (96); atrial fibrillation or flutter was found in 28% of autopsy cases (96) and in 13% of those studied by Lenégre et al. (94). A right-bundle branch block (RBBB) was seen in 15% of patients with massive or submassive PE reported by Stein et al. (94) (Table 1) and in 24% of patients without and 9% in patients with underlying cardiopulmonary disease reported by Lenégre et al. (94) and, respectively, 10% and 16% in the autopsy series (96). Right-axis deviation occurs in only about 5%–10% of patients, and the development of left-axis deviation is equally common (97).

A normal ECG was found in 11% of cases by Lenégre et al. (94), in 20% of the autopsy series, and in 13% of Stein's series (95) including both massive and submassive PE. None of these patients with normal ECG had a history or evidence of cardiac or pulmonary disease. Patients with prior cardiopulmonary disease have more arrhythmias, conduction disorders, and QRS changes, whereas patients with massive PE have more QRS, ST-T segment, and T-wave changes (93).

Miscellaneous Changes

An increase in right atrial pressures and dimensions may be associated with an increased release of atrial natriuretic peptide. Serum or plasma levels of angiotensin-converting enzyme (ACE) activity may decrease for a few days following acute pulmonary embolism (98), and it has been suggested that a chronic decrease in plasma ACE activity may be a marker of endothelial dysfunction in patients predisposed to pulmonary embolism (99).

References

1. Williams MH Jr. Mechanical versus reflex effects of diffuse pulmonary embolism in anesthetized dogs. Circ Res 1956; 4:325–31.
2. Knisley WH, Wallace JM, Mahaley MS Jr, Satterwhite WM Jr. Evidence including in vivo observations, suggesting mechanical blockage rather than reflex vasospasm as the cause of death in pulmonary embolization. Am Heart J 1957; 54:483–97.
3. Parker BM, Smith JR. Pulmonary embolism and infarction. A review of the physiologic consequences of pulmonary arterial obstruction. Am J Med 1958; 24:402–27.
4. Weidner MG Jr, Light RA. Role of the autonomic nervous system in the control of the pulmonary vascular bed. III. Further studies in experimental pulmonary embolism. Ann Surg 1958; 147:895–902.
5. Dalen JE, Haynes FW, Hoppin FG Jr, Evans GL, Bhardwaj P, Dexter L.

Cardiovascular responses to experimental pulmonary embolism. Am J Cardiol 1967; 20:3–9.

6. Okhude K, Nakahara K, Weidner J, Binder A, Staub NC. Lung fluid exchange after uneven pulmonary artery obstruction in sheep. Circ Res 1978; 43:152–61.
7. Dalen JE, Alpert JS. Natural history of pulmonary embolism. Prog Cardiovasc Dis 1975; 17:259–70.
8. Cate WR Jr, Light RA, Daniel RA Jr, Edwards WH. Role of the autonomic nervous system in the control of the pulmonary vascular bed. I. Experimental pulmonary embolism. Surg Forum 1953; 4:190–7.
9. Price KC, Hata D, Smith JR: Pulmonary vasomotion resulting from miliary embolism of the lung. Am J Physiol 1955; 182:183–90.
10. Niden AH, Aviado DM. Effects of pulmonary embolism on the pulmonary circulation with special reference to arteriovenous shunts in the lung. Circ Res 1956; 4:67–73.
11. Nelson JR, Smith JR. The pathologic physiology of pulmonary embolism. A physiologic discussion of the vascular reactions following pulmonary arterial obstruction by emboli of varying size. Am Heart J 1959; 58:916–32.
12. Hyland JW, Piemme TE, Alexander S, Haynes FW, Smith GT, Dexter L. Behavior of pulmonary hypertension produced by serotonin and emboli. Am J Physiol 1963; 205:591–7.
13. Dexter L. Cardiovascular responses to pulmonary embolism. In: AA Sasahara, Stein M, eds. Pulmonary Embolic Disease. New York: Grune and Stratton, 1965:101–9.
14. Caldini P. Pulmonary hemodynamics and arterial oxygen saturation in pulmonary embolism. J Appl Physiol 1965; 20:184–90.
15. Vitolo E, Gola E, Valentini F: Studies on the physiopathology of experimental pulmonary embolism. 1. Pulmonary and systemic hemodynamics. Am Heart J 1965; 69:338–54.
16. Daily PO, Lancaster JR, Moulder PV: The mechanism of pulmonary hypertension following miliary pulmonary embolism. Surg Gynecol Obst 1965; 120:1009–18.
17. Sasahara AA, Sidd JJ, Tremblay G, Leland OS Jr. Cardiopulmonary consequences of acute pulmonary embolic disease. Prog Cardiovasc Dis 1966; 9:259–74.
18. Daily PO, Griffin A, Blackstone E, Moulder PV. The hemodynamic effects of localized pulmonary embolism. Surg Gynecol Obstet 1966; 123:765–73.
19. McIntyre KM, Sasahara AA: Hemodynamic and ventricular responses to pulmonary embolism. Prog Cardiovasc Dis 1974; 17:175–90.
20. Stein M, Levy SE: Reflex and humoral responses to pulmonary embolism. Prog Cardiovasc Dis 1974; 17:167–74.
21. Comroe JH Jr, Van Lingen B, Stroud RC, Roncoroni A. Reflex and direct cardiomyopathy effects of 5-OH-tryptamine (serotonin). Their possible role in pulmonary embolism and coronary thrombosis. Am J Physiol 1953; 173:379–386.
22. Smith G, Smith AN. The role of serotonin in experimental pulmonary embolism. Surg Gynec Obstet 1955; 101:691–700.
23. Cobb B, Nauson EM. Further studies with serotonin and experimental pulmonary embolism. Ann Surg 1960; 151:501–6.
24. Malik AB. Pulmonary microembolism. Physiol Rev 1983; 63:1114–1207.

25. Malik AB, Johnson A. Role of humoral mediators in the pulmonary vascular response to pulmonary embolism. In: Weir K, Reeves J, eds. Pulmonary Vascular Physiology and Pathophysiology. Vol. 23. Lung Biology in Health and Disease. New York: Marcel Dekker, 1989:445–68.
26. Alpert JS, Godtfredsen J, Ockene IS, Anas J, Dalen JE: Pulmonary hypertension secondary to minor pulmonary embolism. Chest 1978; 73:795–7.
27. McIntyre KM, Sasahara AA. The hemodynamic response to pulmonary embolism in patients without prior cardiopulmonary disease. Am J Cardiol 1971; 28:288–94.
28. McIntyre KM, Sasahara AA, Sharma GVRK. Pulmonary thromboembolism: current concepts. Adv Int Med 1972; 18:199–218.
29. Sharma CVRK, McIntyre KM, Sharma S, Sasahara AA. Clinical and hemodynamic correlates in pulmonary embolism. Clin Chest Med 1984; 5:421–37.
30. Haggart GE, Walker AM: The physiology of pulmonary embolism as disclosed by quantitative occlusion of the pulmonary artery. Arch Surg 1923; 6:764–83.
31. Gibbon JH Jr, Hopkinson M, Churchill ED. Changes in the circulation produced by gradual occlusion of the pulmonary artery. J Clin Invest 1932; 11:543–53.
32. Hyland JW, Smith GT, McGuire LB, Harrison DC, Haynes FW, Dexter L: Effect of selective embolization of various sized pulmonary arteries in dogs. Am J Physiol 1963; 204:619–25.
33. Dexter L, Smith GT: Quantitative studies of pulmonary embolism. Am J Med Sci 1964; 247:641–8.
34. Benotti JR, Dalen JE: The natural history of pulmonary embolism. Clin Chest Med 1984; 5:403–10.
35. Leland OS Jr, Sasahara AA. Hemodynamic observations in patients with pulmonary thromboembolism. In: Sasahara AA, Stein M, eds. Pulmonary Embolic Disease, New York: Grune & Stratton, 1965;110–9.
36. McIntyre KM, Sasahara AA. Determinants of cardiovascular responses to pulmonary embolism. In: Moser KM, Stein M, eds. Pulmonary Thromboembolism. Chicago: Year Book, 1973:144–53.
37. Alpert JS, Irwin RS, Dalen JE. Pulmonary hypertension. Curr Probl Cardiol 1981; 5(10) January:1–39.
38. McGinn S, White PD. Acute cor pulmonale from pulmonary embolism. JAMA 1935; 104:1473–80.
39. Wolff L. Pulmonary embolism. Circulation 1952; 6:768–76.
40. Hyman AL, Myers WD, Meyer A. The effect of acute pulmonary embolus upon cardiopulmonary hemodynamics. Am Heart J 1964; 67:313–23.
41. Dunn JS. The effects of multiple embolism of pulmonary arterioles. Q J Med 1919; 13:129–47.
42. Machida K, Rapaport E. Left ventricular function in experimental pulmonary embolism. Jpn Heart J 1971; 12:221–32.
43. Stool EW, Mullins CB, Leshin SJ, Mitchell JH. Dimensional changes of the left ventricle during acute pulmonary arterial hypertension in dogs. Am J Cardiol 1974; 33:868–75.
44. Brinker JA, Weiss JL, Lappe DL, Rabson JL, Summer WR, Permutt S, Weisfeldt ML. Leftward septal displacement during right ventricular loading in man. Circulation 1980; 61:626–33.

45. Rao BS, Cohn KE, Eldridge FL, Hancock EW. Left ventricular failure secondary to chronic pulmonary disease. Am J Med 1968; 45:229–41.
46. Baum GL, Schwartz A, Llamas R, Castillo C. Left ventricular function in chronic obstructive lung disease. N Engl J Med 1971; 285:361–5.
47. Khaja F, Parker JO. Right and left ventricular performance in chronic obstructive lung disease. Am Heart J 1971; 82:319–27.
48. Unger K, Shaw D, Karliner JS, Crawford M, O'Rourke RA, Moser KM. Evaluation of left ventricular performance in acutely ill patients with chronic obstructive lung disease. Chest 1975; 68:135–42.
49. Krayenbuehl HP, Turina J, Hess O. Left ventricular function in chronic pulmonary hypertension. Am J Cardiol 1978; 41:1150–8.
50. Robin ED. Some aspects of the physiologic disturbances associated with pulmonary embolism. Med Clin North Am 1960; 44:1269–78.
51. Robin ED, Forkner CE Jr, Bromberg PA, Croteau JR, Travis DM. Alveolar gas exchange in clinical pulmonary embolism. N Engl J Med 1960; 262:283–7.
52. Sasahara AA, Cannilla JE, Morse RL, Sidd JJ, Tremblay GM. Clinical and physiologic studies in pulmonary thromboembolism. Am J Cardiol 1967; 20:10–20.
53. Kafer ER. Respiratory function in pulmonary thromboembolic disease. Am J Med 1969; 47:904–15.
54. Kapitan KS, Clausen JL, Moser KM. Gas exchange in chronic thromboembolism after pulmonary thromboendarterectomy. Chest 1990; 98:14–9.
55. Henderson Y, Prince AL. The relative discharges of the right and left ventricles and their bearing on pulmonary congestion and depletion. Heart 1914; 5:217–26.
56. Moulopoulos SD, Sarcas A, Stamatelopoulos S, Arealis E. Left ventricular performance during bypass or distension of the right ventricle. Circ Res 1965; 17:484–91.
57. Laks MM, Garner D, Swan HJC. Volumes and compliances measured simultaneously in the right and left ventricles of dogs. Circ Res 1967; 20:565–9.
58. Taylor RR, Covell JW, Sonnenblick EH, Ross JR Jr. Dependence of ventricular distensibility on filling of the opposite ventricle. Am J Physiol 1967; 213:711–8.
59. Bemis CE, Serur JR, Borkenhagen D, Sonnenblick EH, Urschel CW. Influence of right ventricular filling pressure on left ventricular pressure and dimension. Circ Res 1974; 34:498–504.
60. Elzinga GR, van Grondelle R, Westerhof W, van den Bos GL. Ventricular interdependence. Am J Physiol 1974; 226:941–7.
61. Santamore WP, Lynch PR, Meier G, Heckman J, Bove AA. Myocardial interaction between the ventricles. J Appl Physiol 1976; 4:362–8.
62. Glantz SA, Misbach GA, Moores WY, Mathey DG, Lekven J, Stowe DF, Parmley WW, Tyberg JV. The pericardium substantially affects the left ventricular diastolic pressure-volume relationship in the dog. Circ Res 1978; 42:433–41.
63. Ludbrook PA, Byrne JD, McKnight RC. Influence of right ventricular hemodynamics on left ventricular diastolic pressure-volume relations in man. Circulation 1979; 59:21–31.
64. Bove AA, Santamore WP. Ventricular interdependence. Prog Cardiovasc Dis 1981; 23:365–88.

65. Spadaro J, Bing OHL, Gaasch WH, Weintraub RM. Pericardial modulation of right and left ventricular diastolic interaction. Circ Res 1981; 48:233–8.
66. Weber KT, Janicki JS, Shroff S, Fishman AP. Contractile mechanics and interaction of the right and left ventricles. Am J Cardiol 1981; 47:686–95.
67. Kelly DT, Spotnitz HM, Beiser GD, Pierce JE, Epstein SE. Effects of chronic right ventricular volume and pressure loading on left ventricular performance. Circulation 1971; 44:403–12.
68. Alpert JS, Francis GS, Vieweg MC, Thompson SI, Stanton KC, Hagan AD. Left ventricular function in massive pulmonary embolism. Chest 1977; 71:108–11.
69. Janicki JS, Weber KT. The pericardium and ventricular interaction, distensibility and function. Am J Physiol 1980; 238:H494–H503.
70. Hoit BD, Dalton N, Bhargava V, Shabetai R. Pericardial influences on right and left ventricular filling dynamics. Circ Res 1991; 68:197–208.
71. Bernheim PI. De l'asystolie veineuse dans l'hypertrophie du coeur gauche par stenose concomitante du ventricule droit. Rev Med 1910; 30:785–95.
72. Dexter L. Atrial septal defect. Br Heart J 1956; 18:209–225.
73. Singer D, Saltzman PW, Rivera-Estrada C, Pick R, Katz LN. Hemodynamic alterations following miliary pulmonary embolization in relation to the pathogenesis of the consequent diffuse edema. Am J Physiol 1957; 191:437–42.
74. Kabins SA, Fridman J, Neustadt J, Espinosa G, Katz LN. Mechanisms leading to lung edema in pulmonary embolization. Am J Physiol 1960; 198:543–6.
75. Gibbon JH, Churchill ED. The physiology of massive pulmonary embolism. Ann Surg 1936; 104:811–22.
76. Selzer A, Bradley HW. Observations concerning the origin of shock associated with acute cor pulmonale. Am J Med 1957; 22:163–7.
77. Parmley LF Jr, North RL, Pickens GE. Pulmonary embolism as a cause of systemic hypotension and shock. Am J Cardiol 1965; 15:333–44.
78. Schwiegk H. Dehnungentlastung reflex. Pfügers Arch ges Physiol 1935; 236:206–219.
79. Widimsky J. Pressure, flow and volume changes of the lesser circulation during pulmonary artery occlusion in healthy subjects and patients with pulmonary hypertension. Progr Resp Res 1970; 5:224–36.
80. Guzman SV, Chavez FR, Imperial ES. Myocardial blood flow after experimental pulmonary embolism in the intact dog. Am Heart J 1964; 68:66–70.
81. Stein PD, Alshabkhoun S, Hatem C, Pur-Shahriari AA, Haynes FW, Harkem DE, Dexter L. Coronary artery blood flow in acute pulmonary embolism. Am J Cardiol 1968; 21:32–7.
82. Guyton AC, Lindsey AW, Gilluly JJ. The limits of right ventricular compensation following acute increase in pulmonary circulatory resistance. Circ Res 1954; 2:326–32.
83. Brooks H, Kirk ES, Vokonas PS, Urschel CW, Sonnenblick EH: Performance of the right ventricle under stress: relation to right coronary flow. J Clin Invest 1971; 50:2176–83.
84. Spotnitz HM, Berman MA, Epstein SE. Pathophysiology and experimental treatment of acute pulmonary embolism. Am Heart J 1971; 82:511–20.

85. Dunn JS. The effects of multiple embolism of pulmonary arterioles. Q J Med 1920; 13:129–47.
86. Binger CAL, Brow GR, Branch A. Experimental studies on rapid breathing. 1. Tachypnea, independent anoxemia, resulting from multiple emboli in the pulmonary arterioles and capillaries. J Clin Invest 1924; 1:155–180.
87. Megibow RS, Katz LN, Feinstein M. Kinetics of respiration in experimental pulmonary embolism. Arch Int Med 1943; 71:536–46.
88. Whitteridge D. Multiple embolism of the lung and rapid shallow breathing. Physiol Rev 1950; 30:475–86.
89. Bernthal T, Horres AD, Taylor JT III. Pulmonary vascular obstruction in graded tachypneagenic diffuse embolism. Am J Physiol 1961; 200:279–86.
90. Thames MD, Alpert JS, Dalen JE. Syncope in patients with pulmonary embolism. JAMA 1977; 238:2509–11.
91. Hume M, Sevitt S, Thomas DP. Venous Thrombosis and Pulmonary Embolism. Cambridge: Harvard University Press, 1970;290.
92. Petruzzelli S, Palla A, Donna Maria V, Celi A, Giuntini C. Diagnosi di embolia polmonare: ruolo delle tecniche non invasive. G Ital Cardiol 1991; 21:675–82.
93. McFadden ER, Braunwald E. Cor Pulmonale and Pulmonary Thromboembolism. In: Braunwald E, ed. Heart Diseases. Philadelphia: Saunders, 1980;1657.
94. Lenégre J, Gerbaux A, Gay J. L'electrocardiogramme dans l'embolie pulmonaire. In: Denolin H, ed. L'embolie pulmonaire. Paris: Masson, 1970:211.
95. Stein PD, Dalen JE, McIntyre KM, et al. The electrocardiogram in acute pulmonary embolism. Progr Cardiovasc Dis 1975; 17:247–57.
96. Morpurgo M, Schmid C. Clinico-pathological correlations in pulmonary embolism: a posteriori evaluation. Progr Resp Dis 1980; 13:8–15.
97. Rowlands DJ. The resting electrocardiogram. In: Julian DG et al, eds. Diseases of the Heart. London: Bailliere Tindall, 1989:200.
98. Meisel SR, Thaler M, Peleg E, Mekhmandarov S, Rosenthal T. Changes in serum angiotensin-converting enzyme activity after pulmonary embolism. J Lab Clin Med 1990; 115:768–9.
99. Drouet L, Baudin B, Baumann FCH, Caen JP. Serum angiotensin-converting enzyme: an endothelial cell marker. J Lab Clin Med 1988; 112:450–7.

8

Laboratory Recognition of Pulmonary Embolism

HENRI BOUNAMEAUX

University Hospital of Geneva
Geneva, Switzerland

I. Introduction

The present paper reviews the data on the diagnostic potential of plasma measurement of D-Dimer (DD) and thrombin-antithrombin III (TAT) complexes for recognition of pulmonary embolism (PE). A pooled analysis of the studies on the value of plasma measurement of DD in suspected PE (n = 451) revealed a sensitivity of 96.2% (95% CI:93.1–99.3), allowing one to rule out the diagnosis of PE below a given cutoff (500 μg/L for the assay using the monoclonal antibody from Stago), and a specificity of 46.7% (95% CI:40.8–52.6), requiring confirmation by other, more specific examinations. The performances of the TAT measurement are definitely poorer.

The DD assay is of particular interest in patients with an inconclusive lung scan, in whom further investigations can be avoided in 25% of the cases. Thus, this assay should be implemented in the clinical decision-making process that is used for routine diagnosis of PE.

Clinical diagnosis of pulmonary embolism is unreliable. Pulmonary angiography that is the diagnostic gold standard is expensive and not devoid of risks. Therefore, the current diagnostic approach includes chest radiography and ventilation-perfusion (VQ) scintigraphy, for which interpretation criteria are now established (see Chap. 12): a normal VQ scan excludes the diagnosis of pulmonary embolism, whereas a high-probability scan indicates the diagnosis (1,2). However, these two interpretative categories concern only half (3) or even less (4) of the scintigrams that are performed. The remaining examinations are inconclusive because they are classified as "indeterminate" or indicative of a "low or very low probability" of pulmonary embolism, which corresponds to a prevalence of the disease of 4%–46%, depending upon the scintigraphic pattern (1). Even when the scan is combined with clinical assessment as in the PIOPED study (4), noninvasive diagnosis or exclusion of acute pulmonary embolism is possible in a minority of patients. Therefore, there is a need for other noninvasive tests to support or rule out the diagnosis of pulmonary embolism.

II. Plasma Markers of an Activation of Coagulation and/or Fibrinolysis

A potential alternative to radiographic studies is the measurement in blood of markers of an activation of the plasma coagulation and/or fibrinolytic systems, as it was already proposed in the early 1970s by Gurewich et al. (5), who measured fibrin(ogen) degradation products in serum. However, using serum is a notorious source of artifacts, and the method has not been widely used for that purpose. Recently, assays in plasma of other markers were made available. These markers include the DD and the TAT complexes (Fig. 1). Both tests were assessed in the diagnostic approach of pulmonary embolism. The DD is an epitope that is present only after stabilization (cross-linking) of the fibrin network and subsequent lysis by plasmin (6). Assays of DD based on monoclonal antibodies allow measurement in plasma instead of serum, which considerably increases both the sensitivity and practicability of the test (7). Indeed, application of the DD assay to patients with deep venous thrombosis (DVT) (8–11) or myocardial infarction (12) has shown elevated concentrations at presentation. On the other hand, formation of TAT complexes results from the interaction of thrombin with its natural inhibitor, antithrombin III (13). These inactive complexes are rapidly cleared from the circulation. Thus, their presence is a sign of recent thrombin generation and subsequent inactivation; indeed, increased levels have been observed in patients with an inherited risk of venous thrombosis and in patients with disseminated intravascular coagulation (14) as well as in subjects with deep venous thrombosis or pulmonary embolism (15).

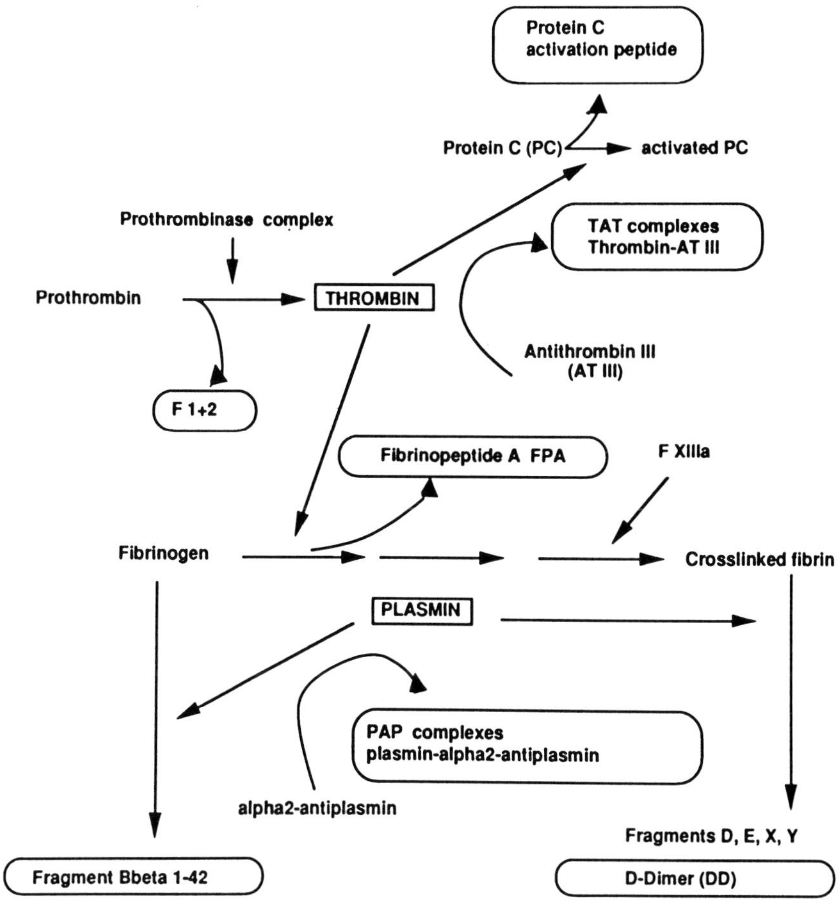

Figure 1 Markers of an activation of plasma coagulation and/or fibrinolysis.

III. Diagnostic Potential of Plasma DD in Suspected PE

In a preliminary report (3), we suggested that measurement of plasma DD might be of diagnostic value, especially in patients with inconclusive lung scans. Because of its excellent sensitivity to the presence of pulmonary embolism, the dosage might allow one to rule out this diagnosis when the level is less than 500 μg/L. However, our suggestion was based on a subgroup of patients, i.e., those with a conclusive lung scan (either normal or indicative of a high probability). Thus, we first confirmed the cutoff of 500 μg/L by studying a series of patients who were submitted to pulmonary angiography (16), and we then prospectively

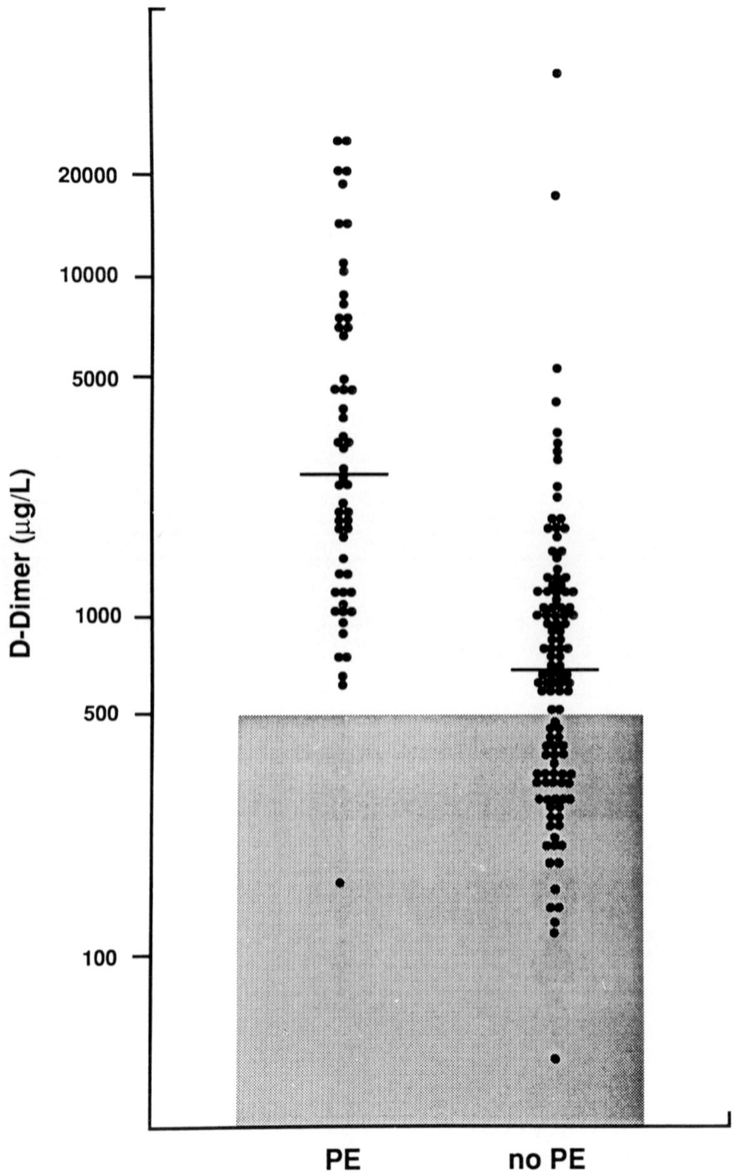

Figure 2 Individual plasma levels (in µg/L) of DD according to the presence (PE) or absence (no PE) of pulmonary embolism in the whole collective ($n = 170$), at the day of presentation. The horizontal bars indicate the median values. The DD levels are significantly higher in the patients with PE ($p < 0.001$). (From Ref. 17.)

investigated 171 consecutive patients who attended the emergency ward of our institution because of suspected pulmonary embolism (17). The patients were followed up until discharge from hospital. Investigations were performed according to a clinical decision-making process (18) that included careful clinical evaluation, VQ lung scanning, and, in some cases, pulmonary angiography or examination of the veins of the lower limbs. The performances (sensitivity, specificity, and positive and negative predictive values) of the test were calculated with respect to the presence of pulmonary embolism, as defined by the final diagnosis at hospital discharge (Fig. 2). The values are comparable with those of the literature (Table 1). By cumulating the data about 541 patients with 184 pulmonary embolisms from these trials, we obtained a sensitivity of 96.2% (95% CI:93.4–99.0) and a specificity of 47.6% (95% CI:42.4–52.8). The excellent sensitivity of the test is also supported by a study in which all patients who had angiographically confirmed pulmonary embolism had DD levels of 900 μg/L or more (22). One study reported a sensitivity of only 84% of the DD-ELISA test in 25 patients with high-probability lung scans (23) with a specificity of 39%. However, the scintigraphic criteria used in that study are questionable because normal and low-probability examinations were pooled together, which is clearly inappropriate (24,25). Moreover, the cutoff was derived from the analysis of a separate group of healthy individuals and not from a receiver operating characteristic (ROC) curve analysis (21,26).

By contrast, the cutoff that was chosen for the ELISA from STAGO (500 μg/L) has clearly been validated (17) by means of such an analysis (Fig. 3). If

Table 1 Diagnostic Performances of the DD and TAT Assays (ELISA) for Diagnosis of PE

Author (ref)	Diagnostic procedure	N (PE)	Sv	Sp	PPV	NPV
DD assay						
Goldhaber et al. (19)	Angiography	69 (19)	89	44	38	92
Bounameaux et al. (3)	Scintigraphy	46 (10)	100	81	59	100
Bounameaux et al. (16)	Angiography	21 (10)	100	36	59	100
Bounameaux et al. (17)	Decision making	170 (55)	98	39	44	98
Rowbotham et al. (20)	Scintigraphy	145 (66)	96	46	26	98
Demers et al. (21)	Scintigraphy	90 (24)	96	52	46	97
TAT assay						
Bounameaux et al. (28)	Scintigraphy	46 (10)	70	42	25	83
Demers et al. (21)	Scintigraphy	71 (24)	96	51	51	96

Abbreviations: DD, D-Dimer; TAT, thrombin-antithrombin III; N (PE), number of patients (number of patients with pulmonary embolism); Sv, sensitivity; Sp, specificity; PPV, positive predictive value; NPV, negative predictive value (all expressed in %).
Cutoffs were set at 500 μg/L (DD) or 4.1 μg/L (TAT).

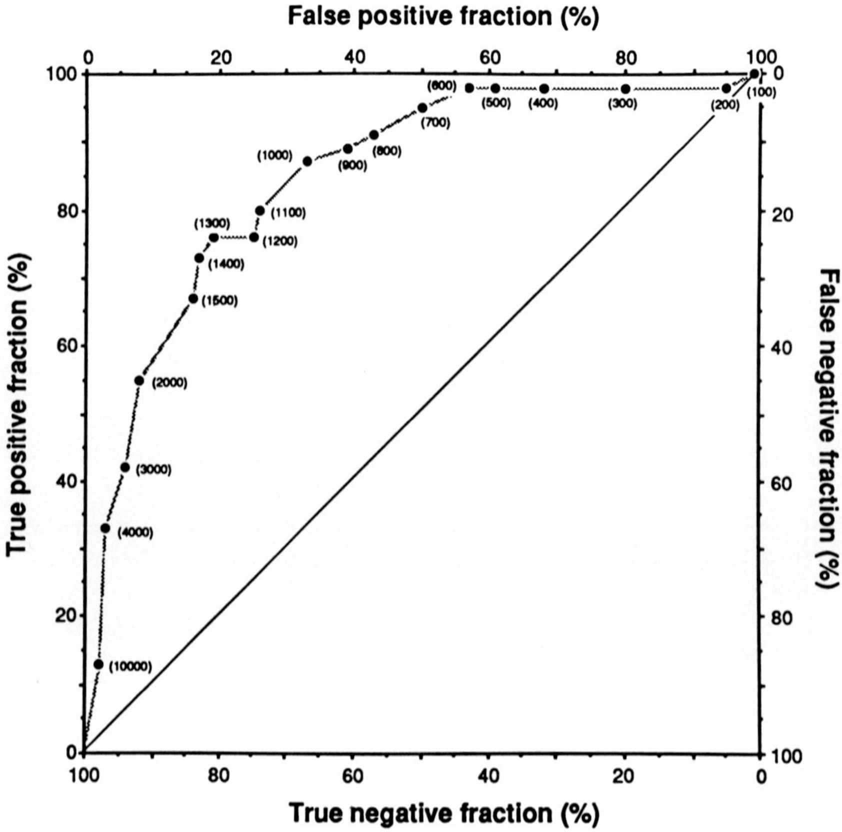

Figure 3 ROC-curve analysis of the accuracy of DD plasma levels for the presence of PE on the day of presentation. The values between brackets represent the respective cutoff levels of Plasma DD. In this analysis, the area under the curve is proportional to the usefulness of a test to discriminate correctly between diseased and nondiseased subjects, the area being 1.0 with the ideal test. (From Ref. 17.)

the utility of the test was assessed by calculating the odds of a patient not being affected given a negative result (27), the odds ratio was 41:1 in the study population with a prevalence of PE of 32% (17) or even 175:1 in a theoretical population with a 10% prevalence of PE. One should, however, remember that only 27% or 35%, respectively, of the results would be negative in the two populations that were considered because of the high prevalence of false-positive results. In practice, in every fourth patient with an inconclusive lung scan, the result of the DD assay would prevent further, invasive investigation.

The sensitivity of the test to the presence of PE decreases with time, but the dosage may be helpful at least up to 3 days after beginning of the symptoms (sensitivity still 96%) (17). This good performance is probably due to the longer half-life (about 3 h) of these compounds and to their continuous generation from the underlying deep venous thrombosis.

Careful examination of the ROC curve (Fig. 2) also revealed that the specificity becomes very high above plasma DD levels of 4000 μg/L. The odds ratio for a patient being affected given a DD level above 4000 μg/L is 5:1 in a population with 32% prevalence of PE. In a population with a lower prevalence (10%), the odds becomes useless (1:1). It should be emphasized that this upper cutoff should be used only in referrals to emergency departments and not in patients who are hospitalized for longer periods, in whom the DD levels are likely to be elevated independently of the presence of PE.

IV. Diagnostic Potential of Plasma TAT in Suspected PE

The performances (sensitivity, specificity, and positive and negative predictive values) of the TAT assay for diagnosing pulmonary embolism were calculated in three studies (21,22,28) in which the values were based on the scintigraphic result (Table 1). In the first study (28), positive and negative predictive values were 25% and 83%, respectively. Thus, measurement of TAT appears to be of no value in the diagnostic procedure of PE. The second study (22) meets similar conclusions with, however, questionable scintigraphic criteria that were discussed earlier—sensitivity and specificity were reported as 72%. However, Demers et al. (21) recently reported a negative predictive value of 96%, which is similar to the performances obtained with the DD assay. Potential explanations for the globally poor performance may include (a) the shorter half-life of these complexes (a few minutes); and/or (b) the presence of heparin, which was already administered in some patients; heparin should immediately prevent thrombin generation by inhibiting prothrombinase formation.

V. Conclusions

The accurate and prompt diagnosis of pulmonary embolism remains a challenge to the clinician. In this diagnostic approach, plasma measurement of DD by ELISA has a definite place, as exemplified in Figure 4: In urgent referrals at emergency departments, when the level is less than 500 μg/L (a cutoff that should be validated for each assay, depending upon the monoclonal antibody used), the diagnosis of pulmonary embolism can be ruled out. This is particularly useful in patients with inconclusive lung scans, a subgroup with a prevalence of PE of 27% (17), which represents about two thirds of all

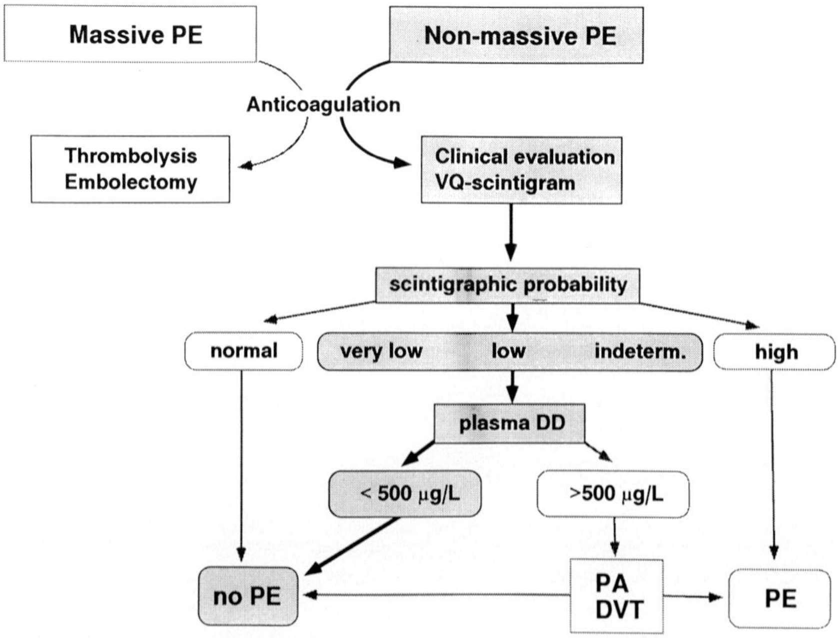

Figure 4 Tentative diagnostic algorithm for patients suspected of having pulmonary embolism, using a clinical decision-making process including clinical evaluation, perfusion-ventilation lung scanning, and plasma DD assay. In few patients, further diagnostic procedures will remain necessary (e.g., pulmonary angiography, PA, or screening for DVT in the lower limbs).

scintigraphic examinations (4,17). However, attempts should be made in order to simplify and shorten the time that is necessary to perform the ELISA before the assay can effectively be used in emergency situations. In this regard, the poor results obtained with latex tests in deep venous thrombosis (9–11) preclude their use for screening purpose in case of suspected pulmonary embolism. On the other hand, the DD assay should be implemented in a clinical decision-making process (18) including an initial clinical assessment, a ventilation-perfusion lung scintigram, and, if necessary, a pulmonary angiogram or an examination of the veins of the lower limbs. Clearly, this combined approach is the only valuable one both from a medical and an economic point of view. In first line, the initial clinical evaluation, which is of paramount importance for the interpretation of any subsequent paraclinical examination, should be reassessed, and the data by Hoellerich et al. (29) and Celi et al. (30) should be confirmed and extended.

References

1. Alderson PO, Martin EC. Pulmonary embolism diagnosis with multiple imaging modalities. Radiology 1987; 164:297–312.
2. Kipper SM, Moser KM, Kortman KE, Ashburn WL. Longterm follow-up of patients with suspected pulmonary embolism and a normal lung scan. Chest 1982; 82:411–25.
3. Bounameaux H, Slosman D, de Moerloose P, Reber G. Diagnostic value of plasma D-dimer in suspected pulmonary embolism. Lancet 1988; ii:628–9.
4. The PIOPED Investigators. Value of the ventilation/perfusion scan in acute pulmonary embolism. Results of the prospective investigation of pulmonary embolism diagnosis (PIOPED). JAMA 1990; 263:2753–9.
5. Gurewich V, Hume M, Patrick M. The laboratory diagnosis of venous thromboembolic disease by measurement of fibrinogen/fibrin degradation products and fibrin monomer. Chest 1973; 64:585–90.
6. Gaffney PJ, Creighton LJ, Callus M, Thorpe R. Monoclonal antibodies to crosslinked fibrin degradation products (XL-FDP). Br J Haematol 1988; 68:83–96.
7. Nieuwenhuizen W. Plasma assays for derivatives of fibrin and of fibrinogen, based on monoclonal antibodies. Fibrinolysis 1988; 2:1–5.
8. Rowbotham BJ, Carroll P, Whitaker AN, Bunce IH, Cobcroft RG, Elms MJ, Masci PP, Bundesen PG, Rylatt DB, Webber AJ. Measurement of crosslinked fibrin derivatives—use in the diagnosis of venous thrombosis. Thromb Haemost 1987; 57:59–61.
9. Bounameaux H, Schneider PA, Reber G, de Moerloose P, Krahenbuhl B. Measurement of plasma D-dimer for diagnosis of deep venous thrombosis. Am J Clin Pathol 1989; 91:82–5.
10. Heaton DC, Billings JD, Hickton CM. Assessment of D dimer assays for the diagnosis of deep vein thrombosis. J Lab Clin Med 1987; 110:588–91.
11. Ott P, Astrup L, Hartving Jensen R, Nyland B, Pedersen B. Assessment of D-dimer in plasma: diagnostic value in suspected deep venous thrombosis of the leg. Acta Med Scand 1988; 224:263–7.
12. Francis CW, Connaghan DG, Scott WL, Marder VJ. Increased plasma concentration of cross-linked fibrin polymers in acute myocardial infarction. Circulation 1987; 75:1170–7.
13. Collen D, De Cock F, Verstraete M. Quantitation of thrombin-antithrombin III complexes in human blood. Eur J Clin Invest 1977; 7:407–11.
14. Hoek JA, Sturk A, ten Cate JW, Lamping RJ, Berends F, Borm JJJ. Laboratory and clinical evaluation of an assay of thrombin-antithrombin III complexes in plasma. Clin Chem 1988; 34:2058–62.
15. Pelzer H, Schwarz A, Heimburger N. Determination of human thrombin-antithrombin III complex in plasma with an enzyme-linked immunosorbent assay. Thromb Haemost 1988; 59:101–6.
16. Bounameaux H, Schneider PA, Slosman D, de Moerloose P, Reber G. Plasma D-dimer in suspected pulmonary embolism: A comparison with pulmonary angiography and perfusion-ventilation scintigraphy. Blood Coag Fibrinol 1990; 1:577–9.

17. Bounameaux H, Cirafici P, de Moerloose P, Schneider PA, Slosman D, Reber G, Unger PF. Measurement of D-dimer in plasma as diagnostic aid in suspected pulmonary embolism. Lancet 1991; 337:196–200.
18. Junod AF, Morabia A. Utilisation rationnelle des différents tests pour le diagnostic d'embolie pulmonaire. Schweiz Med Wschr 1989; 119:1489–92.
19. Goldhaber SZ, Vaughan DE, Tumeh SS, Loscalzo J. Utility of cross-linked fibrin degradation products in the diagnosis of pulmonary embolism. Am Heart J 1988; 116:505–8.
20. Rowbotham BJ, Egerton-Vernon J, Whitaker AN, Elms MJ, Bunce IH. Plasma cross linked fibrin degradation products in pulmonary embolism. Thorax 1990; 45:684–7.
21. Demers C, Ginsberg JS, Johnston M, Brill-Edwards P, Panju A. D-dimer and thrombin-antithrombin III complexes in patients with clinically suspected pulmonary embolism. Thromb Haemostas 1992; 67:408–12.
22. Bridey F, Philipotteau C, Dreyfus M, Simonneau G. Plasma D-dimer and pulmonary embolism. Lancet 1989; i:791–2.
23. Leitha T, Speiser W, Dudczak R. Pulmonary embolism. Efficacy of D-dimer and thrombin-antithrombin III complex determinations as screening tests before lung scanning. Chest 1991; 100:1536–41.
24. Hull RD, Raskob GE. Low-probability lung scan findings: a need for change. Ann Intern Med 1991; 114:142–3.
25. Bounameaux H, Slosman D. Diagnosis of pulmonary embolism. Ann Intern Med 1991; 114:702–3.
26. Hanley JA, McNeil BJ. The meaning and use of the area under the receiving operator characteristic (ROC) curve. Radiology 1982; 143:29–36.
27. Wald N. Rational use of investigations in clinical practice. In: Hopkins A, ed. Appropriate Investigation and Treatment in Clinical Practice. London: Royal College of Physicians, 1989: 7–20.
28. Bounameaux H, Slosman D, de Moerloose P, Reber G. Laboratory diagnosis of pulmonary embolism: value of increased levels of plasma D-dimers and thrombin-antithrombin III complexes. Biomed Pharmacother 1989; 43:385–8.
29. Hoellerich VL, Wington RS. Diagnosing pulmonary embolism using clinical findings. Arch Intern Med 1986; 146:1699–1704.
30. Celi A, Palla A, Petruzzelli S, Carrozzi L, Jacobson A, Cella G, Giuntini C, Sasahara AA. Prospective study of a standardized questionnaire to improve clinical estimate of pulmonary embolism. Chest 1989; 95:332–7.

9

Pulmonary Gas Exchange Abnormalities in Pulmonary Embolism

R. SERGYSELS

Clinique de Pneumologie
Hôpital Universitaire Saint-Pierre
Brussels, Belgium

I. Introduction

Pulmonary embolism clearly affects gas exchange, and both clinical and experimental research report as typical findings a lowering in Pa_{O_2} and in Pa_{CO_2}, with a widening of arterial alveolar gradients for these gases. Furthermore, at least in acute embolism, hyperventilation (1,2) is a common finding that may affect further Pa_{CO_2} and induce respiratory alcalosis.

Obstruction of the vascular bed that does not affect primarily ventilation will increase the dead space (VD) (and, therefore, VD/VT), and this per se does not explain the lowering in Pa_{O_2}, except if alveolar ventilation is reduced to a very large extent.

II. Hypoxia

Despite important clinical and experimental work, the reason for hypoxia in pulmonary embolism remains unclear, and various causes have been suggested. Most authors propose intricateness of these causes at various degrees (Fig. 1).

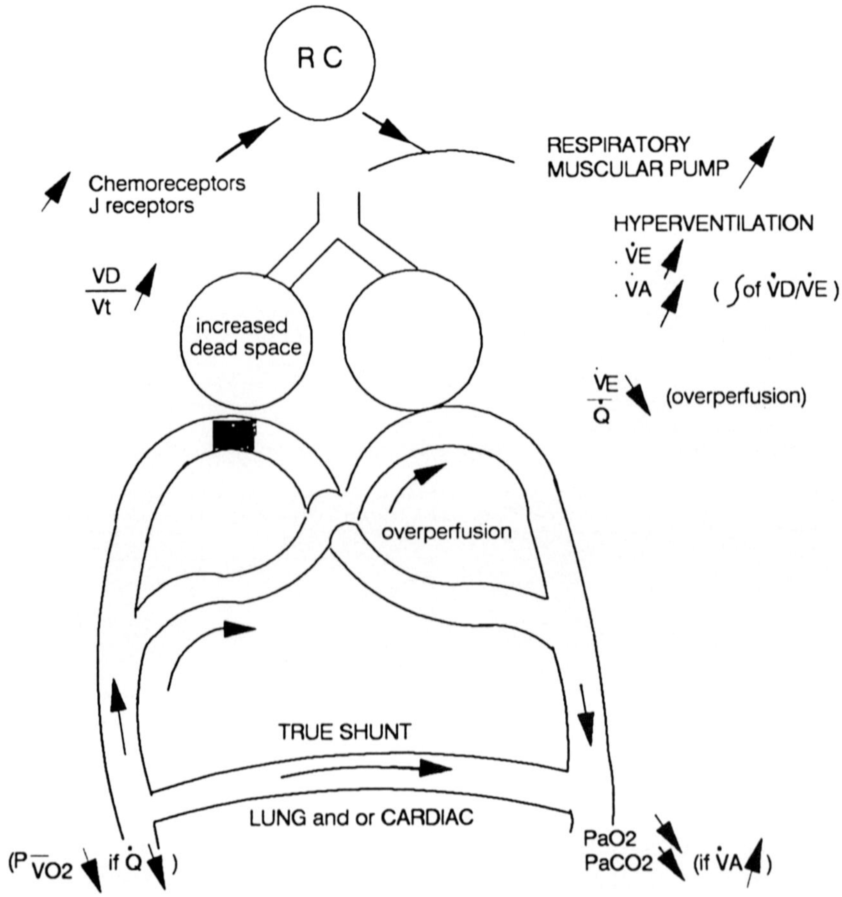

Figure 1 Schematic presentation for the various proposed mechanisms explaining hypoxia in pulmonary emboli. For symbols, see Nomenclature.

A. Ventilation-Perfusion Mismatching

Using the inert gas technique, Huet et al. (3) in a study of seven patients with acute embolism demonstrated that the lowering in Pa_{O_2} could not be solely attributed to a shunt effect and/or by a low Pv_{O_2} but suggested that relative overperfusion of unembolized lung with incomplete oxygenation could better explain hypoxemia. This finding is in contradiction with other clinical studies reported by D'Alonzo and Dantzker (4).

B. Shunting Within the Lung (or the Heart)

This is probably one of the most important and documented mechanisms explaining hypoxia. Shunt has been reported to be as much as 40% of cardiac output (5). By using the inert gas technique, a study was undertaken in two patients with massive embolization. This study confirmed a widening P_{AO_2}-Pa_{O_2} caused by the increased shunt (perfusion of unventilated lung units), while the increase in V_D/V_T was attributed to the increased ventilation of unperfused units.

Animal models of pulmonary embolization (6) showed that intrapulmonary shunt was the major component for a low Pa_{O_2}. This shunt could be due to the opening of preexisting pulmonary arterial venous anastomoses with high pulmonary pressure (7), although Cheney et al. (8) could not confirm this hypothesis.

Other causes of shunt may be the development of areas of atelectasis distal to the embolic obstruction of the vascular bed (6,9) induced by probable loss of surfactant (10), hemorrhage, and pneumoconstriction (11). Finally, shunt could also be explained by the development of a patent foramen ovale (12–14).

In the already quoted study of Huet et al. (3), shunting was only observed when radiological abnormalities of ventilation such as atelectasies, pulmonary infarction, and elevated diaphragm were present.

C. Reduced Mixed Venous Oxygen Saturation

This mechanism has probably been overlooked in most studies, but the reduced cardiac output may lead to low mixed venous oxygen saturation and insufficient time for complete equilibration with alveolar oxygen (3,5). Furthermore, when $\dot{V}E/\dot{Q}$ imbalance and shunt are present, a low $P\bar{v}_{O_2}$ will amplify arterial desaturation.

In most cases, these various mechanisms are probably acting together, their respective importance depending on the possible pulmonary underlying disease, the importance of vascular obstruction, the lowering in cardiac output, and the development of alveolar collapse, edema, or hemorrhage. For instance, in the study of Manier et al. (15) on 10 subjects (mean percentage of obstruction 30% and mean Pa_{O_2} 61.5 mm Hg), all showed a widened P_{AO_2}-Pa_{O_2}, and the authors concluded that (a) 13% was due to a diffusional component, (b) true shunt was on average 9% of the cardiac output, and (c) the fall in mixed venous P_{O_2} accounted for a large part in the explanation of the low Pa_{O_2}.

The importance of hypoxia is reported in some large clinical studies. In 54 patients with angiographically proven acute pulmonary emboli and no previous evidence of cardiopulmonary disease, a compilation of three different studies reported by Dantzker et al. (16) showed a Pa_{O_2} between 60 and 69 mm Hg in 31%, a Pa_{O_2} above 80 mm Hg in 13%, and a Pa_{O_2} below 50 mm Hg in 13%.

These values are quite similar to those reported in two important French studies (17,18).

A consensus conference on this problem, partially reported (19), states that Pa_{O_2} is of limited diagnostic value and recommends that when Pa_{O_2} is normal not to disregard pulmonary embolism, and when Pa_{O_2} is very low to reconsider the diagnosis (differential diagnosis with the ARDS type of disease).

The UPET study (20) showed that using an arterial Pa_{O_2} value of 80 mm Hg or greater results in failure to detect 10%–15% of patients in whom pulmonary embolism was demonstrated by pulmonary angiography. Despite this, Pa_{O_2} has been proven to be correlated with the importance of scintigraphic defect (21) and hemodynamic data such as pulmonary vascular pressure and cardiac index (22).

D. Hypocapnia

Arterial hypocapnia and respiratory alkalosis are commonly seen in patients with acute pulmonary embolism. For instance, among 34 patients, 27 had a Pa_{CO_2} of less than 38 mmHg, and the highest value reported was 44 mm Hg (9,23). In most acute cardiopulmonary diseases caused by hyperventilation, a low Pa_{CO_2} may be found and, therefore, has no diagnostic value (4). The ventilation of unperfused lung results in a widening of the Pa_{CO_2}-PA_{CO_2}, and experimental (24–27) and clinical (28–30) studies have shown that this gradient is enlarged with pulmonary emboli.

Prediletto et al. (21), in a study of 33 patients, could relate Pa_{CO_2} and Pa_{CO_2}-PA_{CO_2} to a score appreciating the importance of scintigraphic defects.

However, the clinical value of measuring Pa_{CO_2}-PA_{CO_2} is questioned because it has been found to be increased in other lung diseases (31–33). Furthermore, it is estimated that at least 20%–30% of lung parenchyma must be unperfused before the P_{CO_2} difference exceeds 6 mm Hg, and compensatory mechanisms restricting ventilation (such as pneumoconstriction) make this test almost valueless within 48 h (34).

It has also been proposed to use the Bohr equation in order to measure VD/VT. This ratio was found to exceed 0.35 in 15 patients out of 23 without underlying disease and proven pulmonary emboli (5,9), but again experimental studies on human subjects by occluding right or left pulmonary artery with a balloon showed minimal increase in the dead space probably because of pneumoconstriction (35).

E. Diagnostic Value of Gas Exchange Abnormalities in Suspected Pulmonary Embolism

It has already been largely stressed that Pa_{O_2}, Pa_{CO_2}, A-a gradients, and calculation of VD/VT have no definite diagnostic value (4,16). Hull et al. (36) stress that the estimation of blood gases in patients with suspected pulmonary embolism should be confined to the management of these patients rather than to the diagnosis.

With this in mind, Cvitanic et al. (37) proposed an improved use of arterial blood gases in suspected pulmonary embolism. In a retrospective study of 78 patients without cardiopulmonary disease, hypoxia was found in 76%, hypoxia or hypocapnia in 93%, an increased PAO_2-PaO_2 in 95%, and an increased PAO_2-PaO_2 or hypocapnia in 77 patients out of 78. The authors suggest that a normal $PaCO_2$ and a normal (A-a) D O_2 gradient can be used as evidence against the diagnosis of pulmonary emboli.

Very recently, Stein et al. (38), in reviewing the data of 117 patients with suspected acute pulmonary embolism (EP), found in air a PaO_2 <80 mm Hg in 74% and a PaO_2-PAO_2 > 20 mm Hg in 86% of the patients. These authors stress that these findings have to be integrated with other clinical and radiological abnormalities in order to help differentiating patients with or without EP.

Additional Problems in Interpretation of Arterial Gas Values in Patients with Suspected Pulmonary Emboli

Most of studies report series of patients without underlying disease that could affect per se PaO_2 and/or $PaCO_2$ such as obesity, pregnancy, chronic lung disease, all situations where a low PaO_2 is completely unrelevant to an hypothetical diagnosis of pulmonary embolism. For the latter disease, it has been suggested that a sudden reduction in $PaCO_2$ may help the diagnosis (39).

Natural History and Gas Exchange Abnormalities Observed in Chronic Lung Emboli

Prediletto et al. (21) followed 33 patients until 6 months after documented embolism. PaO_2 improved within 1 month (close to the normal value) without further improvement after 6 months. A similar pattern was observed for PAO_2-PaO_2, $PACO_2$-$PACO_2$, and VD/VT. After 6 months, PaO_2 and $PaCO_2$ were no longer correlated with an index of scintigraphic defect, although $PACO_2$-$PaCO_2$ and VD/VT still were. Riedel et al. (40,41) reported a group of 87 patients studied 2 months after the last episode: PaO_2 was slightly lower, and VD/VT was slightly higher in the most severe group. In another article, the same authors (42) reported the follow-up of 76 patients for 1–15 years comparing survivors and patients who died from thromboembolic disease. Surprisingly, PaO_2, $PaCO_2$, and PAO_2-PaO_2 could not differentiate the two groups, but this could be done well using hemodynamic criteria and VD/VT. Furthermore, for the 61 patients studied 4.8 years after the acute onset, VD/VT ratio decreased from 32.4% to 27.3%.

Finally, it has also been suggested that in chronic stages, the monitoring of VD/VT during exercise in patients with pulmonary vascular obstruction may show this ratio to increase (43,44). Again, some contradictory results were presented by Riedel et al., showing a fall in VD/VT during exercise in most of their patients.

In conclusion, gas exchange parameters as clinically evaluated by measuring Pao_2, $Paco_2$, and pH may not be used for accurate diagnosis of pulmonary embolism, but they may be helpful because a low Pao_2 and a low $Paco_2$ have to be integrated in the different other diagnostic procedures. Furthermore, these parameters, especially Pao_2, may be of help for the adequate management of the patients.

Nomenclature

Pao_2,$Paco_2$	Partial pressure for oxygen, carbon dioxide in arterial blood
Pvo_2,$Pvco_2$	Partial pressure for oxygen, carbon dioxide in venous blood
PAO_2-Pao_2	Oxygen partial pressure difference between alveolar gas and arteriel blood
$Paco_2$-$PACO_2$	Carbon dioxide partial pressure differences between arterial blood and alveolar gas
$\dot{V}E$	Expired ventilation
$\dot{V}A$	Alveolar ventilation
VD	Dead space
Vt	Tidal volume
$\dot{V}E/\dot{Q}$	Ventilation perfusion ratio

References

1. Llamas R, Swenson EW. Diagnostic clues in pulmonary thromboembolism evaluated by angiographic and ventilation-blood flow studies. Thorax 1965; 20:327.
2. Sasahara AA, Stein M, Simon M, et al. Pulmonary angiography in the diagnosis of thromboembolic disease. N Engl J Med 1964; 270:1075.
3. Huet Y, Lemaire F, Brun-Buisson C, Knaus WA, Teisseire B, Payen D, Mathieu D. Hypoxemia in acute pulmonary embolism. Chest 1985; 88:829–36.
4. D'Alonzo GE, Dantzker DR. Gas exchange alterations following pulmonary thromboembolism. Clin Chest Med 1984; 5:411–19.
5. D'Alonzo GE, Bower JS, Dehart P, Dantzker R, et al. The mechanisms of abnormal gas exchange in acute massive pulmonary embolism. Am Rev Respir Dis 1983; 128:170.
6. Caldini P. Pulmonary hemodynamics and arterial oxygen saturation in pulmonary embolism. J Appl Physiol 1965; 20:184.
7. Niden AH, Aviado DM. Effects of pulmonary embolism on the pulmonary circulation with special reference to arteriovenous shunts in the lung. Circ Res 1956; 4:67–73.

8. Cheney FW, Pavlin J, Ferens BS, et al. Effect of pulmonary microembolism on arteriovenous shunt flow. J Thorac Cardiovasc Surg 1978; 4:473–7.
9. Wilson J, Pierce AK, Johnson RL, et al. Hypoxemia in pulmonary embolism. J Clin Invest 1971; 50:481–91.
10. Chernick V, Hodson WH, Greenfield LJ. Effects of chronic pulmonary artery ligation on pulmonary mechanisms and surfactant. J Appl Physiol 1966; 21:1315–20.
11. Levy SE, Simmons DH. Redistribution of alveolar ventilation following pulmonary thromboembolism in dogs. J Appl Physiol 1974; 36:60–8.
12. Alexander JA, Rembert JC, Sealy WC, et al. Shunt dynamics in experimental atrial septal defects. J Appl Physiol 1975; 39:281–6.
13. Moorthy SS, Losasso AM. Patency of the foramen ovale in the critically ill patient. Anesthesiology 1974; 41:405–7.
14. Moorthy SS, Losasso AM, Gibbs AS. Acquired right to left intracardiac shunts in severe hypoxemia. Crit Care Med 1978; 6:28–31.
15. Manier G, Castaing Y, Guenard H. Determinants of hypoxemia during the acute phase of pulmonary embolism in humans. Am Rev Respir Dis 1985; 132:332–8.
16. Dantzker DR, Bower JS. Alterations in gas exchange following pulmonary thromboembolism. Chest 1982; 4:495–501.
17. Dalen JE. Pulmonary embolism, diagnostic problem. In: Dequinot, ed. Problèmes de réanimation et de biotechnologie en chirurgie cardiaque. Paris: Arnette, 1976:87–97.
18. Even P, Sors H, Safran D, et al. Diagnostic des embolies pulmonaires. Analyse critique à propos de 338 observations. La maladie thrombo-embolique. Paris: Masson, 1981:45–94.
19. Conférence de consensus. Diagnostic de l'embolie pulmonaire. Rev Mal Resp 1991; 8:319–23.
20. National cooperative study. The urokinase pulmonary embolism trial. Circulation 1973; 47-48(suppl 2);1–108.
21. Prediletto R, Paoletti P, Fornai E, et al. Evaluation of perfusion lung scintigraphy, gas exchange and chest roentgenogram. Chest 1990; 97:554–61.
22. McIntyre KM, Sasahara AA. Pulmonary angiography, scanning and hemodynamics in pulmonary embolism: critical review and correlations. Crit Rev Radiol Sci 1972; 3:489–521.
23. Stanek V, Riedel M, Widimsky J. Hemodynamics monitoring in acute pulmonary embolism. Bull Eur Physiopathol Resp 1978; 14:561–72.
24. Julian D, Travis D, Robin ED, et al. Effect of pulmonary artery occlusion upon end-tidal Co_2 tension. J Appl Physiol 1960; 15:87–91.
25. Levy SE, Stein M, Totten RS, et al. Ventilation-perfusion abnormalities in experimental pulmonary embolism. J Clin Invest 1965; 44:1699–1707.
26. Marshall R, Sabiston DC, Allison PR, et al. Immediate and late effects of pulmonary embolism by large thrombi in dogs. Thorax 1963; 18:1–9.
27. Stein M, Forkner CE, Robin ED, et al. Gas exchange after autologous pulmonary embolism in dogs. J Appl Physiol 1961; 16:488–92.
28. Colp CR, Williams MH. Pulmonary function following pulmonary embolism. Am Rev Respir Dis 1962; 85:799–807.

29. Robin ED, Forkner CE, Bromberg PA, et al. Alveolar gas exchange in clinical pulmonary embolism. N Engl J Med 1960; 262:283–7.
30. Robin ED, Julian DG, Travis DM, et al. A physiologic approach to the diagnosis of acute pulmonary embolism. N Engl J Med 1959; 60:586–91.
31. Hatle L, Rokseth R. The arterial to end-expiratory carbon dioxide tension gradient in acute pulmonary embolism and other cardiopulmonary diseases. Chest 1974; 66:352–7.
32. Herzog H, Staub H, Richterich R: Gas-analytical studies in severe pneumonia. Lancet 1959; i:593–7.
33. Nutter DO, Massumi RA. The arterial-alveolar carbon dioxide tension gradient in diagnosis of pulmonary embolus. Chest 1966; 50:380.
34. Sasahara AA. Clinical studies in pulmonary thromboembolism. In: Sasahara, Stein, eds. Pulmonary Embolism Disease. New York: Grune & Stratton, 1965:256–64.
35. Swenson EW, Finley TN, Guzman SV. Unilateral hypoventilation in man during temporary occlusion of one pulmonary artery. J Clin Invest 1961; 40:835.
36. Hull RD, Raskob GE, Hirsh J. Pulmonary thromboembolism. In: Flenley, Petty, eds. Recent Advances in Respiratory Medicine. Churchill Livingstone. No 4. 1986;156–72.
37. Cvitanic O, Marino PL. Improved use of arterial blood gas analysis in suspected pulmonary embolism. Chest 1989; 95:48–51.
38. Stein PD, Terrin ML, Hales CA, Palevsky HI, Saltzman HA, Thompson BT, Weg JG. Clinical, laboratory, roentgenographic and electrocardiographic findings in patients with acute pulmonary embolism and no-pre-existing cardiac or pulmonary disease. Chest 1991; 100:598–603.
39. Lippman M, Fein A. Pulmonary embolism in the patient with chronic obstructive pulmonary disease. A diagnostic dilemma. Chest 1981; 79.
40. Riedel M, Stanek V, Widimsky J. Spirometry and gas exchange in chronic pulmonary thromboembolism. Bull Eur Physiopathol Resp 1981; 17:209–21.
41. Riedel M, Widimsky J, Stanek V. Steady-state pulmonary transfer factor in chronic thromboembolic disease. Bull Eur Physiopathol Resp 1980; 16:469–77.
42. Riedel M, Stanek V, Widimsky J. Longterm follow-up of patients with pulmonary thromboembolism. Late prognosis and evolution of hemodynamic and respiratory data. Chest 1982; 81:151.
43. Jones NL, Goodwin JF. Respiratory function in pulmonary thromboembolic disorders. Br Med J 1965; 1:1089–93.
44. Nadel J, Gold W, Burgess JH. Early diagnosis of chronic pulmonary vascular obstruction. Am J Med 1968; 44:16–25.

10

Prognosis of Pulmonary Embolism

JIŘÍ WIDIMSKÝ

Postgraduate Medical Institute
Prague, Czech Republic

I. Introduction

Prognosis of acute pulmonary embolism depends on several factors. Among the most important ones are the presence of concomitant disease, especially malignancy, previous cardiac or pulmonary disease, patient's age, size, localization and age of pulmonary embolism, and degree of pulmonary hypertension. Diagnosed and treated acute pulmonary embolism is accompanied with markedly better short-term prognosis than undetected and, thus, untreated pulmonary embolism.

II. The Effect of Concomitant Disease and Age

The presence of concomitant disease and age is among the most important prognostic factors (1–4). Pulmonary embolism often accompanies advanced illnesses that predispose patients to thromboembolism, venous stasis, hypercoagulate states, or vascular injury (3). Already in 1959, Coon and Coller (5) stated that in little more than 50% of patients, prognosis had been hopeless because of advanced malignancy or the like. Morpurgo and Schmid (6) in 1980 reviewed 538 autopsies and disclosed that 39% of patients would probably have died within weeks or months from their concomitant disease.

In a recent multicentric study including 399 patients with pulmonary embolism (3), most patients dying of pulmonary embolism were already quite ill, and pulmonary embolism was often the final event in a setting of serious cardiopulmonary disease or cancer (3). Most of the deaths caused by acute pulmonary embolism itself occurred early in the follow-up period (3). While the 1-year mortality in this group of patients was nearly 24%, death from pulmonary embolism itself occurred in only 2.5%. Thus, the presence of a severe concomitant disease markedly influences both the short- and long-term prognoses (3).

From the concomitant diseases, most important predictors of death are cancer (relative risk 3.8), left heart failure (relative risk 2.7), and history of chronic lung disease (relative risk 2.2) (3). Age greater than 60 years also negatively influences the prognosis of acute pulmonary embolism, with relative risk being 2.2 (3).

In the acute stage, the presence of another cardiac or pulmonary disease has a marked impact on the prognosis (2,4,7). In many older patients, coronary artery disease is usually present. The presence of damaged and ischemic myocardium can especially have a negative influence on the short-term prognosis, and malignant arrhythmias and cardiac arrest (8) occur more frequently, as stated elsewhere in this volume (Chap. 11).

On the other hand, we should be aware of the fact that many patients have a favorable prognosis in the absence of pulmonary embolism. From the autopsy data of Morpurgo and Schmid (6), it appears that approximately 21% of patients had had a favorable prognosis in the absence of pulmonary embolism, and another 39% would probably have survived without pulmonary embolism.

III. The Effect of Treatment

The acute prognosis of pulmonary embolism depends primarily on whether the embolism has been detected and treated (4). Treatment exerts a major effect on the short-term prognosis of acute pulmonary embolism (see also Chap. 16). Mean 1-month mortality rates of treated and untreated pulmonary embolism are 8% and 30%, respectively (9).

An early start of treatment leads to a quick decrease of pulmonary hypertension. The later the treatment is started (late correct diagnosis), the slower the pulmonary artery pressure decreases (10,11).

Regression of thromboembolic pulmonary vascular obstruction also depends on the type of treatment, with thrombolytic therapy resulting in far more rapid removal of the vascular obstruction than with the heparin administration (12–16).

A. Extent of Acute PE

In acute stage the chief prognostic factor is the extent of pulmonary embolism reflected by the degree of pulmonary hypertension (10) and the presence of another cardiac or pulmonary disease (1,9–17). In patients without preexisting cardiac or pulmonary disease, the acute mortality is low, ranging from 3% to 9% (2,7).

B. The Effect of Pulmonary Hypertension

In patients without previous cardiopulmonary disease, the degree of pulmonary hypertension caused by acute pulmonary embolism is a significant prognostic factor (10,18).

While the mortality of treated patients with severe pulmonary hypertension concomitant with acute pulmonary embolism (mean pulmonary artery pressure ≥40 mm Hg) was 31.2%, it was as low as 5.7% in treated patients with moderate or mild pulmonary hypertension (mean pulmonary artery pressure 20–39 mm Hg) (18).

C. Resolution of Acute PE

Thrombi can be removed from the pulmonary vasculature by fibrinolysis and by fragmentation. Fibrinolytic dissolution of the thromboembolism is accomplished by the fibrinolytic activity of blood and endothelial cells of pulmonary arteries. However, there are interindividual variations in the degree of the fibrinolytic activity of pulmonary vessels. For reasons still unclear, the emboli do not resolve completely in some patients; rather, they flow an aberrant path of organization and recanalization and leave endothelialized residua that obstruct or significantly narrow major (main lobar or segmental) pulmonary arteries (19,20) (see Chap. 5).

Another factor affecting the natural course of acute pulmonary embolism includes age of the embolus. Fresh thrombi tend to dissipate into pieces on passage through the right ventricle, thereby causing minor embolisms. Older, organized thrombi pass unaltered into the pulmonary circulation and frequently get stuck on the pulmonary main branch, causing obstruction of major pulmonary arteries (10,21).

Other factors influencing the resolution of the embolus include size of the embolus, presence of other cardiac or pulmonary disease, and the type of treatment.

IV. Trends in the Diagnosis and Mortality of Acute PE

In 1975, Dalen and Alpert (9) estimated the total annual prevalence of acute pulmonary embolism in the United States at 630,000. Eleven percent of patients with acute pulmonary embolism die suddenly (in less than 1 h) according to these authors. In the early 1980s, the percentage of well-diagnosed (and, hence, treated) cases of pulmonary embolism (surviving more than 1 h) in the United States was 29%. This attests to an improving diagnostic capability compared with the 1950s and 1960s, when the proportion of correct diagnoses of pulmonary embolism was as low as 10%–11% (22).

Trends in mortality from pulmonary embolism in the United States between 1962 and 1984 were studied by Lilienfeld et al. (23). Age-adjusted pulmonary embolism mortality increased by 67 to 100% between 1962 and 1974 for white and nonwhite men and women. From 1975 to 1984, these rates declined by 20%–28%. This pattern might reflect improved ascertainment of cases and better prevention of the disease (23).

A. The Natural Course of Unrecognized Acute PE

According to data released by Dalen and Alpert (9), pulmonary embolism is not recognized and, as a result, remains untreated in 71% of patients. The mortality of these patients averages 30%. The implication is that 280,000 persons survive undetected and untreated acute pulmonary embolism in the United States each year. The fate of these patients is not clear. Dalen and Alpert 1975 (9) believe that recurrent thromboembolic attacks and gradual development of pulmonary hypertension can be expected in many of these patients. According to many authors, however, patients with detected and properly treated acute pulmonary embolism are highly unlikely to develop chronic thromboembolic pulmonary hypertension (10,15,23,24).

B. Recurrent PE

Pulmonary embolism tends to recur in some treated patients. The Urokinase study (15,16) revealed that 15% of patients with acute massive pulmonary embolism had had two or more previous minor attacks before massive attack, and 20% of treated patients were found to have signs of recurrent pulmonary embolism within the first 2 weeks.

According Carson et al. (3), symptomatic recurrent pulmonary embolism occurs in 8.3% of patients with properly diagnosed and treated disease. Pulmonary embolism recurs most frequently during the first week of follow-up (3). Such recurrence was associated with a case fatality rate of 45% during the follow-up, and 9 of 10 deaths from this condition in the series of Carson et al.

(3) were in patients with embolic recurrences. Therefore, recurrent pulmonary embolism often has lethal consequences.

Recurrences are more frequent in patients with free-floating thrombus on venography (25). Venography seems, according to Monreal et al. (25), mandatory in patients with pulmonary embolism, because it recognizes a subgroup of patients at a high risk of recurrences.

C. The Prognosis of Subacute PE

Our understanding of the course of subacute pulmonary embolism is more limited (24). Subacute pulmonary embolism is characterized by dyspnea, persisting longer than in the acute form and, more important, progressing over 1–4 weeks without an acute attack or syncope. However, on follow-up at 4–6 years (7,24), a small proportion of these patients is found to have pulmonary hypertension, and the condition tends to progress slowly. This may be due to the fact that therapy was started late.

V. Chronic Thromboembolic Pulmonary Hypertension

Recurrent pulmonary embolism can be seen in treated patients with acute pulmonary embolism before therapy initiation and during the acute stage. However, acute as well as massive treated pulmonary embolism does not usually result in chronic thromboembolic pulmonary hypertension (10,26,27).

Which patients with acute pulmonary embolism are then hypothetically most likely to develop chronic thromboembolic pulmonary hypertension? First, they are those with undiagnosed and, hence, untreated acute pulmonary embolism (28) and, also patients with recurrent minor embolism most often from the area of pelvis veins (so-called silent recurrent pulmonary embolism), and perhaps even those with unsuccessful lysis of acute embolism (e.g., because of late start of therapy) (19). Development of chronic thromboembolic hypertension may also be due to endothelial dysfunction.

According Palla et al. (28), many patients with pulmonary embolism who develop chronic thromboembolic pulmonary hypertension are not diagnosed and, thus, untreated because clinical symptoms and signs of acute pulmonary embolism have not been recognized. In some of these cases, clinical assessment (including chest radiograph, ECG, and blood gas analysis) may show a quite characteristic pattern useful for diagnosis (28).

Quite surprisingly, chronic thromboembolic pulmonary hypertension is not a frequent condition, and its prevalence in autopsy studies has not changed over the past 50 years! Owen et al. (29) found a 0.15% prevalence (12 deaths in a total of 8,000 autopsies) of chronic thromboembolic hypertension over the years 1933–1953. Urbanová and Staněk (30) reported only 3 deaths with the same diagnosis in the series of 720 postmortem examinations in the Department of Cardiology of the Institute for Clinical and Experimental Medicine in Prague in the years 1979–1988. The prevalence of 0.38% found in the group of Urbanová and Staněk (30) thus, is, virtually consistent with the data furnished by Owen et al. (29).

Prognosis of chronic thromboembolic pulmonary hypertension relates to the degree of pulmonary hypertension. Prognosis is serious in all patients with a mean pulmonary artery pressure ≥30 mm Hg (24). The worst prognosis was observed in patients with an elevated right atrial pressure (≥6 mm Hg). While 82% of those patients with a mean right atrial pressure <6 mm Hg were surviving after 4.8 years, only 18% were alive of those with an elevated right atrial pressure (right atrial pressure ≥6 mm Hg) (24).

No relationship between chronic thromboembolic pulmonary hypertension and the clinical signs, number, and extent of previous pulmonary embolism or the extent of a residual defect after acute pulmonary embolism on the pulmonary perfusion scan has been found (13,24). Thus, only a small proportion of patients with acute pulmonary embolism develops pulmonary hypertension; no explanation for this finding is yet available. Presumably, the functional properties of the pulmonary vascular endothelium (e.g, the degree of individual fibrinolytic activity) may play a key role.

Neither a high resting PAI-1 activity nor a blunted t-PA response to venous occlusion can be invoked as an etiology for chronic thromboembolic pulmonary hypertension (31). Relatively common deficiencies classically associated with thrombosis (i.e., antithrombin III, protein C, protein S) (32–34) have been observed only in 2 of 32 patients with chronic thromboembolic pulmonary hypertension (31).

Mechanisms responsible for poor thrombus dissolution may involve local abnormalities in the regulation, activity, inhibition, or release of t-PA as well as intrinsic properties of the embolus itself that may render it resistant to lysis (i.e., size, platelets, age) (31).

However, no method has been developed allowing us to identify these patients at risk.

Immunological dysfunction may also play a role in the pathogenesis of recurrent pulmonary embolism (35). According these authors, HLA-CW 4 are increased and HLA-Bw22 completely absent in patients with chronic thromboembolic disease.

Many patients with chronic thromboembolic pulmonary hypertension recall an episode of unexplained dyspnea, "pneumonia," or "asthma"; a minority have had acute embolic disease diagnosed by scan or pulmonary angiography (19). After the initial embolic event, the patient improves and according to Moser et al. (19,36), a "honeymoon" period appears during which the patient receives limited medical attention; if anticoagulants were administered, they are usually discontinued. Rarely are follow-up lung scans performed (19). Sometimes the "honeymoon" period lasts for several months, sometimes for several years.

Preliminary observations from lung biopsy material indicate that these patients develop classic pulmonary hypertensive changes in the "open"—as well as in the obstructed-pulmonary vascular bed (19). These pulmonary hypertensive changes further increase pulmonary vascular resistance and, therefore, right ventricular afterload (19).

Proximal extension of pulmonary emboli, possibly promoted by turbulence caused by downstream obstruction, is suggested by observations at thrombo-endarterectomy of reddish granulation tissue proximal to the obstructive white, organized thrombi (19).

It can be reasonably concluded that a single attack of massive pulmonary embolism does usually not lead to chronic pulmonary hypertension. The long-term fate of patients with undetected and untreated pulmonary embolism (if they survive it, because the mortality is 30%) depends rather on concomitant diseases (1,3,37). Chronic thromboembolic pulmonary hypertension is a relatively rare condition when compared to acute embolism, which is third most frequent cardiac cause of death.

The likelihood that acute pulmonary embolism will produce pulmonary hypertension depends largely on the total volume of emboli and on whether these are fragmented in transit through the right heart to be disbursed in multiple smaller vessels or remain intact to occlude major proximal vessels (19). A relatively small dose of injected emboli may block the vascular bed to a much greater extent than is generally presumed.

In patients with acute pulmonary embolism who are free of other cardiopulmonary disease, the value of pulmonary artery pressure is related to the degree of embolic obstruction as shown by pulmonary angiography (15,16,17).

References

1. Benotti JR, Dalen JE. The national history of pulmonary embolism. Clin Chest Med 1984; 5:403–10.
2. McIntyre D, et al. Pulmonary embolism—a long-term follow-up. Postgrad Med J 1982; 58:222–5.
3. Carson JL, et al. The clinical course of pulmonary embolism. N Engl J Med 1992; 326:1240–5.
4. Widimský J. The prognosis of pulmonary embolism. Cor et Vasa 1979; 21:221–7.
5. Coon WW, Coller FA. Some epidemiological considerations on thromboembolism Sur Gynecol Obstet 1959; 109:487–93.
6. Morpurgo M, Schmid C. Clinico-pathological correlations in pulmonary embolism: a-posteriori evaluation. Prog Respir Dis 1980; 13:8–15.
7. Sutton GC, et al. Clinical course and late prognosis of treated subacute massive,

acute minor, and chronic pulmonary thromboembolism. Br Heart J 1977; 39:1135–42.

8. Morpurgo M, Marzegalli M, Casazza F. L'embolia polmonare in Unità di Cure Coronariche. Cardiologia 1991; 36(suppl 1):179–85.
9. Dalen JE, Alpert JS. National history of pulmonary embolism. Progr Cardiovasc Dis 1975; 17:259–70.
10. Widimský J. Advances in clinical diagnosis of pulmonary embolism. Acta Univ Carol Med Monogr (Praha) 1983; 29:401–84.
11. Staněk V, et al. Haemodynamic monitoring in acute pulmonary embolism. Bull Europ Physiopathol Resp 1978; 14:561–72.
12. Goldhaber SZ. Thrombolysis in venous thromboembolism. An international perspective. Chest 1990; 97(suppl):176S–181S.
13. Meyer G, et al. Effect of intravenous urokinase versus alteplase on total pulmonary resistance in acute massive pulmonary embolism. A European multicenter double-blind trial. JACC 1992; 19:239–45.
14. Tibbut DA, et al. Comparison by controlled clinical trial of streptokinase and heparin in treatment of life-threatening pulmonary embolism. Br Med J 1974; 1:343–47.
15. Urokinase Pulmonary Embolism Trial. Phase 1 results: a cooperative study. JAMA 1970; 214:2163–72.
16. Urokinase-Streptokinase Embolism Trial Phase 2 results. JAMA 1974; 219:1606–13.
17. McIntyre KM, Sasahara AA. Haemodynamic and ventricular responses to pulmonary embolism. Progr Cardiovasc Dis 1974; 3:175–90.
18. Widimský J, Staněk V. Clinical diagnosis of haemodynamically significant pulmonary embolism in a coronary care unit. Cor et Vasa 1985; 27:337–45.
19. Moser KM, et al. Chronic major-vessel thromboembolic pulmonary hypertension. Circulation 1990; 81:1735–43.
20. Murphy ML, Bullock RT. Factors influencing the restoration of blood flow following pulmonary embolization as determined by angiography and scanning. Circulation 1968; 38:1116–26.
21. Messer JV. Thromboembolic pulmonary hypertension. In: Weir EK, Reeves JT, eds. Pulmonary Hypertension. Mount Kisco, NY: Futura Publishing Company, 1984; 169–250.
22. Goldhaber SZ, Hennekens Ch. Time trends in hospital mortality and diagnosis of pulmonary embolism. Am Heart J 1982; 104:305–6.
23. Lilienfeld DE, et al. Mortality from pulmonary embolism in the United States 1962 to 1984. Chest 1990; 89:1067–72.
24. Riedel M, et al. Long-term follow-up of patients with pulmonary thromboembolism. Late prognosis and evolution of hemodynamic and respiratory data. Chest 1982; 81:151–8.
25. Monreal M, et al. Recurrent pulmonary embolism. A prospective study. Chest 1989; 95:976–9.
26. Hall RJC, et al. Long-term prognosis of treated acute massive pulmonary embolism. Br Heart J 1977; 39:1128–34.
27. Paraskos JA, et al. Late prognosis of acute pulmonary embolism. N Engl J Med 1953; 289:55–8.

28. Palla A, et al. From not detected pulmonary embolism to diagnosis of chronic thromboembolic pulmonary hypertension. A retrospective study. Respiration 1993; 60:9–14.
29. Owen WR, et al. Unrecognized emboli to the lungs with subsequent cor pulmonale. N Engl J Med 1953; 249:919–26.
30. Urbanová D, Staněk V. Thromboembolic attacks in cardiological departement. Čas Lék čes 1990; 129:747–50.
31. Olman MA, et al: Endogenous fibrinolytic system in chronic large-vessel thromboembolic pulmonary hypertension. Circulation 1992; 86:1241–8.
32. Comp PC, Esmon CT. Recurrent venous thromboembolism in patients with a partial deficiency of protein S. N Engl J Med 1984; 311:1525–8.
33. Griffin JH, et al. Deficiency of protein C in congenital thrombotic disease. J Clin Invest 1981; 68:1370–3.
34. Marciniak F. Familiar thrombosis due to antithrombin III deficiency. Blood 1974; 43:209–11.
35. Ivašková E, et al. Venous thromboembolism and HLA antigen. Eur Heart J 1981; 2(suppl A):P52.
36. Moser K. Venous thromboembolism. State of the art. Am Rev Respir Dis 1990; 141:235–49.
37. Ansari A. Acute and chronic pulmonary thromboembolism: current perspectives. Part I. Glossary of terms, historic evolution and prevalence. Clin Cardiol 1986; 9:398–402.

11

Death in Pulmonary Embolism

MARIO MORPURGO and MAURIZIO MARZEGALLI

San Carlo Borromeo Hospital
Milan, Italy

And death shall be no more;
Death thou shalt die.

—J. Donne, 1573–1631

Why and how do the victims of pulmonary embolism (PE) die? The question has rated relatively little attention in recent literature. Yet as far back as 1846, von Virchow (1) wrote, ". . . we confirm to a high degree the ancient observation, that interruption of the pulmonary circulation paralyzes primarily the heart rather than respiration . . . in turn, cardiac paralysis might result from alterations of the coronary blood flow." At about the same time, Panum (2) stated "In pulmonary embolism, sudden death is caused by a reduced blood flow to the brain."

Many years later, in a booklet devoted entirely to PE, Bardin (3) suggested that the disorder under discussion might result in sudden death through a reflex arc starting from pulmonary nerve endings, reaching vagus, sympathetic or phrenic nerve fibers, the posterior cervical roots, and from there the respiratory and cardiac centers: "something akin to an inhibitory phenomenon."

In another monograph on the subject, published in 1947, Lériche (4) concluded his paragraph on the immediate causes of death by saying that "the patient with pulmonary embolism dies as well from cardiac as from respiratory causes; yet he also dies from cerebral causes . . . a mechanical factor should be viewed as prominent. . . ."

Pilcher (5) distinguished three modes of death in PE, i.e., sudden (instant, within 10 minutes), rapid (10 minutes to 1 h), and gradual (more than 1 h). Concerning the last-named mode, in a review of 88 cases from his autopsy files, Neuhof (6) found that fully 48 cases yielded evidence suggesting one or more episodes of PE occurring hours, days, or weeks before the fatal event, something that we have been able to confirm in our own autopsy study of 538 cases (7). A broader interpretation of death in the course of PE was offered by Chiche (8), who argued that we should not expect to discover a straightforward cause of death in all cases—most, in fact being hard to attribute to a definite mechanism. He wrote, Death is usually produced by a mechanical factor; yet it may result suddenly from ventricular fibrillation or asystole, or conversely from peripheral shock leading to coma or collapse of some duration. In non-massive PE several events are possible. In the experimental animal the passage of thrombus through the right ventricle may trigger runs of extrasystoles, ventricular tachycardia, and cardiac arrest. Similar events may occur in human patients with atherosclerotic heart disease or acute myocardial ischemia.

About animal experiments designed to elucidate pathogenesis, it must be said that such studies raised more questions than they answered. Many experiments were not above criticism. First of all, in most cases, pulmonary embolization was produced by injecting particles and materials quite foreign into the living organism, signally with physicochemical properties very different from those of blood. Secondly, experimental embolization is usually produced in a very short time, whereas spontaneous PE in man may occur in the form of a slowly progressive event. And last, humoral and vasomotor responses to PE are apt to vary not only between different animal species but also between different subjects of the same species.

Again in more recent times, a good deal of debate was generated to determine whether the effects of PE reflect the obstruction of pulmonary vasculature in merely mechanical terms or involve the intervention of reflex and/or humoral mechanisms as well (see Chap. 7). According to Hume et al. (9), "the mechanics of sudden death in cor pulmonale is unclear, but it seems likely that a combination of factors are involved, including mechanical and humoral effects." The contributory role of severe bronchoconstriction and posthypoxic lesions of vital organs (as in shock kidney) was stressed by other authors (10). Another recent study (11) speaks of a "circadian rhythm of sudden death from pulmonary emboli with a peak incidence from 9.00 hours to 14.30 hours"—not to mention "a circannual rhythm with a peak incidence from

December to April." The circadian rhythm is attributed to changes of blood clottability; the circannual, tentatively to disturbance of both coagulation and cardiovascular reactivity to external, chiefly seasonal factors. The chances of pulmonary embolism resulting in a picture of acute cor pulmonale and its major sequels depend essentially on the total volume of embolus materials and also on whether said materials are torn and fragment as they go through the right heart, hence to obstruct many small vessels, or remains whole and so obstruct a bigger proximal artery (12). We must, however, note that the size and location of emboli seen at autopsy are not necessarily equal to in vivo findings.

In massive PE the clots are for the most part of considerable size, but not always occlusive—especially if V-shaped or folded over (see Chap. 5). When clot material rests astride an arterial bifurcation (saddle embolus), occlusion may be incomplete and sudden death be avoided. Conversely, Neuhof (6) reports cases where "embolism of peripheral branches of the pulmonary arteries, leaving the main branches free, may produce symptoms of marked severity and may even cause death." In a review of 49 PEs from our files (13), where death had been sudden and unexpected, we found that in about one fifth of cases embolization involved only peripheral and unilateral branches (Table 1). Likewise, Hoagland (14) states that only one half the cases of fatal PE fit a description of anatomically "massive" embolization, whether death occurred suddenly or not.

This is one reason why in modern parlance, a PE is called *massive* not so much according to its anatomical extent or location as on the basis of hemodynamic criteria: Thus, massive EP is defined as one characterized by severe hemodynamic repercussions, such as shock and cardiac arrest (14).

At this point it is relevant to understand how cardiac arrest develops in the acute stage of PE. To that end we have reviewed the anatomoclinical data relative to a group of patients with massive or submassive PE who suffered a total of 39

Table 1 Localization of Pulmonary Embolism in Subjects Who Were Victims of Sudden and Unexpected Death (48 Cases)

	Total	Percent
Main pulmonary artery	8	16.1
Right and left branches	10	20.4
Right branch	7	14.2
Left branch	2	4.1
Lobar and segmental arteries (unilateral)	7	14.2
Lobar and segmental arteries (bilateral)	5	10.2
Subsegmental arteries (unilateral)	3	6.1
Subsegmental arteries (bilateral)	7	14.2

From Ref. 13.

documented episodes of cardiac arrest (Table 2). There, and more specifically in 31 patients who were already under continuous ECG monitoring at the time of cardiac arrest, it turned out that the latter was invariably caused by electromechanical dissociation (EMD). In turn, this circumstance invites the following comments.

Most episodes of cardiac arrest (CA), reversible or otherwise, that occur in the acute stage of PE, are the consequence of EMD, i.e., the presence of organized cardiac electrical activity in the absence of femoral or carotid pulses (15), in a clinical setting of cardiac arrest. This event is more likely to occur next to cardiogenic shock (Table 3) but may also strike suddenly in a clinical context of acute cor pulmonale. With EMD at least momentarily reversible, the heart rate measured during dissociation is usually higher than 50 beats/min, and QRS complexes are narrow. From the pathogenetic point of view, EMD is generally termed *primary* if there is a failure of heart muscle to produce an effective contraction in response to normal electrical excitation (16), and it is termed *secondary* when abrupt changes in the loading conditions of the heart result in marked reduction of cardiac output despite preserved cardiac function. If we were to apply these criteria to our cases of EMD in the course of PE, we would be obliged to classify most of them as "mixed" forms, because the sudden pressure overload imposed on the right ventricle by the onset of PE was very often superimposed on a previous intrinsic myocardial deficit—indeed, of 26 autopsy cases in our series, in addition to confirmatory signs of PE, 9 revealed

Table 2 Cardiac Arrest in Acute Pulmonary Embolism

Patients	
Deceased	26
Survived	2
Total	28
Episodes of cardac arrest	
Reversible	13
Due to EMD	12
Due to asystole	1
Irreversible	
Due to EMD	22
Due to asystole or bradycardia	3
Due to VF after AV block	1
Total	39

Abbreviations: EMD, electromechanical dissociation; VF, ventricular fibrillation; AV, atrio-ventricular.
From Dept. of Cardiology and Dept. of Pathology, San Carlo Borromeo Hospital, Milan.

Table 3 Presentation of Cardiac Arrest in Acute Pulmonary Embolism (39 Episodes)

	Reversible	Irreversible	Total
Electromechanical dissociation			
Sudden	7	5	12
After shock <2 h	5	11	16
After shock >2 h	—	6	6
Asystole or extreme bradycardia			
Sudden	1	1	2
After shock <2 h	—	—	—
After shock >2 h	—	2	2
Ventricular fibrillation after shock >2 h	—	1	1
Totals	13	26	39

From Dept. of Cardiology, San Carlo Borromeo Hospital, Milan.

a fresh or old myocardial infarct, 11 showed moderate or severe coronary lesions, and 4 gave evidence of congestive heart failure and/or dilated cardiomyopathy.

According to some authors (17), in massive PE complicated by cardiac arrest caused by EMD, external cardiac massage may sometimes result in prompt and dramatic restoration of blood pressure and consciousness, because the embolus breaks up and migrates distally, thereby permitting improved pulmonary blood flow and cardiac output.

On the other hand, external cardiac massage is generally regarded as a relative contraindication to thrombolytic therapy because of the risk of severe bleeding. Yet, recent observations (18) suggest that in the more threatening cases of PE, thrombolysis may prove lifesaving even if administered in the course of prolonged cardiopulmonary resuscitation. In our own patients treated with cardiac massage for as long as 40 minutes and receiving bolus fibrinolytic therapy only a few minutes later (19), the absence of clinical or anatomical evidence of bleeding goes to confirm those observations.

The prognosis of PE is discussed elsewhere in this book (see Chap. 10). Here we only want to stress that the importance of PE as a cause of death depends very largely on the underlying disease (20): In other words, the PE episode does not always represent the coup de grace that kills a patient already fated to die. A few examples follow: In 1959 Coon and Coller (21) reviewed 388 autopsy cases in which PE was regarded as sole or contributory cause of death. In little more than half the cases, prognosis had been hopeless on account of advanced malignancy or the like; in 22% of cases, the underlying disease condition was not much influenced by the onset of PE of lesser severity; yet in another 21% of cases, the prognosis would have been excellent were it not on account of supervening PE. From our own review of 538 autopsies (7), it emerged that approximately 21% of patients would have rated a favorable prognosis in the absence of PE, 39% would probably have survived, and another 39% would probably have died within weeks or months from their basis diseases (unavoidable deaths). Rightly, therefore, does Even (22) argue that fatal PE does not have the unpredictable and inevitable character that has been attributed to it—quite the contrary, PE is predictable and must be avoided.

Now the problem is how to avoid cardiac arrest and death in patients rated "nonresponders" by Greenfield (23), i.e., those responding only partly and fleetingly to fibrinolytic and positive inotropic drugs, and such as are not amenable to traditional embolectomy on short order, or only so with inordinate risk. Future expectations lie in two directions, one being the removal or fragmentation of embolus material with special catheters, and the other being the implementation of biventricular mechanical supports affording correction of the shock situation pending further, resolutive interventions.

Catheter pulmonary embolectomy was attempted by Greenfield et al. (24) more than 20 years ago; the idea was revived recently by other authors (see also Chap. 17). For Timsit and associates (25), the best indication is massive PE of not more than 48–72 h standing, with mean pulmonary artery pressure less than 50 mm Hg. If thrombus is already organized, fragment removal may result in a definite increment of pulmonary blood flow (23). The method may be perfected by creating a partial bypass in the angiography room or at the bedside in the more severe cases, and by effecting embolectomy under visual control from a fiberoptic system run through the same catheter device. Other authors (26,27) have tried breaking up embolus material mechanically with the same catheter used for angiographic localization of the obstruction, apparently with good results. More recently, rotational catheters of various description have been tested in animals with encouraging preliminary results. Some of these devices, like the Kensey catheter, are somewhat rigid and lack a guidewire; others, like the Angiocor Thrombolizer, have a guidewire and convey a soft, flexible centrifugal spiral apparently suitable for "pulverizing" embolus materials. These new-fashioned instruments and techniques, currently undergoing multicenter testing in humans, are claimed to be effective also in PE of some standing, and they are allegedly not unduly traumatic to pulmonary artery walls.

In the same spirit, modern continuous-flow centrifugal pumps that are portable, can operate transcutaneously, and will work for 48–72 h at a stretch, may permit the bypassing of pulmonary circulation, giving support to the right ventricle and insuring adequate oxygenation. These characteristics make such devices suitable for use in intensive care units and in hospitals not equipped for cardiac surgery. Their use in cases of shock from massive PE (28) may afford survival until the patient can receive resolutive treatment such as traditional or catheter embolectomy.

References

1. von Virchow R. Weitere Untersuchungen ueber die Verstopfung der Lungenarterien und ihre Folge. Traube's Beitraege der Path u Physiol 1846; 3:303.
2. Panum A. Experimentelle Beitraege zur Lehre von der Embolie. Virchow's Archiv 1862; 25:310–8.
3. Bardin P. L'embolie pulmonaire. Paris: Masson, 1937.
4. Leriche R. Les embolies de l'artères pulmonaire et des artères des membres. Paris: Masson, 1974.
5. Pilcher R. The role of obstruction in fatal pulmonary embolism. Lancet 1939; 256:1257–63.
6. Neuhof H. Venous thrombosis and pulmonary embolism. New York: Grune & Stratton, 1948.
7. Morpurgo M, Schmid C. Clinico-pathological correlations in pulmonary embolism: a-posteriori evaluation. Prog Respir Dis 1980; 13:8–15.
8. Chiche P. La maladie thromboembolique pulmonaire. Paris: L'Expansion Scientifique Française, 1969.
9. Hume N, Sevitt S, Thomas DP. Venous thrombosis and pulmonary embolism. Cambridge: Harvard University Press, 1970.
10. Marion P, Binet JP. Embolies pulmonaires. Paris: Masson, 1974.
11. Gallerani M, Manfredini R, Ricci L, et al. Sudden death from pulmonary thromboembolism: chronobiological aspects. Eur Heart J 1992; 13:661–5.
12. Widimsky J. Mechanisms in embolic pulmonary hypertension. In: Wagenvoort CA, Denolin H, eds. Pulmonary Circulation. Advances and Controversies. Amsterdam: Elsevier 1989; 75–86.
13. Morpurgo M, Rustici A. Lo spettro dell'embolia polmonare. Cardiologia 1988; 33:1105–8.
14. Hoagland PM. Massive pulmonary embolism. In: Goldhaber SZ, ed. Pulmonary Embolism and Deep Vein Thrombosis. Philadelphia: Saunders, 1985; 179–208.
15. Bocka JJ, Overton DT, Hauser A. Electromechanical dissociation in human beings: an echocardiographic evaluation. Ann Emerg Med 1988; 17:450–2.
16. Charlap S, Kahlam S, Lichstein E, Frishman W. Electromechanical dissociation: diagnosis, pathophysiology and management. Am Heart J 1989; 18:355–60.
17. Benotti JR, Dalen JE. Pulmonary embolism. In: Horwitz LD, Groves BM, eds. Signs and Symptoms in Cardiology. Philadelphia: Lippincott, 1985; 277–97.
18. Gulba DC, Claus G, Daniel WG, Lichtlen PR. Thrombolysis in acute submassive and life-threatening pulmonary embolism. Eur Heart J 1992; 13(suppl):30(A304).
19. Morpurgo M, Marzegalli M, Casazza F. L'embolia polmonare in Unità di Cure Coronariche. Cardiologia 1991; 6(suppl 1):179–85.
20. Carson JL, Kelley MA, Duff A, et al. The clinical course of pulmonary embolism. N Engl J Med 1992; 326:1240–5.
21. Coon WW, Coller FA. Some epidemiological considerations on thromboembolism. Surg Gynecol Obstet 1959; 109:487–93.
22. Even Ph. Histoire naturelle de l'embolie pulmonaire. In: La maladie thromboembolique. Paris: Expansion Scientifique Française, 1984;33–8.
23. Greenfield LJ. Catheter pulmonary embolectomy. Chest 1991; 100:593–4.

24. Greenfield LJ, Kimmell GD, McCardy WC. Transvenous removal of pulmonary emboli by vacuum-cup catheter technique. J Surg Res 1969; 9:347–52.
25. Timsit JF, Reynaud P, Meyer G, Sors H. Pulmonary embolectomy by catheter device in massive pulmonary embolism. Chest 1991; 100:655–8.
26. Brady AJ, Crake T, Oackley CM. Percutaneous catheter fragmentation and distal dispersion of proximal pulmonary embolus. Lancet 1991; 338:1186–9.
27. Horstkotte D, Heintzen MP, Strauer BE, Leschke M. Aggressive nonsurgical management of massive pulmonary embolism with cardiogenic shock. XIII Congr Eur Soc Cardiol, Amsterdam, Aug 18–22, 1991 (abstr 370).
28. Bennett J, Hill J, Long W, et al. Biocompatible circuits: an adjunct to noncardiac extracorporeal cardiopulmonary support. J Extracorporeal Technol 1992; 24:6–11.

Part Three

IMAGING TECHNIQUES

12

Imaging of Pulmonary Embolism

ANTONIO PALLA and CARLO GIUNTINI

University of Pisa
Pisa, Italy

I. Introduction

The ultimate diagnosis of pulmonary embolism (PE) would require pulmonary arteriography; however, it is invasive for the patient, costly, and hardly available. Therefore, the diagnosis should be pursued with the use of simpler and noninvasive techniques of imaging.

II. Planar Chest Radiography

Planar chest radiography is currently employed in PE to rule out diseases mimicking PE, such as pneumothorax, rib fractures, pleural diseases, and lung neoplasm (1); or to support ventilation/perfusion studies in order to increase their diagnostic probability (2,3). In fact, as will be made clearer later in this review, it may show abnormalities that match defects appreciable in perfusion studies.

However, the role of chest radiography in PE should be reviewed by starting with a simple consideration: In patients with PE, chest radiography does not show only parenchymal densities but also several findings often characteristic of diagnosis of PE appears the role to raise (along with other noninvasive tools such as history, electrocardiogram [ECG], blood gas analysis) the suspicion of PE, or to reinforce the clinically raised suspicion (4). This is an uncomparably useful role because more than one half of patients with PE still go undetected because it is not suspected (5,6).

The technique of performing chest radiography should be very accurate to obtain good-quality pictures. Indeed, radiographic signs of lung parenchyma focal hyperlucency (e.g., the so-called Westermark sign visible in some patients with PE) may be simulated by an excessive number of kilovolts, while differences of density between two contiguous vascular structures (e.g., descending pulmonary arteries [DPAs] and their branches) may not be appreciated if the number of kilovolts is insufficient. Other signs may go undetected when the exposure time, exceedingly long, allows the movements of thoracic or cardiovascular structures to be recorded. Finally, the technique must be standardized in order to make possible the comparison of pictures taken at different times.

A list of the signs commonly associated with PE is reported in Table 1.

The enlargement of descending pulmonary arteries is a frequent sign that is often reported in the literature (7–11); its clinical reliability has been evaluated in a retrospective study demonstrating that this sign is present in almost 65% of patients in whom the suspicion of PE has been clinically raised (Fig. 1) (11). This sign is due to the acute occlusion of a vessel section with the ensuing exclusion of a part of vascular bed from blood flow; as a consequence, pulmonary vascular resistances increase, and that causes increase in pulmonary artery pressure; the increase of transmural pressure may cause dilatation of vascular section above the obstruction (12). Also, in the literature (14) a modification of shape of the above artery following acute PE is reported (7,13). This sign has been documented by measuring four different diameters of this vessel (at superior venous angle, and 1, 2, and 3 cm distally) in patients with PE; indeed, by comparing diameters of acute and resolution phases, the two upper diameters

Table 1 Radiological Signs of Pulmonary Embolism

Descending pulmonary artery: normal, enlarged, "sausage-like"
Level of diaphragm: normal, elevated (on one side or bilaterally)
Cardiac shadow: normal, enlarged (right-side, left-side, or both sides enlargement)
Atelectasis lines: large, curvilinear, above diaphragm, single, or rectilinear, peripheral, above diaphragm, multiple, bilateral
Lung densities compatible with pulmonary infarction: dense, truncated cone areas; lightly, homogeneous opacity with no sharp borders; "Hampton hump"
Radiolucent areas: zones with markedly reduced density and vessels (Westermark sign)
Pleural effusion: small and large effusion
Azygos vein: normal or enlarged

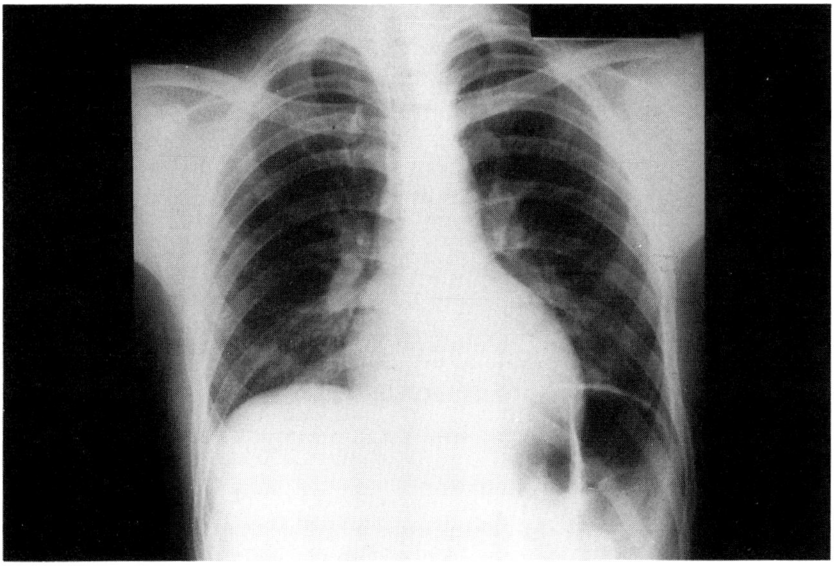

(A)

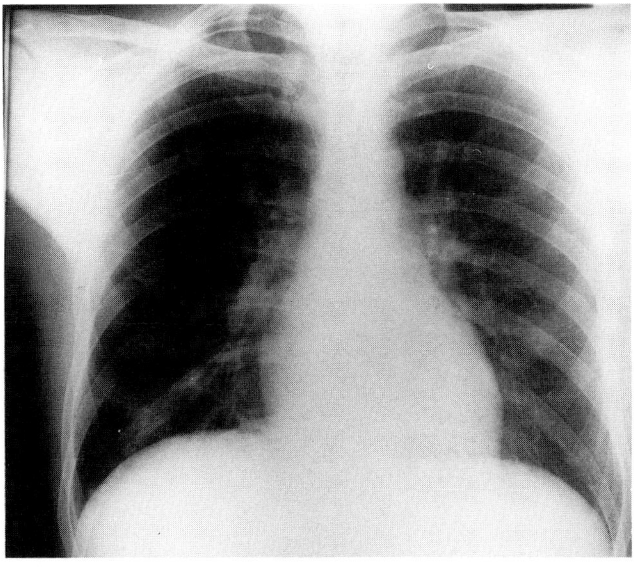

(B)

Figure 1 Chest radiography of embolic patient. (A) Right descending pulmonary artery (DPA) is enlarged and dense. (B) 30 days later; right DPA size and density have markedly decreased.

were found to be significantly wider than the two lower diameters (12). This different behavior of the upper and lower artery sections is responsible for the shape modification of the artery, from an irregular cone appearance in the acute phase to a regular cone shape some 3 weeks later (12). In about one fourth of cases, this enlargement is so extreme that the artery takes the typical appearance of a "sausage" (12); this is due to the prevailing increase of proximal sections of the artery and reflects the increased flow impedance at the major pulmonary arteries with the attendant hydraulic power increment, compatible with the right ventricular performance. In these patients the proximal localization of large emboli causes both extreme vessel dilatation and poor visualization of the branches directed to the lower and middle lobes (Fig. 2). "Sausage" descending pulmonary artery is visible early in the embolization, but, if PE is not readily treated, the artery may keep this appearance later on. Modifications of width and shape of descending pulmonary artery also allow the selection of patients with more serious embolization; indeed, patients with markedly enlarged DPA are the most seriously ill because they show a severe vascular obstruction (as demonstrated by the number of unperfused lung segments on perfusion lung scintigraphy) while patients with normal or mildly enlarged artery are less impaired by PE (15). Interestingly, patients with extreme increase of descending pulmonary

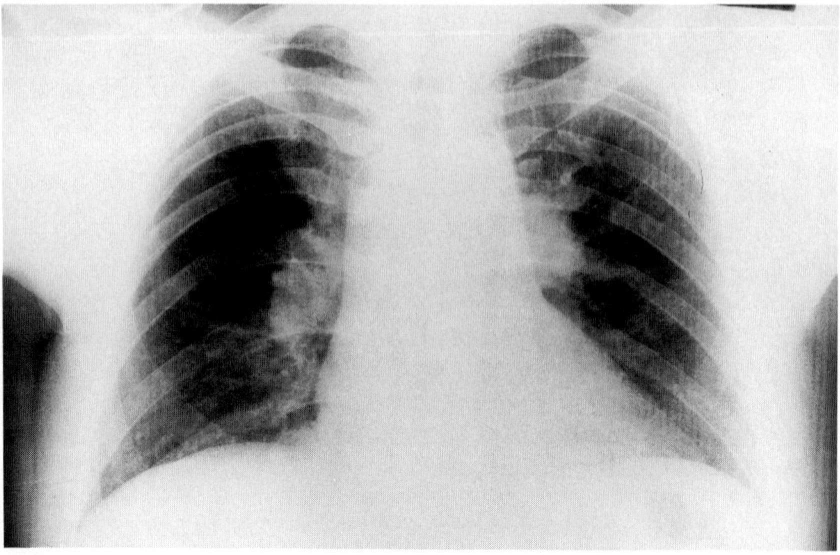

Figure 2 Chest radiography of embolic patient showing "sausage-like" DPA: The artery is very enlarged and dense with clear-cut borders and ends abruptly. Branches for middle and lower lobes are poorly visible and distorted.

artery, which takes the "sausage" appearance, show a mean vascular obstruction of 10 unperfused segments (corresponding to 56% of total vascular bed), while patients with normal arteries show a mean obstruction of 5 segments (26% of total vascular bed). From a pathophysiological point of view, in patients with "sausage" artery, large emboli are lodged above the segmental arteries (Fig. 3); therefore, the proximal vascular obstruction induces increase of flow impedance at the entry of pulmonary circulation, and this increases the transmural pressure of main arteries that dilate, thus causing them to take the "sausage" appearance (12). In patients with normal arteries, emboli are lodged into peripheral branches of pulmonary circulation and, therefore, are distributed over a much wider cross-sectional area of pulmonary bed; the obstructed vascular area is proportionally smaller, and the increase in pulmonary artery pressure, if any, is limited. In the resolution, a contemporary reduction of the artery width and of the vascular obstruction occurs, and this property may be utilized in monitoring the effect of fibrinolytic or anticoagulant treatment (15).

The enlargement of the right heart section has been frequently described

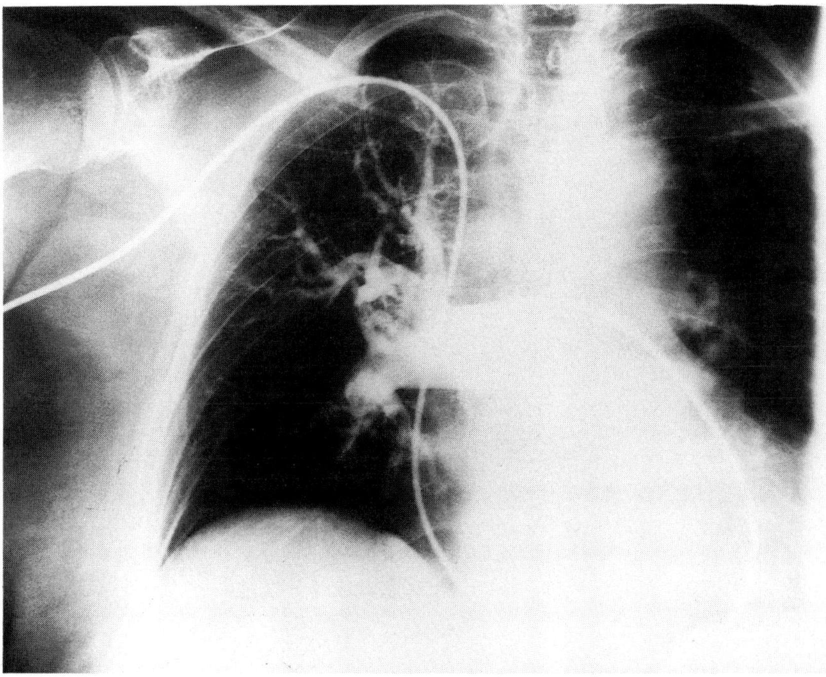

Figure 3 Pulmonary arteriography demonstrates multiple proximal filling defects in the patient with "sausage" appearance of right DPA shown in Fig. 2.

in PE (16,17) but never definitely demonstrated. This is likely due to the fact that modifications of heart shadow are difficult to detect for several reasons: Heart dimensions vary from subject to subject, and standard measures are not available; in PE, moreover, elevation of diaphragm may overlay the heart shadow whose detection is often made difficult by the poor quality of pictures obtained with portable units (18); finally, the supine position, often the only one possible in hemodynamic unstable patients, does not allow a quantification of heart dimensions (18). To overcome this limitation, four heart diameters (Fig. 4) were compared in acute and resolution (assumed as normal) phases of PE: The previous diameters were demonstrated to be slightly greater in acute PE, but the difference between the two phases was not significant (19). Moreover, an hemodynamic adaptation takes place early after PE, bringing back cardiac indices to normal levels (20). Accordingly, it is likely that a modest heart enlargement is transient and, thus, not visible on chest radiograph. Paradoxically, the lack of visualization of the entire cardiac silhouette hidden by the marked elevation of both emidiaphragms, the so-called drowned heart (13), is the only feature of the heart shadow suggestive of PE (Fig. 5).

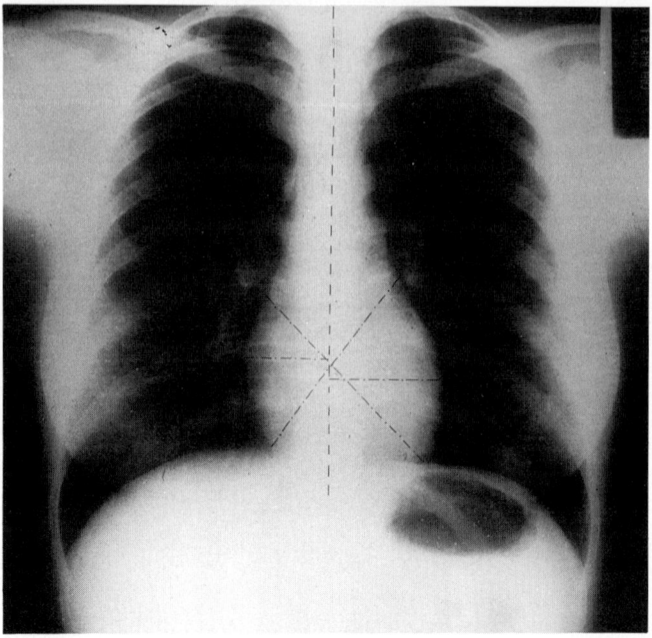

Figure 4 Method employed to measure heart dimensions: schematic representation of longitudinal, basal (right and left), and transverse diameters is reported. (From Ref. 11.)

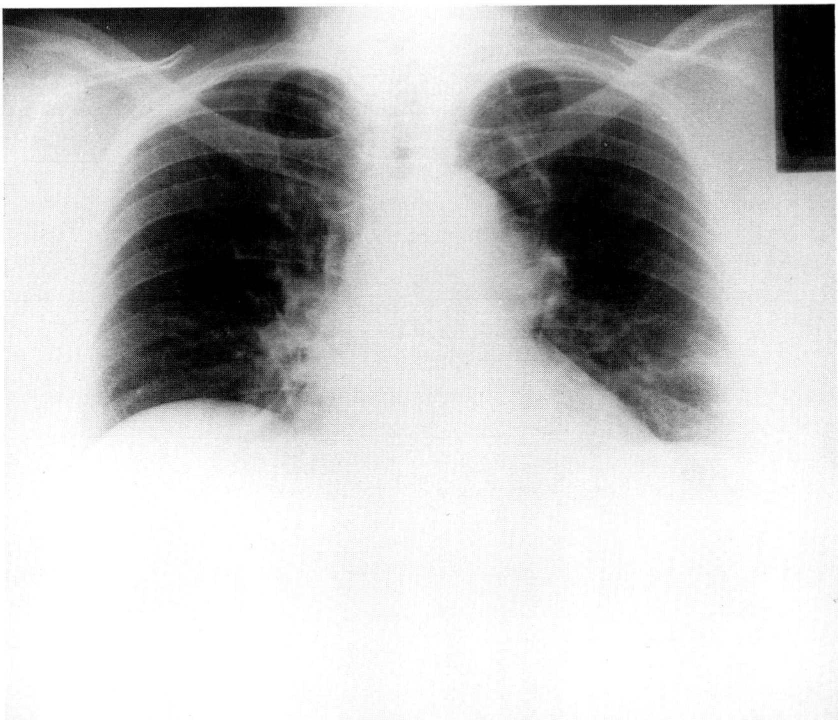

Figure 5 Appearance of "drowned heart" as originally described by Fleischner (13). (From Ref. 11.)

The azygos vein, enlarged in venous engorgement of the superior caval venous system, may be expected to be enlarged in PE too. Indeed, an increased diameter of the vein (more than 5 mm) is frequent in PE (62% of cases) (19); however, this is a difficult sign to be detected in these patients (19), and it is present in many other cardiopulmonary diseases.

Reduction of lung volume caused by the elevation of diaphragm, most often bilateral, is frequent in PE. It is likely associated to the presence of signs such as dyspnea and chest pain and is due to the loss of surfactant that follows the reduction of pulmonary perfusion. This sign usually appears in the early phase of PE, probably along with the previous symptoms. Its detection is easy when monolateral (21), but this is a rare event; on the contrary, the bilateral elevation of diaphragm is much more frequent although sometimes difficult to detect. This explains why its frequency in different series is largely variable (14,21–23). A way to overcome, a posteriori, the undetection of this sign is to measure the height of diaphragmatic dome both in the acute and resolution phases of PE, thus avoiding the large individual variations. A consolidated method of measure is to take the distance between the diaphragmatic dome and the inferior margin of the posterior tract of the fourth rib (11); by using this method, a statistical elevation of both diaphragms has been demonstrated between the two phases of disease (11). In PE the elevation of both emidiaphragms is frequent (74% of cases) (16) and characteristic of this disease when associated to other radiographic signs, such as pulmonary densities (22); thin linear atelectases at the lung bases (13); or large, curvilinear, oblique atelectases always positioned over the diaphragms (11).

Pulmonary hyperlucencies caused by the marked reduction of pulmonary vessels, the so-called Westermark sign, is a characteristic sign of PE (Fig. 6) (24). The frequency is variable in different series of patients reported in the literature (25–28), and this can be explained by the relatively difficult detection of the sign, i.e., in technically poor radiographies. When carefully searched for, the Westermark sign is present in 16% of patients with PE (11) and is very rare in pathological conditions other than PE (11). Its appearance is very early (24 h or so), as is its disappearance (24–36 h) (29).

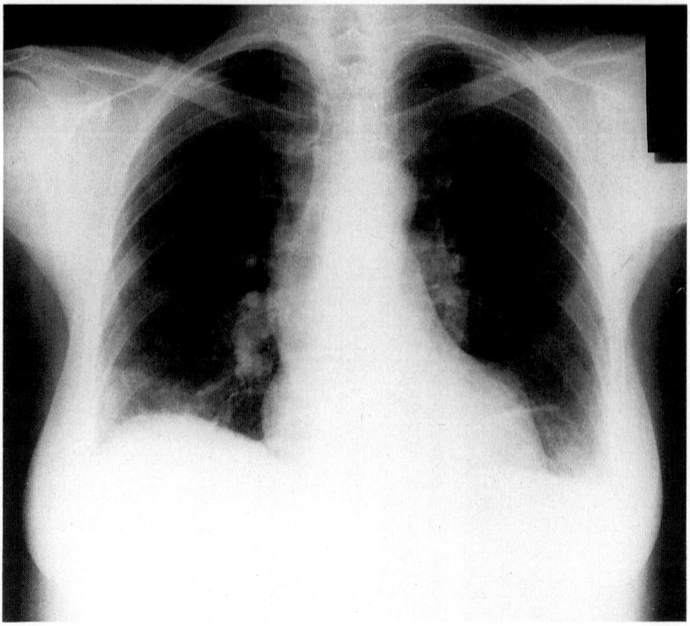

Figure 6 Chest radiography showing the Westermark sign in both upper lobes in a patient with PE: pulmonary density is markedly reduced and vessels are poorly represented in the above regions. Incidentally, "sausage" right DPA is also present. Other densities, described in details in Figs. 7–9, are also present.

Pulmonary densities compatible with pulmonary infarction may be associated with PE (30–33). These pulmonary densities are present in 14% of patients and may appear as cone-shaped areas described by Hampton and Castleman (33) in 1940, but more frequently they take the shape of an opacity positioned into the costophrenic angle, the so-called Hampton hump (Fig. 7) or the shape of a rounded density with blurred margins, often over the diaphragm. The shape usually appears homogenous and modestly dense in the early embolization and more dense in the following days; air bronchogram is very rare, thus allowing it to be distinguished from infectious diseases (34). Dimensions vary from 0.3 to 10 cm depending upon the dimensions of the occluded vessel (35), with an average of 2–5 cm. Localization is, in the large majority of cases, in the lower lung lobes (8,33). They appear early in PE; after 2–4 days their consolidation is complete (13), after 7 days they are reduced (7), and after 20 days they have disappeared (7).

Linear pulmonary consolidations may be also present in PE. Two main types of lines may be distinguished: large, curvilinear, oblique lines, 5–15 mm thick and 2–6 cm long, dense, with well-defined margins, located in lower lobes over the diaphragms that have been considered by some authors typical of PE

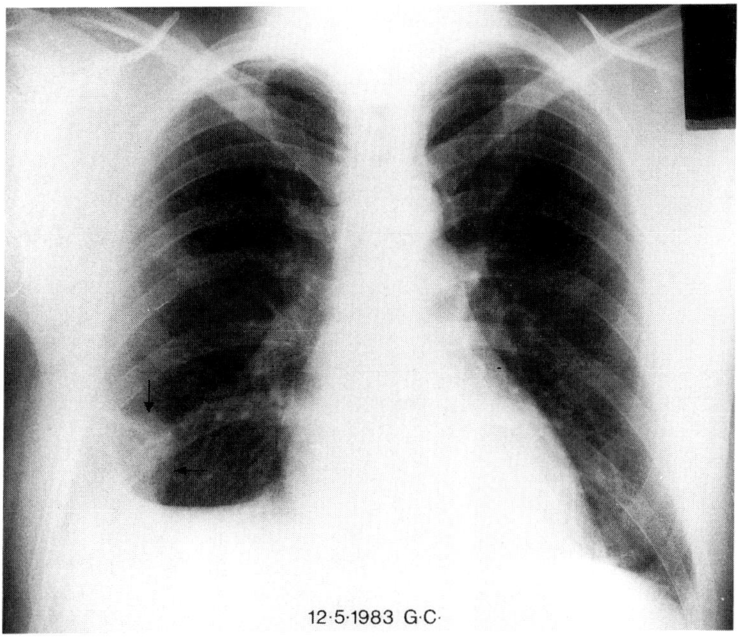

Figure 7 Typical appearance of the "Hampton hump" density positioned into the right costo-phrenic angle in a patient with pulmonary embolism. (From Ref. 11.)

(Fig. 8) (36); or laminar horizontal opacities, 2–5 mm thick, 1–4 cm long, multiple, often bilateral (Fig. 9) (37). The frequency of the former type is 8% (11), and the latter type is 23% (11). Both appear early in PE and disappear completely after few days, at the same time that perfusion improves (11).

The presence of pleural effusion in PE has been described by many authors (13,21,23,38,39). They are small effusions, often unilateral, more visible in the lateral view of the chest radiography; the frequency is variable with the different series (13,21,23,38,39), but a figure of about 30% of cases seems reasonable. The association with lung densities is frequent (21,26,39). Small pleural effusions appear early in PE and disappear within 7 days.

The previously described signs are reliable, frequent, and, to some extent, characteristic of this disease, as demonstrated by the following studies.

By applying the Kappa analysis, a statistical method that measures the agreement over the chance, the concordance between two readers in detecting the previous signs in a series of 265 patients with suspicion of PE (118 of them were really affected by this disease) was estimated. For most signs the concordance was good, i.e., more than 0.4 (Table 2), and, therefore, the subjectivity of reading can be considered relatively low (18).

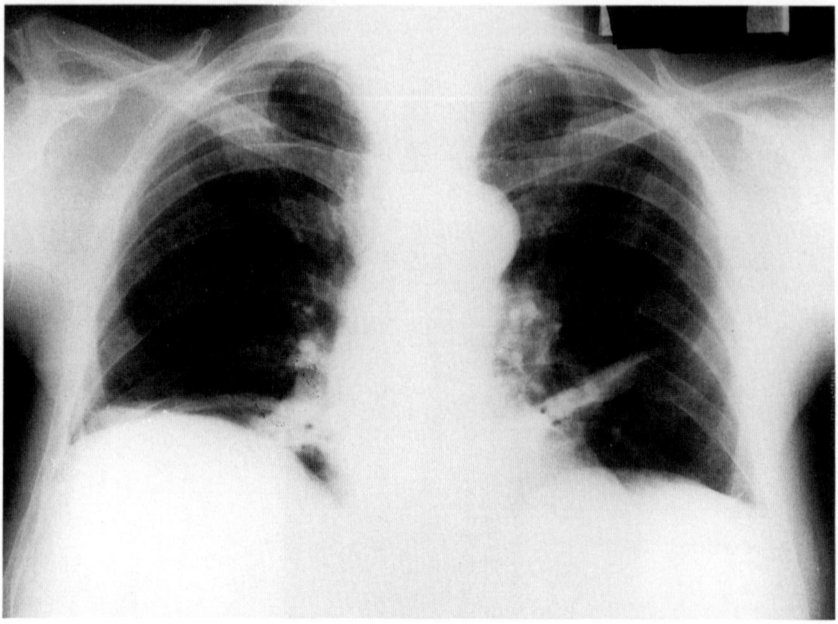

Figure 8 Chest radiography showing large, dense atelectasis line with sharp borders located over the left diaphragm. The "Hampton hump" is also present in the right cardiophrenic angle.

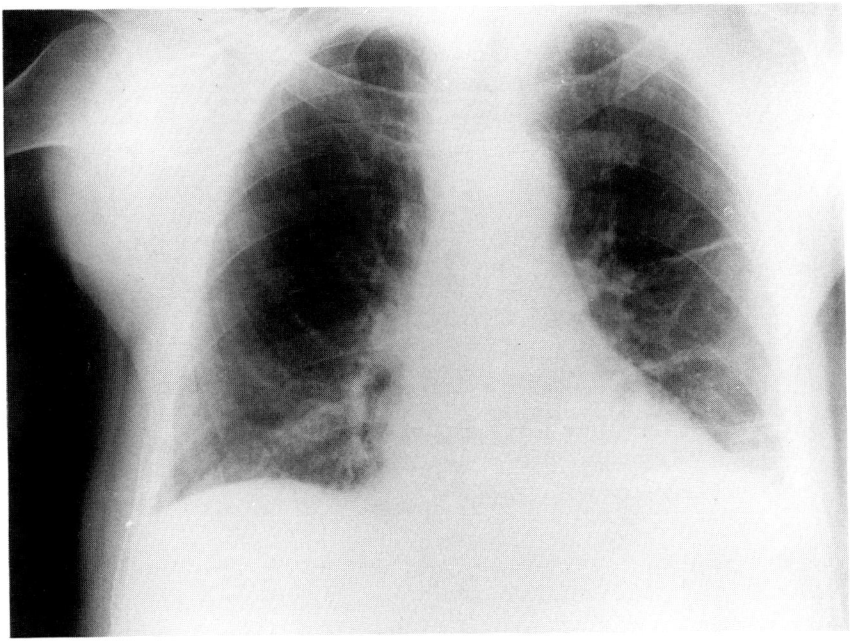

Figure 9 Chest radiography showing thin, multiple, horizontal opacities located in the left lower lobe. (From Ref. 11.)

Table 2 Agreement "*K*" Between Two Observers

Sign	Kappa[a]
Descending pulmonary artery	0.551
Diaphragm	0.550
Heart shadow	0.435
Pulmonary infarction	0.642
Atelectasis lines	0.477
Westermark sign	0.190
Pleural effusion	0.390
Azygos vein	0.505

[a] $K > 0.6$ = high agreement; $0.2 > K < 0.6$ = good agreement; $K < 0.2$ = poor agreement.

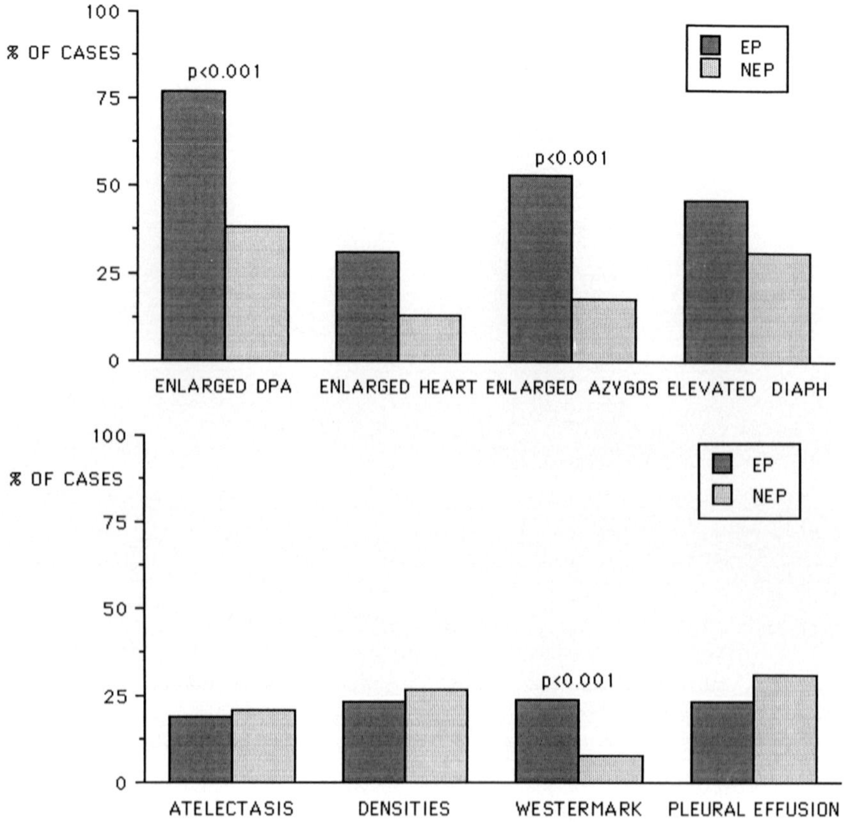

Figure 10 Frequency of radiographic signs in patients with confirmed (EP) and unconfirmed (NEP) PE.

In a series of 196 patients with suspicion of PE (98 had angiography-confirmed PE, and 98 age-matched patients had perfusion-excluded PE), several signs (such as the enlargement of DPA, elevation of diaphragm, enlargement of the azygos vein) were found frequently associated with PE, and, therefore, they should alert one to the presence of PE (Fig. 10) (40).

In the same study, through a multivariate statistical method, the relative risk of patients in this series of being affected by PE on the basis of radiographic signs was tested. The presence of enlarged or "sausage"-shaped DPA gave these patients a risk of being embolic that was four times greater than those without the sign (relative risk [RR] = 3.6); the presence of enlarged azygos vein gave a risk three times greater (RR = 3.3); the presence of elevated diaphragms and of the Westermark sign gave a risk of about two times greater (RR = 1.7 and 2.2, respectively) (40).

III. Perfusion Scintigraphy

Perfusion scintigraphy represents by far the most important technique for the screening and diagnosis of PE. Indeed, perfusion scintigraphy is noninvasive, increasingly available, and inexpensive. The diagnosis of PE on this basis is made likely by the detection of clear-cut perfusion defects reproducing one or more pulmonary segments. Depending on their size, pulmonary emboli may cause subsegmental, segmental, or lobar perfusion defects. Emboli are usually multiple and most often bilateral. Peripheral defects may be seen when emboli are small. Central, large emboli may completely block perfusion of several segments, lobes, or even a whole lung. Perfusion scintigraphy makes use of radiopharmaceuticals, human albumin macroaggregates or microspheres, labeled with Tc-99m; these radiopharmaceuticals range in size from 15 to 70 μm and, once injected intravenously, lodge in the pulmonary arterioles and capillaries, giving a map of the pulmonary circulation. The recommended injection is about 60,000 labeled particles, which occludes transiently 1 out of 1500 arterioles in the lung; a dose of 2–4 mCi (74–148 MBq) of Tc-99m pertechnetate is used to label radiopharmaceuticals. Radiopharmaceutical is injected through the antecubital vein; its distribution to lungs will follow the relative distribution of pulmonary blood flow and is nearly even apex to base in supine subjects.

Perfusion scintigraphy has a high sensitivity but an unsatisfactorily low specificity. Indeed, a normal scan virtually excludes the diagnosis of PE while lung pathologies other than PE may cause perfusion defects. However, the specificity of perfusion lung scan depends greatly on the technical requirements employed.

Imaging acquisition needs a rectilinear scanner, or a large field of view Anger scintillation camera or a single photon emission computed tomography (SPECT) camera.

The rectilinear scanner equipped with a cylindrical crystal of sodium iodide was the first instrument employed to detect the activity from the lungs. The crystal, with a diameter of 5 in. and 2 in. thick, is shielded all around with some 5 cm of lead. The collimator is of the focusing type with 91 holes. This instrument has an excellent distribution of count efficiency, which gives it good in vivo resolution in identifying perfusion defects (Fig. 11). However, the length of the procedure, the impossibility to obtain more than three views of the lungs, and the impossibility to obtain ventilation studies limited use of this instrument in the clinical practice.

The Anger scintillation camera is equipped with a parallel-hole collimator (low energy, high resolution). It allows one to collect eight pulmonary views in

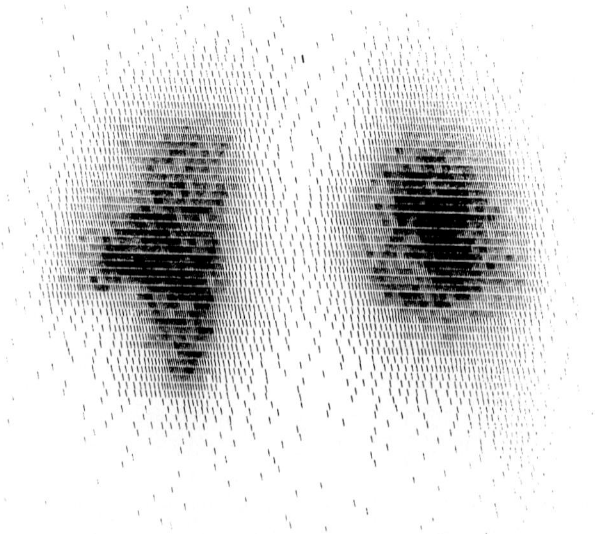

(A)

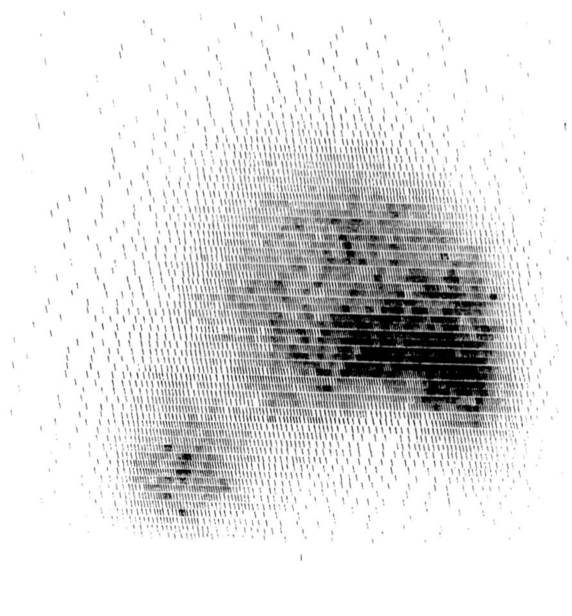

(B)

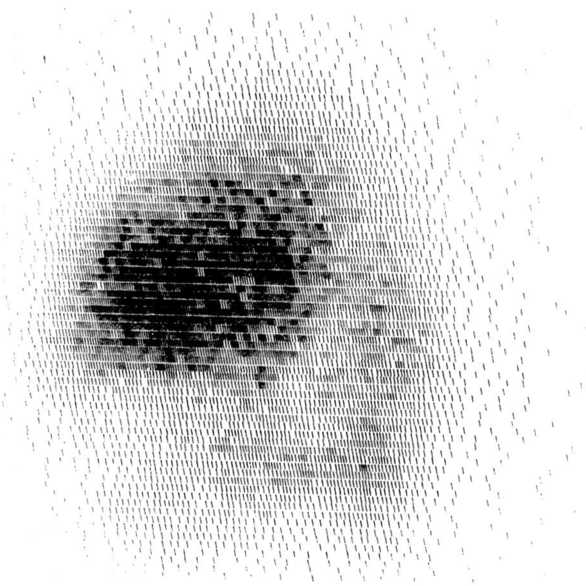

(C)

Figure 11 Perfusion lung scan of embolic patient in anterior (A), right (B), and left (C) lateral views obtained with a rectilinear scanner. Multiple segmental perfusion defects involving lower lobes of both lungs and middle lobe of right lung are visible.

a reasonable lot of time (around 15 min): anterior, posterior, right and left lateral, right and left posterior oblique (45 degrees) views should be always obtained, while the right and left anterior oblique views might be often omitted. The importance of the posterior oblique views is underlined by the necessity of better identifying the posterior and lateral segments of the lower lobes, thus avoiding artifacts caused by the "shine-through" phenomenon from the opposite lung that is frequent in the lateral views (Fig. 12).

Several advantages over planar imaging, and some disadvantages are offered by SPECT scintigraphy of the lungs, a relatively new technique. It has an actual tomographic effect that gives better contrast, edge definition, and separation of target from background, thereby providing information on size, shape, and distribution of perfusion in patients suffering from PE. Furthermore, SPECT permits quantitative measurement of radionuclide uptake in a defined volume of the lung. However, acquiring SPECT imaging takes longer (20–25 min) than planar scintigraphy and, therefore, requires the patient to stay still for a longer period of time. Technical apparatus for SPECT includes a large-field-of-view camera with a rotating head, equipped with a low-energy, all-purpose collimator and dedicated computed and software. By acquiring a 360-degree

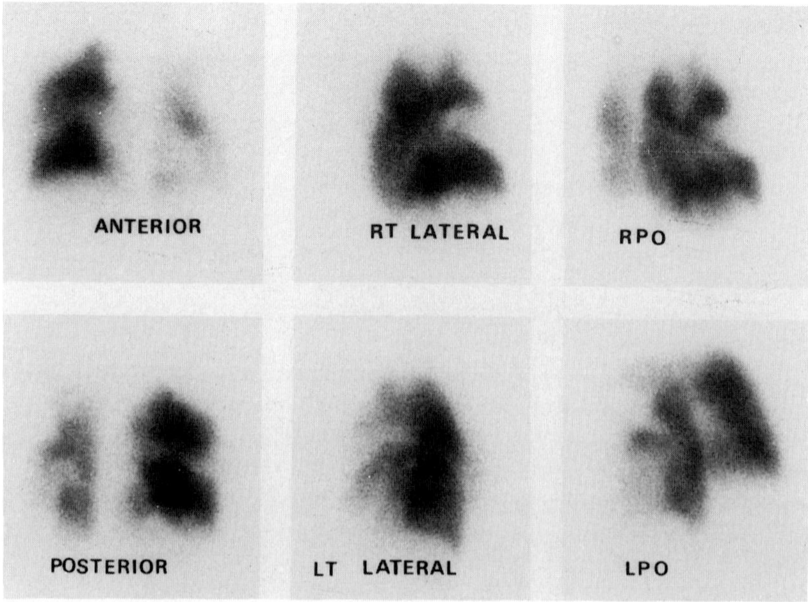

Figure 12 Perfusion lung scan of embolic patient obtained with a planar gamma-camera. From left to right: anterior, right lateral, right posterior oblique in the upper row and posterior, left lateral, and left posterior oblique in the lower row are visible. Several perfusion defects that are detectable in oblique views would be missed by looking only at lateral views.

circular orbit around the thorax of the patient, it allows one to get 64 projections in a 64 × 64 matrix on three different planes (transaxial, sagittal, coronal) (Fig. 13).

In a study done in 30 patients with suspicion of PE (10 with normal perfusion scintigraphy and 20 with angiographically demonstrated PE), perfusion imaging by SPECT appeared to be more sensitive than planar imaging in identifying segmental defects (Fig. 14). But it was poorly specific for PE because of the high number of defects erroneously interpreted as embolic and actually caused by normal endothoracic structures, such as hila, heart, fissures, etc. (41). Therefore, a new study was undertaken to show the normal segmental lung anatomy on SPECT and normal structures that mimic perfusion defects. Each normal pulmonary segment was visualized by both angiography and planar and SPECT perfusion scintigraphy (Fig. 15) (42). Results of this study may help in increasing the specificity of SPECT diagnosis of PE.

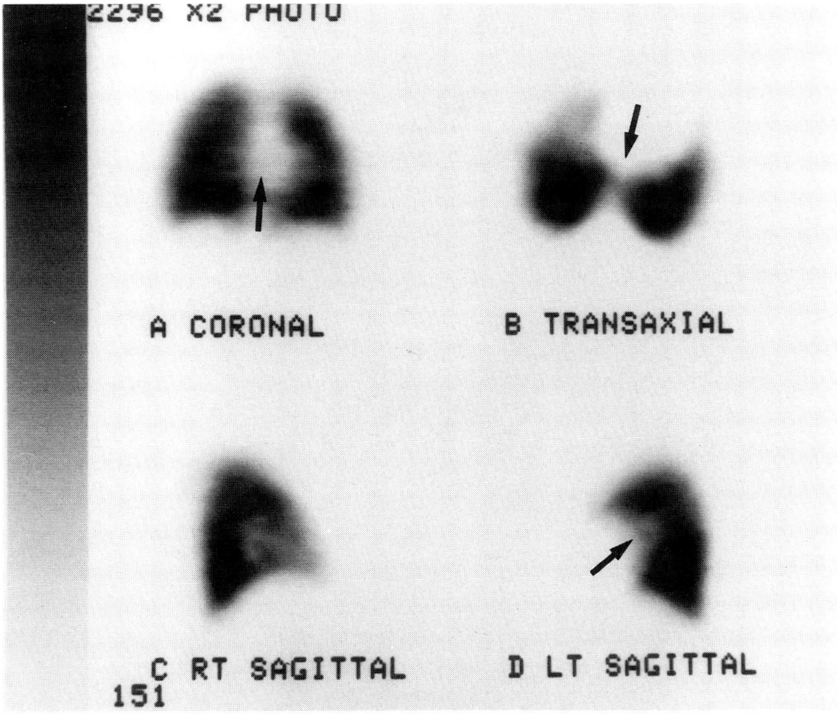

Figure 13 Normal SPECT perfusion scintigraphy showing the four views routinely used. The arrows point to the photopenic area caused by the heart silhouette. (From Ref. 41.)

IV. Ventilation Scintigraphy

The introduction of pulmonary ventilation in addition to perfusion in the diagnosis of PE was based on the rationale that ventilation would be normal in unperfused areas, and, thus, the ventilation/perfusion mismatch should be diagnostic of PE (43). To this end, the inert gases Xe-133 (81 KeV, t1/2 = 5.2 days), Xe-127 (172,203,375 KeV, t1/2 = 36 days), or Kr-81m (190 KeV, t1/2 13 s) are used in many nuclear medicine departments. Single inhalation of Xe-133 is followed by a 20-s breath hold (single-breath image) and by a 45-s tidal breathing (areas of abnormal ventilation may be documented as decreased activity in this phase); after 3–5 min of tidal volume, patients reach the equilibrium phase, followed by the wash-out phase (patients breath room air) during which several images are acquired that may show areas of Xe retention (44). Xe-127 has the advantage of higher photon energy, which allows the contemporary use of Tc-99m (140

(A)

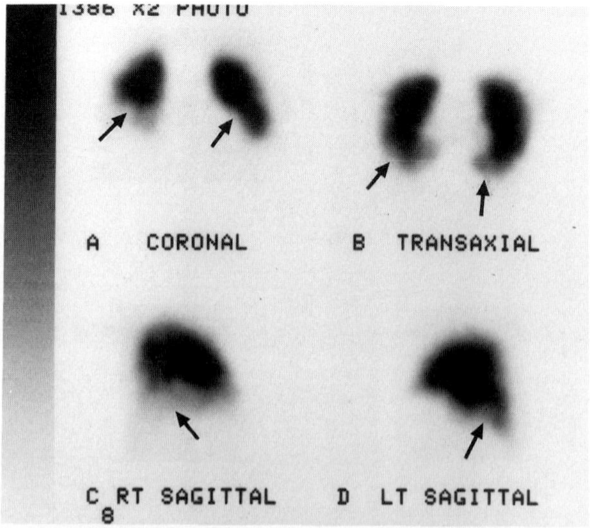

(B)

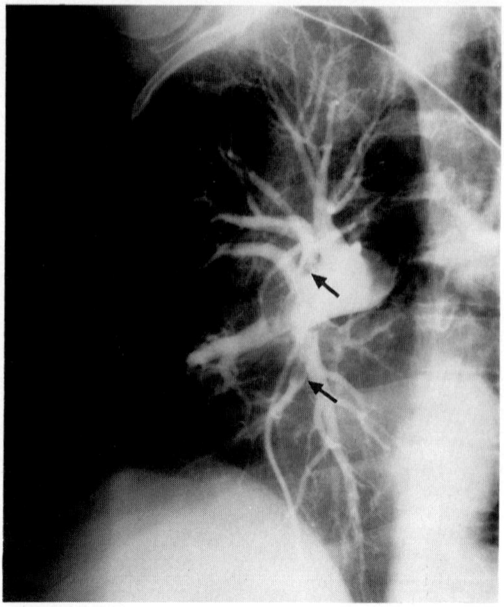

Figure 14 (A) SPECT perfusion scintigraphy showing multiple segmental defects in lower lobes bilaterally (arrows). (B) Pulmonary arteriography of the same patient shows filling defects corresponding to perfusion defects. (From Ref. 41.)

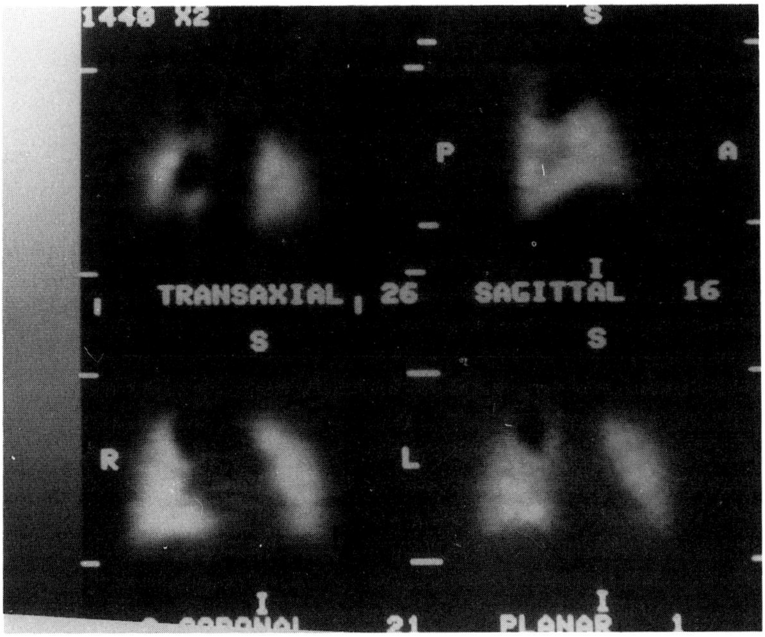

Figure 15 SPECT images in the transaxial, sagittal, and coronal planes showing apical segment of right upper lobe after subtraction of the activity of this segment from the activity of the rest of the lung; accordingly, the segment appears as a photopenic area. For comparison, planar imaging in anterior view is reported near the coronal slice.

KeV, t1/2 = 6 h) for perfusion studies, but it is expensive and poorly available. Kr-81m (190 KeV, t1/2 = 13 s) thanks to its short half-life and low radiation dose, permits many ventilation views to be obtained during normal tidal ventilation (45). However, it is costly and hardly available because a cyclotron needs to be obtained.

Nebulized aerosols have also been introduced for the same purpose (46). Various radiopharmaceuticals have been administered by aerosol using positive pressure. These aerosols may or may not contain preformed particles. Tc-99m-labeled diethylentriaminepentaacetate (DTPA) and sulfur colloid are probably the most extensively used (47); smaller-sized particles (about 0.7 μm geometric diameter) such as human albumin minimicrospheres (HAMM) (48) labeled with Tc-99m or with In-113m may be employed. With proper aerosol administration, particle size may be made small enough to reach the alveoli (49). Recently, inhalation of ultrafine carbon particle Tc-99m aerosol (Technegas) seems to offer an overall improved approach in the diagnosis of PE, including ease of administration, high counting rate obtainable also in very dyspnoic patients, and possibility of obtaining multiple views (50).

Whatever the nuclide used, scintillation cameras with appropriate collimator are generally used to image ventilation: Cameras with a large field of view are equipped with a low-energy parallel-hole collimator for Xe-133 and medium-energy collimator for Xe-127. The routine view for performance of this study is the posterior view; however, if the patient has recently undergone perfusion scintigraphy, his or her position should be correlated with the affected areas on the lung perfusion image. If one is using Kr-81m, a large-field-of-view Anger camera equipped with a low-energy, parallel-hole collimator is to be employed, and all the eight pulmonary views can be obtained to be compared with the previously made perfusion. If aerosols are being employed, gamma-camera with a parallel-hole, medium- or high-resolution collimator should be used. Also in this case all the traditional views may be achieved. However, because the isotope employed is the same as for perfusion, the patient should inhale higher doses of radiopharmaceuticals or should undergo ventilation before perfusion.

Based upon its ability to separate target organ from background activity, SPECT also has been employed to image ventilation in conjunction with radiolabeled aerosols or Kr-81m. Available results suggest that SPECT finds regions of abnormal deposition of tracer not seen on conventional imaging (51); these data, however, need to be confirmed in larger clinical studies.

Imaging interpretation is more difficult with ventilation than with perfusion because anatomy is not as clear-cut on ventilation images. Xenon ventilation images are limited to one view, usually chosen from the perfusion study to demonstrate the defects to best advantage. One of the main advantages of a gas wash-out study is that it detects regions of airway obstruction by showing retention of the gas during the clearance phase, while aerosols and krypton do not. However, because of the very short half-life of Kr-81m, inhalation studies using this gas may be repeated to match the six-eight-view lung perfusion study (Fig. 16); on the other hand, the use of aerosols allows a direct comparison of perfusion and ventilation in multiple views (Fig. 17). Compared with Kr-81m, aerosols are less expensive and more readily available. Ventilation studies with aerosols should be obtained before the perfusion because both are done with the same radionuclide. However, accurate computer techniques of subtraction may obviate the overlap of activity from the perfusion and ventilation studies.

V. Ventilation/Perfusion Patterns

A normal-lung scintigraphy virtually excludes the diagnosis of PE (52). On the contrary, many lung pathologies may cause perfusion defects. About two decades ago, the addition of ventilation was suggested to increase the specificity of perfusion (2,3). Nevertheless, although a large trial comparing the diagnostic

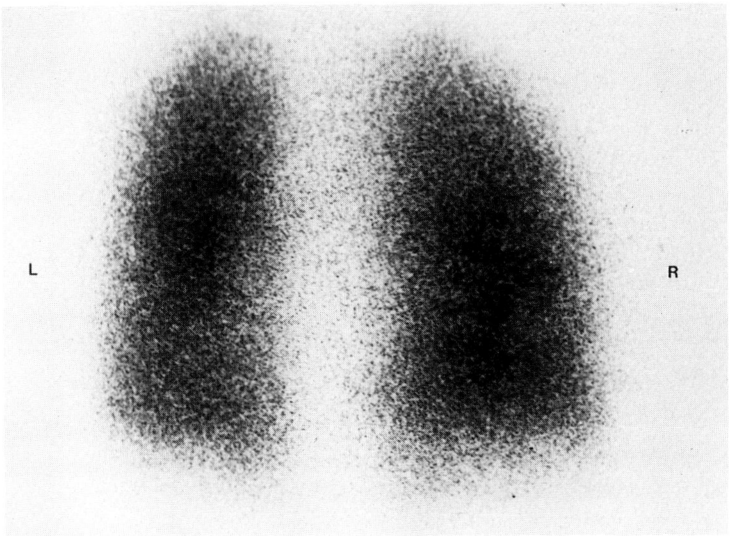

(A)

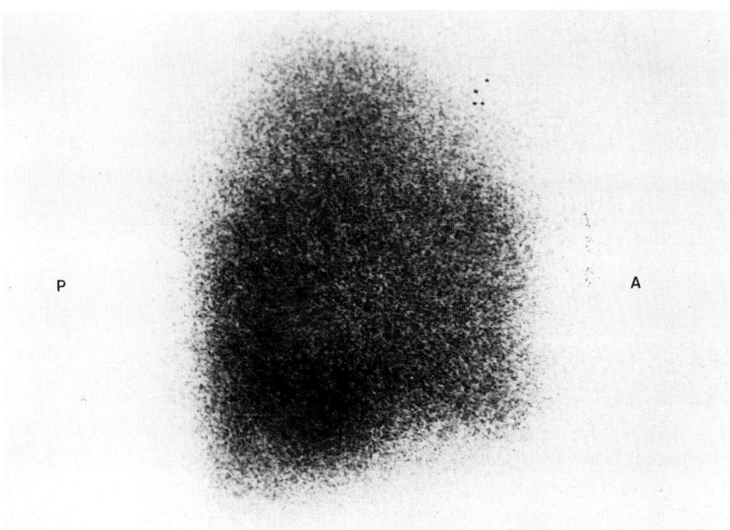

(B)

Figure 16 Kr-81m ventilation images of a normal subject demonstrate uniform distribution of gas to both lungs. Multiple views may be obtained; only two are shown here for sake of brevity: (A) posterior view. (B) right lateral view. (Pictures courtesy of Dr. AM Santolicandro.)

(A)

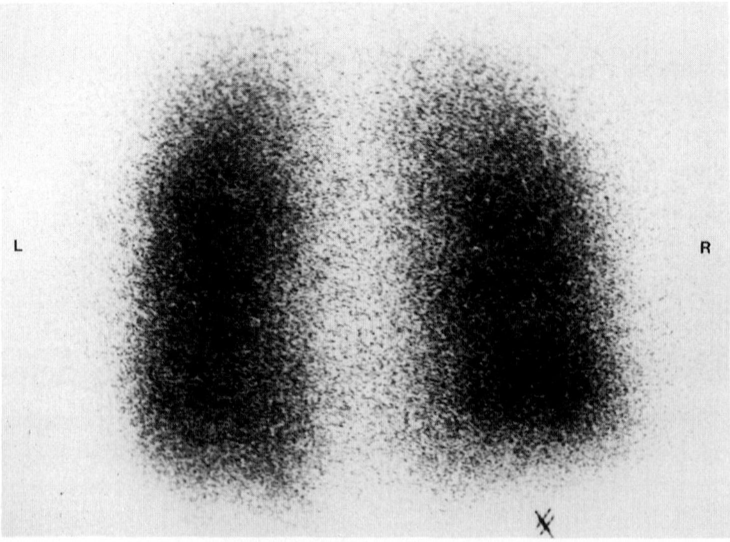

(B)

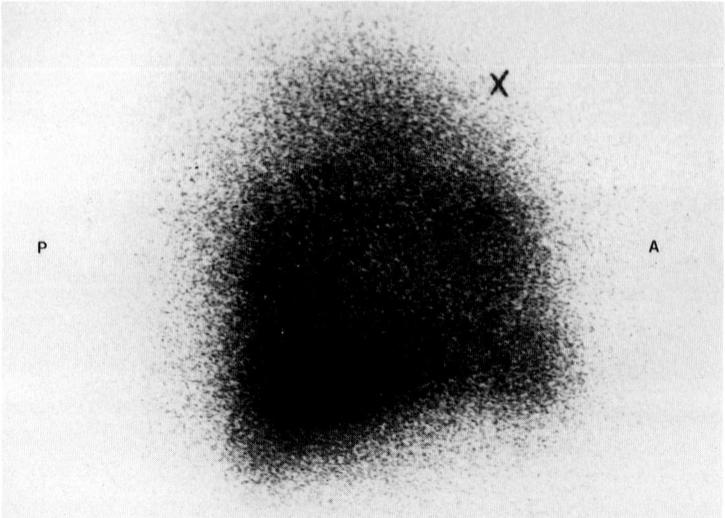

Figure 17 Tc-99m minimicrospheres (HAMM) ventilation images of a normal subject showing uniform distribution of tracer to both lungs. Multiple views may be obtained; only two are reported here for the sake of brevity: (A) posterior view, (B) right lateral view. (Pictures courtesy of Dr. AM Santolicandro.)

efficacy of ventilation-perfusion lung scan (V/Q scan) in comparison with the perfusion scan (Q scan) alone does not exist, the experience of almost two decades suggests that ventilation does not add specificity to perfusion in most patients.

Indeed, in considering the results of the PIOPED (53), the last NIH-sponsored trial with the aim of evaluating the role of V/Q scintigraphies in the diagnosis of PE, in only 13% of patients, the ones with high-probability V/Q scan, the ventilation, and the perfusion together allow one to obtain a specificity of 97%. In all other instances, the specificity of V/Q scan is either equal to the chance (intermediate or indeterminate probability) or even worse (low probability) (Table 3) and presumably worse than with perfusion alone, once patients have been selected on the basis of an accurate clinical assessment. Moreover, the adjunct of ventilation determines a decrease of sensitivity of perfusion scintigraphy in the vast majority of cases; this latter observation, which may be ascribed to actual decrease of ventilation in embolized lung zones, is particularly worrying because perfusion lung scan is the most important screening test in patients with suspicion of PE thanks to its high sensitivity.

In addition, the technique of ventilation suffers from several limitations that may have further discouraged its use in most European countries. In fact, in patients with PE, complications such as pleural effusion or pulmonary infarction often occur that may impair ventilation as well as perfusion; however, the demonstration of a chronic obstructive pulmonary disease does not exclude per se the presence of PE. Furthermore, no agreement exists about the technique to be used to perform the ventilation study, and this contributes to making the results of the centers difficult to compare with each other. Moreover, irrespective to the method used, ventilation often requires cumbersome equipment that makes the technique not readily available in many nuclear medicine centers. Finally, a very important limitation of ventilation is the fact that the V/Q diagnostic strategies suggested are all very complicated and impractical in the routine clinical practice under the emergency pressure. Accordingly, in a realistic diagnostic strategy, ventilation should be considered in a minority of patients.

In conclusion, the following practical guidelines should be taken into

Table 3 Comparison of Ventilation/Perfusion Lung Scan Categories with Angiogram Findings in the PIOPED Study

	Number	Percent	Sens	Spec
High	124	13	41	97
Inter.	364	39	82	52
Low	312	34	98	10
Normal	131	14	—	—
Total	931	100		

consideration in the diagnostic process of PE. Clinical assessment, chest radiography, blood gas analysis, ECG, and echocardiography may allow one to suspect PE early and accurately (54,55). A high-probability scan (either based on X-ray/perfusion or ventilation/perfusion studies) is highly specific for PE and should be followed by immediate therapy. In uncertain cases (either intermediate or low probability), a pulmonary angiography may be performed to confirm or rule out the diagnosis. Otherwise, the therapy may be started or excluded according to the level of clinical suspicion. In these uncertain cases, the study of the veins of the lower limbs may help with the decision making. Indeed, approximately 35%–50% of patients with deep vein thrombosis (DVT) proximal to the calf develop PE, while the risk is lower, 15%–30%, when DVT is confined to calf veins. Sasahara et al. (56) demonstrated a high prevalence of DVT of lower limbs in patients with angiographically proven PE (95%), and, even more important, a high probability of positive angiogram for PE in patients with proven DVT (56).

Several recent flow charts have been proposed that take into account this strategy, such as the one from Bone (57) in 1990 or the one from Giuntini in 1985 (Fig. 18) (58).

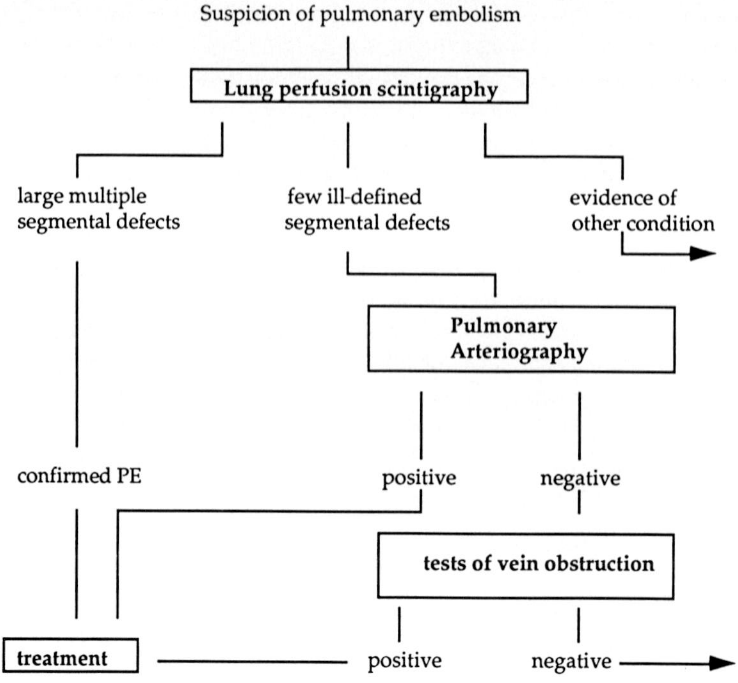

Figure 18 Flow chart for the diagnosis of pulmonary embolism. (Modified from C. Giuntini, Ref. 58.)

VI. Techniques for Detection of DVT

Contrast venography is accepted as the reference standard for diagnosing venous thrombosis because it is able to outline the entire venous system of the lower limbs including the external and common iliac veins in most patients. However, contrast venography requires expensive, complicated equipment and considerable experience to execute and interpret it; moreover, it is unconfortable for patients (59). Radionuclide venography is a simple and accurate diagnostic technique using a radioactive bolus (Tc-99m pertechnetate or Tc-99m albumin macroaggregates) injected into symmetrical pedal dorsal veins. The venographic images are visualized by means of a gamma camera connected with a computer, which allows one to record images sequentially. The accuracy of radionuclide venography in the assessment of lower extremity veins is high, and it is greatly enhanced by observing the transit of the bolus and comparing legs each other (Fig. 19) (59,60).

A practical, noninvasive approach to diagnose clinically suspected venous thrombosis is based on impedance plethysmography (IPG). It is a method that detects volume changes in the leg when a pneumatic thigh cuff is inflated and deflated, resulting in changes in electrical resistance (impedance). The IPG is a sensitive and specific test for thrombosis of the popliteal, femoral, or iliac vein (proximal veins); however, because it detects only thrombi that produce obstruction to venous outflow, it will not detect calf vein thrombi (59,61). Another noninvasive diagnostic technique for diagnosing DVT is Doppler ultrasonography. It was introduced and developed at about the same time as IPG and has similar advantages and limitations. In expert hands, Doppler ultrasonography is a sensitive method for detecting proximal vein thrombosis, but it is less sensitive for detecting calf vein thrombosis. Interpretation of results is subjective and requires considerable experience. B-mode ultrasonography or duplex sonography is a recently introduced diagnostic procedure that is being used with increasing frequency in the diagnosis of venous thrombosis. Like IPG and Doppler ultrasonography, B-mode ultrasonography is highly sensitive and specific for proximal vein thrombosis but is of limited sensitivity in the detection of calf vein thrombosis (59,62).

VII. New Diagnostic Modalities

Recent nuclear medicine techniques have been tested to improve the diagnosis of DVT and PE. Platelets accumulate at the site of tissue injury during the process of thrombus formation. Hence, these cells represent a potential target for radioisotopic imaging of thrombi. Autologous platelets labeled with In-111 have been successfully used to identify thrombotic and thromboembolic diseases (63,64).

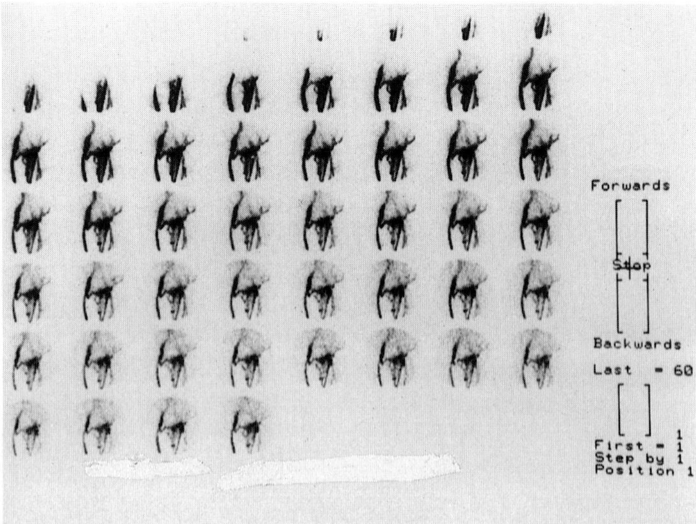

(A)

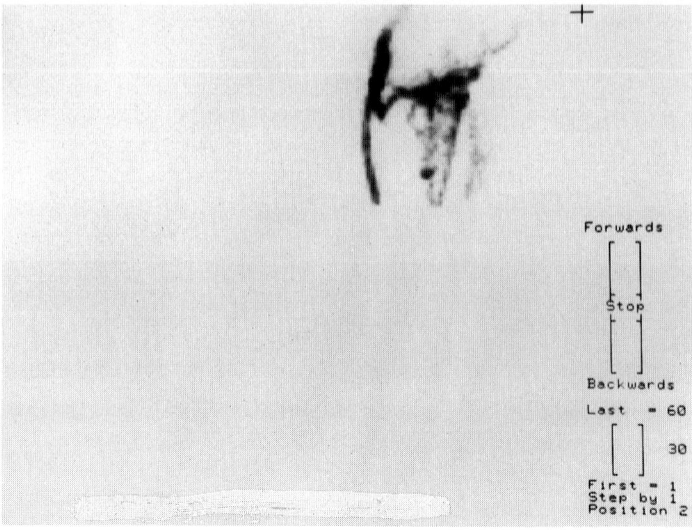

(B)

Figure 19 (A) Radionuclide venography of the lower limbs obtained by simultaneously injecting 99mTc into each pedal dorsal vein after applying a tourniquet to both ankles in order to visualize the deep venous system. The dynamic images show a complete obstruction of the left iliac vein (demonstrated by the abrupt termination of the radioactive column with collateral circulation). (B) Particular of the above pattern.

However, despite promising preliminary reports, this technique has failed to gain widespread clinical use. A number of reasons can explain the limited success of this approach. The isolation of platelets from the patient's blood, and their subsequent labeling, must be carried out in rigorously sterile and pyrogen-free conditions, which makes it a complex and time-consuming process. To overcome this limitation, the possibility to use universal donor's platelets, previously labeled and readily available at the time of symptoms' presentation, has been investigated in a dog model (65). The sensitivity of the technique was significantly reduced when platelets isolated and labeled 24 h prior to injection were used (44% thrombi visualized versus 67% using freshly isolated platelets). Another potential limitation of the use of In-111–labeled platelets is the effect of heparin, which has been reported to reduce the adhesion of platelets to the growing thrombus (66). This is of major practical importance, because heparin is administered as soon as clinical suspicion of pulmonary embolism arises. In a dog model, indium-labeled platelets failed to image thrombi in the animals pretreated with heparin, while the scans became positive in all but one case when repeated 4 h later, when the heparin effect was essentially absent (65).

More recently, the use of radiolabeled antiplatelet monoclonal antibodies has been proposed to reduce some of the limitations described earlier (67). A monoclonal antibody to the platelet glycoprotein complex GPIIbIIIa (7E3) was labeled with In-111 and incubated with whole blood rather than washed platelets (67). Following subsequent reinjection of the cells into the circulation, experimental thrombi in a dog model were visualized within 1 h, with a thrombus:blood pool ratio greater than 2:0 and no need for subtraction techniques. The authors propose that part of the superiority of this approach compared to In-111–labeled platelet scintigraphy is due to the faster blood disappearance of the unbound In-111 antibody that accounts for the lower background. In the same study, thrombus imaging was obtained, in a subset of animals, with direct injection of In-1117E3, without prior incubation with blood (67). These observations have been confirmed in preclinical human studies (68,69) and are currently undergoing a more rigorous clinical evaluation.

Platelets circulate in a resting form and become activated at the site of thrombus formation. Thus, the potential exists for a more thrombus-specific targeting using antibodies specific to activated platelets. P-selectin (CD62), previously known as PADGEM and GMP-140, is a platelet glycoprotein that is translocated from an internal location to the cell membrane upon platelet activation (70). Accordingly, antibodies to P-selectin only bind to activated platelets. Based on these considerations, Palabrica et al. (71) used I-123–labeled polyclonal anti–P-selectin antibodies in a baboon model. By using an ex vivo dacron shunt, the kinetics of antibody uptake by thrombus were studied. Thrombus associated radioactivity reached half-maximum levels as early as 10 min after injection and approached maximal levels within 30 min, with a thrombus:blood pool ratio of 33:1. In vivo thrombi, obtained by stasis in the femoral vein, were visualized within 15 min after injection of I-123 anti–P-selectin antibodies; the images were optimal between 30 and 60 min, with a thrombus:blood pool ratio greater than 3:1. These data, although very promising, are still awaiting verification in human studies.

Fibrin has also been used as a target for immunoscintigraphy of thrombi. Upon cleavage of soluble fibrinogen by thrombin, epitopes are exposed on the newly formed fibrin molecule that are not available on the parent molecule. Several monoclonal antibodies that react with fibrin and cross-react only very weakly with circulating fibrinogen have been generated and radiolabeled for thrombus imaging (72–74). In animal models, thrombus:blood pool ratios greater than 7:1 have been obtained. Preliminary clinical trials suggest that these reagents are of great potential interest; however, optimal images seem to be available only several hours after injection (74,75).

Radiological techniques, such as computed tomography (CT) and magnetic resonance (MR), have been employed to detect thrombi in pulmonary arteries. The former proved useful in showing wedge-shaped pulmonary densities compatible with pulmonary infarction (76–78) and, more recently, in detecting thrombi in central pulmonary arteries (Fig. 20) (79–80) but not for evaluating

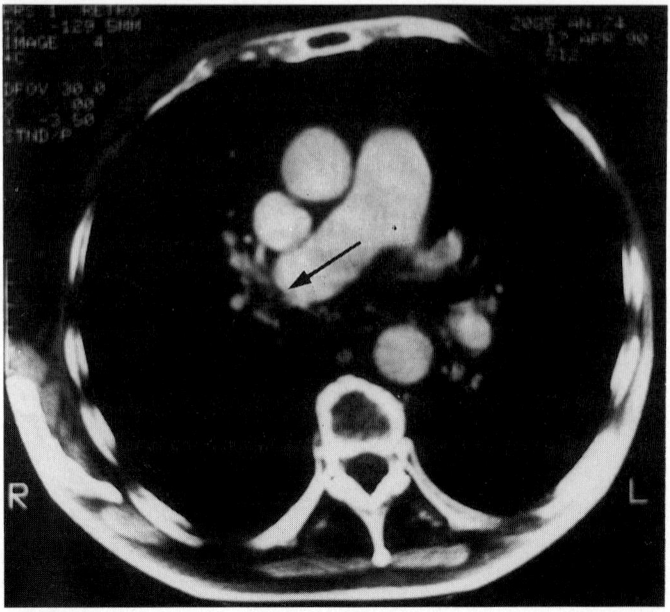

Figure 20 Thorax CT showing a large embolus lodged into the right main pulmonary artery (arrow) in a patient with acute pulmonary embolism.

thrombi in the periphery of the lung. More promising, this technique appears in the evaluation of pulmonary circulation in chronic thromboembolic pulmonary hypertension. In fact, in patients with this disease, CT shows emboli lodged into main pulmonary arteries, thus helping with the diagnosis; moreover, it may show findings characteristic of pulmonary hypertension, such as the increase of artero:bronchial (A:B) ratio (Fig. 21), the dilatation of bronchial arteries, and the presence of zones of tissue densities higher in the central than in the middle and peripheral lung compartments (80).

Vascular imaging by MR seems useful in detecting centrally positioned emboli (81–83) and slow flow in main pulmonary arteries caused by pulmonary hypertension (84); most of these data were confirmed in experimental studies (85–87). Unlike CT, MR appears capable also of imaging submillimeter vessels (88). However, the technique employed to image thrombi is critical because the differential diagnosis of the thrombus itself and the slow blood flow proximal to the obstruction can be equivocal. Techniques such as the electrocardiographically gated MR (81) or, better, the multiphasic, double spin-echo, or gradient-echo imaging (84) may allow the differentiation between pulmonary emboli and pulmonary arterial hypertension. Recently, fast-acquisition, high-resolution tech-

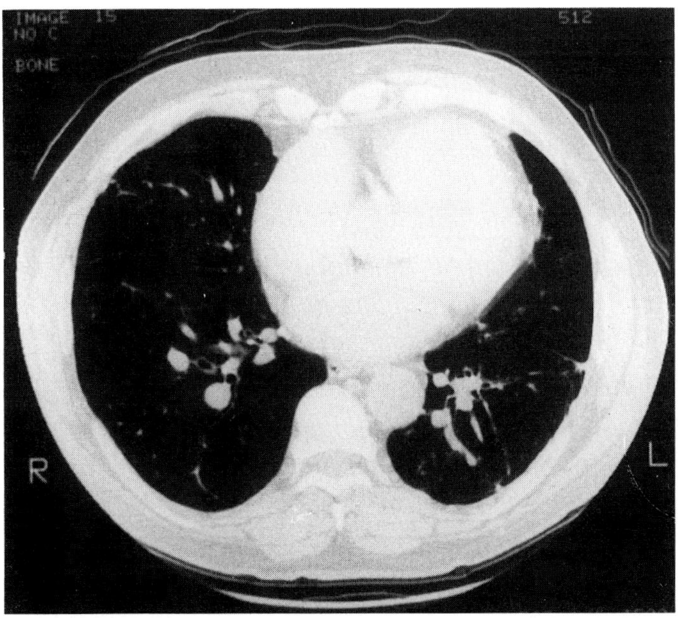

Figure 21 Thorax CT showing increased (>1) artero:bronchial (A:B) ratio in a patient with chronic thromboembolic pulmonary hypertension.

niques have been employed to image small pulmonary vessels. The gradient-echo acquisition in a steady state (GRASS) with breath holding in association with ECG gating in diastole and the cine gradient-echo MR imaging, which has high temporal resolution, may allow one to diagnose accurately pulmonary hypertension and to appreciate the different appearance of arteries and veins, supporting the possibility that cine MR may help in giving both morphological and functional information on the pulmonary vasculature (89,90).

A great deal of interest has been most recently raised by MR angiography of the pulmonary vessels (91,92), as a potential tool for diagnosing PE and pulmonary hypertension. This technique allows the visualization of pulmonary vessels thanks to the method called time of flight (TOF), which increases the signal intensity coming from protons inside arteries and veins and the method called maximum intensity projection (MIP), which allows one to observe the pulmonary vascular tree from multiple angles. Moreover, the use of ultrafast sequences (GRASS, FLUSH), ECG gating, and surface coils permit one to obtain well-defined images free from artifacts caused by cardiac or respiratory movements.

For the present time, however, MR represents a promising technique for the future, but at the moment it cannot be considered a reliable diagnostic tool in the diagnosis of PE or pulmonary hypertension.

VIII. Techniques for Evaluation of Severity

Along with blood gas analysis, perfusion scintigraphy represents the best technique to evaluate the severity of embolization. By simply counting the number of unperfused lung segments on lateral views of rectilinear scanner (15) or on all six views available on gamma camera (93), it is possible to obtain a reliable index of severity of disease, both acutely and after appropriate therapy. In a series of over 1000 patients affected by PE, the mean number of unperfused lung segments (ULS) was 9.22, which corresponds to an average obstruction of the total pulmonary vascular bed of about 51%. Distribution of ULS in patients with PE reproduces the normal error frequency function, the so-called Gauss bell (Fig. 22). This distribution suggests that PE has a continuous spectrum of severity from the case with only 2 or 3 to the case with 15–18 ULS (58).

SPECT scintigraphy has the technical characteristic of allowing semiquantitative volumetric analysis of perfusion defects, which could be more accurate than the evaluation based upon the count of number of ULS. However, this possibility has been denied so far by difficulties of outlining the area of abnormal perfusion on tomographic images because there are fewer landmarks in a section than in a planar image; moreover, because of photon variable attenuation in the chest, quantitative intensity measurements may be inaccurate.

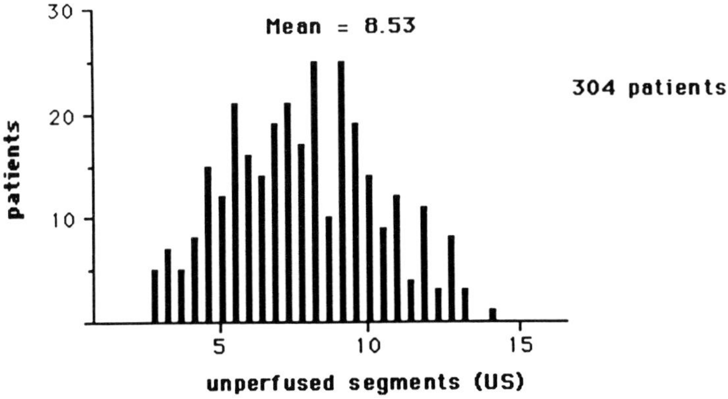

Figure 22 Distribution of unperfused lung segments that takes a "gaussian" appearance in patients with PE.

IX. Techniques for Evaluation of Recovery

Perfusion defects caused by PE change with the time. Reperfusion may be rapid or delayed, according to patient's age, promptness of treatment, preexistence of cardiopulmonary disease, or recurrences. Therefore, an accurate follow-up of patients, both in the early stages after embolization and later on, is clinically helpful. Methods already described of counting ULS on pulmonary scintigraphy allow one to monitor the evolution of PE under proper treatment both in early and late phases. In a group of 69 patients with PE, perfusion impairment decreased from the beginning from 50% of the total vascular bed to less than 20% after 6 months from acute embolization. The majority of recovery occurred during the first month, but it kept improving slowly during the first 6 months of follow-up (94). Recovery of arterial blood gases was parallel to the increase in perfusion (Table 4).

Table 4 Evolution of Blood Gases in PE

	Mean ± SE (mm Hg)			
	Pa_{O_2}[a]	Standard Pa_{O_2}[a]	Pa_{CO_2}[a]	pH[a]
At diagnosis	65.8 ± 1.6	54.8 ± 2.1	33.4 ± 0.6	7.43 ± 0.006
After 7 days	74.3 ± 1.4[b]	65.0 ± 1.6[b]	34.6 ± 0.6	7.43 ± 0.006
After 30 days	85.1 ± 1.5[b]	78.0 ± 1.7[b]	35.6 ± 0.4	7.40 ± 0.005[b]
After 180 days	85.1 ± 1.4	80.2 ± 1.5	37.3 ± 0.4[b]	7.38 ± 0.004
After 365 days	81.5 ± 1.2	76.1 ± 1.2	37.2 ± 0.4	7.39 ± 0.005

[a]Highly significant, $P < 0.001$ for the cumulative variance.
[b]Significant, $P < 0.05$ for the given subset.

During the follow-up, clinically guided scintigraphies allowed the detection of recurrences, thus avoiding further episodes that could be fatal. Recurrences of PE mainly occur in the late phases of follow-up (after months from acute embolization), and this should reinforce the careful evaluation of the patient's compliance to the anticoagulant therapy.

Perfusion damage evaluated on perfusion scintigraphy correlates with the impairment of pulmonary gas exchanges, and, thus, it can give information about the functional conditions of patients during the follow-up, e.g., under treatment. In fact, hypoxemia is related to the perfusion impairment, and the recovery of pulmonary defects is accompained by the recovery of hypoxia (94).

In a subsequent study, 33 patients were followed for 6 months with perfusion lung scintigraphy, gas exchange, and chest roentgenogram (95). Accurate functional evaluation of patients demonstrated good correlation between ULS, on the one hand, and the increase of the standardized oxygen tension of Pa_{O_2}, the reduction of both Pa_{O_2}-P_{AO_2} and P_{ACO_2}-Pa_{CO_2} on the other hand. Therefore, it can be concluded that simple measurement of gas exchange may be sufficient to assess the functional recovery of patients with PE (95).

X. Final Remarks

Pulmonary embolism is still known as the "great masquerader" because of difficulties in making the diagnosis. To reduce the possibility of underdiagnosis, the first and necessary step is to raise suspicion: To this purpose, an accurate clinical assessment is essential followed by the careful use of noninvasive, routinely available techniques. Among them, planar chest radiography should be always considered.

Among screening tests for diagnosis, perfusion lung scan still has a paramount importance, because it is highly sensitive, increasingly available, and easily repeatable. Regardless of the instrument employed, it represents the central tool for all diagnostic strategies and also the most accurate and safe way to monitor the early efficacy of fibrinolytic treatment and late protective effect of anticoagulants. The use of chest radiography and ventilation scan should be pursued whenever possible in association with perfusion scan to increase its specificity, provided the chosen diagnostic strategy to obtain a noninvasive diagnosis of PE should be as simple as possible to be effective.

In cases where the diagnosis remains doubtful after pulmonary scintigraphies, the study of the veins of the lower limbs should be performed; radionuclide venography is almost as accurate as the contrast venography without being so invasive.

New techniques of imaging using isotopes (labeled platelets, monoclonal antibodies), X-rays (high-resolution CT), or magnetic properties (MR) look promising for the future but have not gained enough credit for the present.

References

1. Greenspan RH, Ravin CE, Polansky SM, et al. Accuracy of the chest radiograph in diagnosis of pulmonary embolism. Invest Radiol 1982; 17:539–43.
2. Mc Neil BJ. A diagnostic strategy using ventilation-perfusion studies in patients suspect for pulmonary embolism. J Nucl Med 1976; 17:613–6.
3. Biello DR, Mattar AG, McKnight RC, et al. Ventilation perfusion studies in suspected pulmonary embolism. Am J Roentgenol 1979; 133:1033–7.
4. Celi A, Palla A, Petruzzelli S, et al. Prospective study of a standardized questionnaire to improve clinical estimate of pulmonary embolism. Chest 1989; 95:332–7.
5. Dalen JE, Alpert JS. Natural history of pulmonary embolism. Prog Cardiovasc Dis 1975; 17:259–70.
6. Morpurgo M, Schmid C. Clinico-pathological correlations in pulmonary embolism: a posteriori evaluation. Prog Resp Res 1980; 13:8–15.
7. Figley MF, Gerdes AJ, Ricketts HJ. Radiographic aspects of pulmonary embolism. Semin Roentgenol 1967; 2:389–405.
8. Fleischner FG. Pulmonary embolism. Can Med Assoc J 1958; 78:653–60.
9. Sasahara AA, Cannilla JE, Morse RL, Sidd JJ, Tremblay GM. Clinical and physiologic studies in pulmonary thromboembolism. Am J Cardiol 1967; 20:10–20.
10. Silver D. Pulmonary embolism. Surg Clin North Am 1974; 54:1089–1106.
11. Palla A, Petruzzelli S, Giuntini C. L'embolia polmonare. In: Marano P, ed. La radiologia funzionale del torace. Verona: Libreria Cortina, 1986:87–120.
12. Palla A, Donnamaria V, Rossi G, Riccetti G, Giuntini C. Enlargement of the right descending pulmonary artery in pulmonary embolism. Am J Roentgenol 1983; 141:513–7.
13. Fleischner FG. Pulmonary embolism. Clin Radiol 1962; 13:169–82.
14. Urokinase Pulmonary Embolism Trial: a national cooperative study. Circulation 1973; 47(suppl II):81–5.
15. Palla A, Petruzzelli S, Donnamaria V, Rossi G, Maltinti G, Giuntini C. Radiographic assessment of perfusion impairment in pulmonary embolism. Eur J Radiol 1985; 5:252–5.
16. Laur A. Roentgen diagnosis of pulmonary embolism and its differentiation from myocardial infarction. Am J Roentgenol 1963; 90:632–7.
17. Sasahara AA. Current problems in pulmonary embolism: introduction. Prog Cardiovasc Dis 1974; 17:161–5.
18. Donnamaria V, Palla A, Petruzzelli S, Carrozzi L, Pugliesi O, Giuntini C. Early and late follow-up of pulmonary embolism. Respiration; 1993; 60:15–20.
19. Palla A, Petruzzelli S, Donnamaria V, Bronzini R, Giuntini C. Modificazioni dell'aspetto radiografico dell'ombra cardiaca in corso di embolia polmonare. Minerva Pneumol 1991; 30:115–20.
20. McIntyre KM, Sasahara AA. Hemodynamic and ventricular responses to pulmonary embolism. Prog Cardiovasc Dis 1974; 17:175–90.
21. Barritt DW, Jordan SC. Clinical features of pulmonary embolism. Lancet 1961; 1:729–32.
22. Kerr IH, Simon G, Sutton MB. The value of the plain radiograph in acute massive pulmonary embolism. Br J Radiol 1971; 44:751–7.

23. Moses DC, Silver TM, Bookstein JJ. The complementary roles of chest radiography, lung scanning, and selective pulmonary angiography in the diagnosis of pulmonary embolism. Circulation 1974; 49:179–88.
24. Westermark N. On the roentgen diagnosis of lung embolism. Acta Radiol 1938; 19:357–72.
25. Stein GN, Chen JT, Goldstein F, Israel HL, Finkelstein A. The importance of chest roentgenography in the diagnosis of pulmonary embolism. Am J Roentgenol 1959; 81:255–63.
26. Fleischner FG. Recurrent pulmonary embolism and cor pulmonale. N Engl J Med 1967; 276:1213–20.
27. Talbot S, Worthington BS, Roebuck EJ. Radiographic signs of pulmonary embolism and pulmonary infarction. Thorax 1973; 28:198–203.
28. Wiener SN, Edelstein J, Charms BL. Observations on pulmonary embolism and the pulmonary angiogram. Am J Roentgenol 1966; 98:859–73.
29. Wolfe WG, Sabiston DC Jr. A study of changes in the roentgenogram of the chest in experimental pulmonary embolism. Surg Gynecol Obstet 1968; 127:492–8.
30. Freiman DG, Suyemoto J, Wessler S. Frequency of pulmonary thromboembolism in man. N Engl J Med 1965; 272:1278–80.
31. Smith GT, Dammin GJ, Dexter L. Post-mortem arteriographic studies of the human lung in pulmonary embolization. JAMA 1964; 188:143–51.
32. Tsao MS, Schraufragel D, Wang NS. Pathogenesis of pulmonary infarction. Am J Med 1982; 72:599–606.
33. Hampton AO, Castleman B. Correlation of post-mortem chest teleroentgenogram with autopsy findings. AJR 1940; 43:305–26.
34. Bachynsky JE. Absence of the air bronchogram sign: a reliable finding in pulmonary embolism with infarction or hemorrhage. Radiology 1971; 100:547–52.
35. Dalen JE, Affajee CI, Alpert JS, et al. Pulmonary embolism, pulmonary hemorrhage, and pulmonary infarction. N Engl J Med 1977; 296:1431–5.
36. Baron MG. Fleischner lines and pulmonary emboli. Circulation 1972; 45:171–8.
37. Fleischner F, Hampton AO, Castleman B. Linear shadows in the lung. Am J Roentgenol 1941; 46:610–8.
38. Uhland H, Goldberg LM. Pulmonary embolism: a commonly missed clinical entity. Dis Chest 1964; 45:533–6.
39. Williams JR, Wilcox WC. Pulmonary embolism: roentgenographic and angiographic considerations. Am J Roetgenol 1963; 89:333–42.
40. Petruzzelli S, Palla A, Donnamaria V, Cipriani S, Viegi G, Giuntini C. Clinical features in suspected pulmonary embolism: a multivariate analysis of 196 cases. Am Rev Respir Dis 1992; 145:A718. Abstract.
41. Palla A, Tumeh SS, Nagel JS, Meyerovitz MF, Goldhaber SZ, Holman BL. Detection of pulmonary perfusion defects in man by single photon emission computed tomography (SPECT). J Nucl Med Allied Sci 1988; 32:27–32.
42. Palla A, Singer SJ, Tumeh SS, et al. Segmental pulmonary anatomy in man: a method of study with angiography and single photon emission computed tomography. J Nucl Med Allied Sci 1989; 33:247–51.
43. De Nardo GL, Goodwin DA, Ravasini R, Dietrich PA. The ventilatory lung scan in the diagnosis of pulmonary embolism. N Engl J Med 1970; 282:1334–6.

44. Alderson PO, Lee H, Summer WR, et al. Comparison of Xe-133 washout and single breath imaging for the detection of ventilation abnormalities. J Nucl Med 1979; 20:917–22.
45. Fazio F, Lavender PJ, Steiner RE. Kr-81m ventilation and Tc-99m perfusion scans in chest disease: comparison with standard radiographs. Am J Roentgenol 1978; 130:421–8.
46. Taplin GV, Poe ND, Greenberg A. Lung scanning following radioaerosol inhalation. J Nucl Med 1966; 7:77–87.
47. Alderson PO, Biello DR, Gottschalk A, et al. Tc-99m DTPA aerosol and radioactive gases compared as adjuncts to perfusion scintigraphy in patients with suspected pulmonary embolism. Radiology 1984; 153:515–21.
48. Santolicandro AM, Ruschi S, Fornai E, Giuntini C. Imaging of ventilation in chronic obstructive pulmonary disease. J Thorac Imag 1986; 1(2):36–53.
49. Santolicandro A, Giuntini C. Patterns of deposition of labelled monodispersed aerosols in obstructive lung disease. J Nucl Med Allied Sci 1979; 23:115–27.
50. Murray IP. Clinical experience with technegas. Clin Nucl Med 1991; 16:247–50.
51. Touya JJ, Corbus HF, Savala KM, et al. Single photon emission computed tomography in the diagnosis of pulmonary thromboembolism. Semin Nucl Med 1986; 16:306–36.
52. Kipper MS, Moser KM, Kortman KE, Ashburn WL. Longterm follow-up of patients with suspected pulmonary embolism and a normal lung scan. Chest 1982; 82:411–5.
53. The PIOPED investigators. Value of the ventilation/perfusion scan in acute pulmonary embolism. JAMA 1990; 263:2753–9.
54. Petruzzelli S, Palla A, Citi M, Giuntini C. Improvement of screening for pulmonary embolism with a standardized questionnaire. Respiration 1990; 57:329–37.
55. Petruzzelli S, Palla A, Donnamaria V, Pieraccini F, Giuntini C. Routine electrocardiography in screening for pulmonary embolism. Respiration 1986; 50:233–43.
56. Sasahara AA, Sharma GVRK, Parisi AF. New developments in the detection and prevention of venous thromboembolism. Am J Cardiol 1979; 43:1214–24.
57. Bone RC. Ventilation/perfusion scan in pulmonary embolism. "The emperor is incompletely attired." JAMA 1990; 263:2794–5.
58. Giuntini C. Do radioisotope techniques fulfil their role in the diagnosis of pulmonary embolism? J Nucl Med Allied Sci 1985; 29:1–6.
59. Hirsh J. Diagnosis of venous thrombosis and pulmonary embolism. Am J Cardiol 1990; 2:45c–49c.
60. Ennis JT, Elmes RJ. Radionuclide venography in the diagnosis of deep vein thrombosis. Radiology 1977; 125:441–9.
61. Wheeler HB, Mullick SC, Anderson JN, Searson D. Diagnosis of occult deep vein thrombosis by non-invasive bed-side technique. Surgery 1971; 70:20–4.
62. Sigel B, Felix WR Jr, Popky GL, et al. Diagnosis of lower limb venous thrombosis by Doppler ultrasound technique. Arch Surg 1972; 104:174–9.
63. McIlmovle G, Davis HH, Welch MJ, Primeau JL, Sherman LA, Siegel BA. Scintigraphic diagnosis of experimental pulmonary embolism with ^{111}In-labeled platelets. J Nucl Med 1977; 18:910–4.
64. Goodwin DA, Bushberg JT, Doherty PW, Lipton MJ, Conley FK, Dimanti CL,

Meares CF. Indium-111-labeled autologus platelets for location of vascular thrombus in humans. J Nucl Med 1978; 19:626–34.
65. Cella G, Palla A, Tow DE, Cunningham T, McCracken L, Godin PF, Sasahara AA. Indium-111 autologus platelets in the detection of experimental pulmonary emboli. Effect of heparin and aged platelets. J Nucl Med Allied Sci 1986; 30:133–40.
66. Thomas DP, Gurewich V, Asford TP. Platelet adherence to thromboemboli in relation to the pathogenesis and treatment of pulmonary embolism. N Engl J Med 1966; 274:953–6.
67. Oster ZH, Srivastava SC, Som P, et al. Thrombus radioimmunoscintigraphy: an approach using monoclonal antiplatelet antibody. Proc Natl Acad Sci USA. 1985; 82:3465–8.
68. Peters AM, Lavender JP, Needham SG. Imaging thrombus with radiolabelled monoclonal antibody to platelets. Br Med J 1986; 293:1525–7.
69. Stuttle AWJ, Peters AM, Loutfi I, Lumley P, George P, Lavender JP. Use of an anti-platelet monoclonal antibody $F(ab')_2$ fragment for imaging thrombus. Nucl Med Comm 1988; 9:647–55.
70. Celi A, Furie B, Furie BC. PADGEM: an adhesion receptor for leukocytes on stimulated platelets and endothelial cells. Proc Soc Exp Biol Med 1991; 198:703–9.
71. Palabrica TM, Furie BC, Konstam MA, et al. Thrombus imaging in a primate model with antibodies specific for an external membrane protein of activated platelets. Proc Natl Acad Sci USA 1989; 86:1036–40.
72. Hui KY, Haber E, Matsueda GR. Monoclonal antibodies to a synthetic fibrin-like peptide bind to human fibrin but not fibrinogen. Science 1983; 222:1129–32.
73. Rosebrough SF, Kudryk B, Grossman ZD, et al. Radioimmunoimaging of venous thrombi using iodine-131 monoclonal antibody. Radiology 1985; 156:515–7.
74. Wasser MNJM, Koppert PW, Arndt JW, Emeis JJ, Feitsma RIJ, Pauwels EKJ, Nieuwenhuizen W. An antifibrin monoclonal antibody useful in immunoscintigraphic detection of thrombi. Blood 1989; 74:708–14.
75. Knight LC. Imaging thrombi with radiolabeled anti-fibrin monoclonal antibodies. Nucl Med Comm 1988; 9:823–9.
76. Sinner WN. Computed tomographic patterns of pulmonary thromboembolism and infarction. J Comput Assist Tomogr 1978; 2:395–9.
77. Lourie GL, Pizzo SV, Ravin C, Putman C, Thompson WM. Experimental pulmonary infarction in dogs: a comparison of chest radiography and computed tomography. Invest Radiol 1982; 17:224–32.
78. Chiantapalli K, Thorsen MK, Olson DL, Goodman LR, Gurney J. Computed tomography of pulmonary thromboembolism and infarction. J Comput Assist Tomogr 1988; 12:553–9.
79. Godwin JD, Webb WR, Gamsu G, Ovenfors CO. Computed tomography of pulmonary embolism. Am J Roentgenol 1980; 135:691–5.
80. Falaschi F, Palla A, Formichi B, Sbragia P, Petruzzelli S, Giuntini C, Bartolozzi C. CT evaluation of chronic thromboembolic pulmonary hypertension. J Comput Assist Tomogr 1992; 16(6):897–903.
81. Fisher MR, Higgins CB. Central thrombi in pulmonary arterial hypertension detected by MR imaging. Radiology 1986; 158:223–6.

82. Thickman D, Kressel HY, Axel L. Demonstration of pulmonary embolism by magnetic resonance imaging. Am J Roentgenol 1984; 142:921–2.
83. Moore EH, Gamsu G, Webb WR, Stulbarg MS. Pulmonary embolus: detection and follow-up using magnetic resonance. Radiology 1984; 153:471–2.
84. White RD, Winkler ML, Higgins CB. MR imaging of pulmonary arterial hypertension and pulmonary emboli. Am J Roentgenol 1987; 149:15–21.
85. Gamsu G, Hirji M, Moore EH, Webb WR, Brito A. Experimental pulmonary emboli detected using magnetic resonance. Radiology 1984; 153:467–70.
86. Rapoport S, Sostman HD, Pope C, Camputaro CM, Holcomb W, Gore JC. Venous clots: evaluation with MR imaging. Radiology 1987; 162:527–30.
87. Stein MG, Crues JV III, Bradley WG Jr., Kortman KE, Andrues TA, Waxman AD, Henderson RW. MR imaging of pulmonary emboli: an experimental study in dogs. Am J Roentgenol 1986; 147:1133–7.
88. Haacke EM, Lenz GW. Submillimiter flow imaging. Radiology. 1986; 161(P):127. Abstract.
89. Hatabu H, Gefter WB, Kressel HY, Axel L, Lenkinsky RE. Pulmonary vasculature: high-resolution MR imaging. Radiology 1989; 171:391–5.
90. Gefter WB, Hatabu H, Dinsmore BJ, et al. Pulmonary vascular cine MR imaging: a noninvasive approach to dynamic imaging of the pulmonary circulation. Radiology 1990; 176:761–70.
91. Foo TKF, Mac Fall JR, Hayes CE, Sostman HD, Slayman BE. Pulmonary vasculature: single breath-hold MR imaging with phased-array coils. Radiology 1992; 183:473–7.
92. Wielopolski PA, Haace EM, Adler LP. Three-dimensional MR imaging of the pulmonary vasculature: preliminary experience. Radiology 1992; 183:465–72.
93. Parker JA, Markis JE, Palla A, et al. Pulmonary perfusion after rt-PA therapy for acute embolism: early improvement assessed with segmental perfusion scanning. Radiology 1988; 166:441–5.
94. Palla A, Donnamaria V, Petruzzelli S, Giuntini C. Follow up of pulmonary perfusion recovery after embolism. J Nucl Med Allied Sci 1986; 30:23–8.
95. Prediletto R, Paoletti P, Fornaie E, et al. Natural course of treated pulmonary embolism. Evaluation by perfusion lung scintigraphy, gas exchange, and chest roentgenogram. Chest 1990; 97:554–61.

13

Echocardiography in Pulmonary Embolism

ADAM TORBICKI

Medical Academy
Warsaw, Poland

I. Introduction

The definite diagnosis of pulmonary embolism requires positive pulmonary angiography or high-probability lung scan accompanied by suggestive clinical picture (1,2). Pulmonary arteriography is invasive and not always readily available (3), while high-probability lung scans are found only in a minority of patients with suspected pulmonary embolism (2). Thus, early management of a patient with suspected pulmonary embolism is often based on highly unreliable clinical evidence only.

While echocardiography is a potent diagnostic tool in many cardiovascular disorders, its role in the management of patients with suspected pulmonary embolism has been less extensively studied. Potentially, this noninvasive, available at the bedside, and relatively inexpensive method has much to offer: It provides important data regarding morphology and function of the right heart, including a reliable estimate of pulmonary arterial pressure. It makes visualization of intraluminal thrombi possible. Finally, alternative cardiovascular diseases mimicking the clinical picture of pulmonary embolism may be found or excluded by echocardiography.

This chapter discuss current knowledge and future perspectives regarding the role of echocardiography in the work-up of patients with suspected pulmonary embolism.

II. Echocardiographic Changes in Patients with Pulmonary Embolism

A. Character and Prevalence of Echocardiographic Changes in Patients with Pulmonary Embolism

Kasper et al. (4) found M-mode echocardiographic abnormalities in the majority of 105 consecutive patients with acute (n = 72), subacute (n = 22), or chronic recurrent (n = 11) pulmonary embolism confirmed by angiography (n = 48), autopsy (n = 6), or high-probability lung perfusion scan (n = 51). Echocardiographic findings consisted of increased right ventricular end diastolic dimension (defined as RVEDD > 27 mm) seen in 75% of cases and of reduced left ventricular end diastolic dimension (LVEDD < 36 mm) seen in 42% of cases. Dilated right pulmonary artery (RPA > 11.4 mm/m^2) was seen in 77% of the patients, but assessment of the diameter of right pulmonary artery was technically difficult, often requiring registration from the suprasternal notch with a specially designed transducer. Abnormal septal motion was observed in 44% of the patients and decreased EF slope of the mitral valve (<50 mm/s), suggesting compromised left ventricular filling in 50%. However, in 19 out of 105 (18%) patients, all the previous parameters were within the normal range. Because the study population consisted of patients with confirmed pulmonary embolism, specificity of the echocardiographic changes for pulmonary embolism could not be assessed.

In a recent, study Jardin et al. (5) found that among 61 patients admitted to an intensive care unit for suspected acute pulmonary embolism, 6 out of 13 had normal two-dimensional (2-D) echocardiographic examination despite angiographically confirmed pulmonary embolism. On the other hand, all 48 patients with right ventricular dilation and flattening of the interventricular septum had also positive pulmonary angiograms for pulmonary embolism. In a subsequent discussion, Jardin (6) admitted that the study population was limited to patients free of previous cardiopulmonary disorders.

B. Echocardiography in the Assessment of the Severity of Pulmonary Embolism

To verify whether echocardiographic changes could reflect the degree of hemodynamic compromise, Kasper et al. (4) developed a score and used it to establish an echocardiographic severity index of pulmonary embolism. The score was based on the presence and severity of five echocardiographic signs: right ventricular enlargement, decreased left ventricular dimension, flattened mitral EF slope, dilated right pulmonary artery, and abnormal interventricular septum motion. Significant correlation was found when this echocardiographic score was compared to the angiographic severity index of embolic obstruction according to Walsh et al. (7) (n = 36, $r = 0.72$, $P < 0.001$) (Fig. 1). Similar correlation was reported recently between the ratio of diastolic dimensions of the two ventricles (RVEDD/LVEDD) and Miller index of angiographic obstruction ($r = 0.75$, $P < 0.01$) (8,9). All but one patient with occlusion exceeding 40% of pulmonary arterial bed had enlarged right ventricles on echocardiography (Fig. 2).

Jardin et al. (10) followed 14 patients with acute massive pulmonary embolism with both echocardiography and direct right heart hemodynamic measurements. They noticed enlarged right heart chambers, dilated pulmonary artery, and inferior vena cava as well as decreased fractional area contraction of the right ventricle, decreased left ventricular dimensions, and flattened interventricular septum. These changes resolved simultaneously with the regression of directly assessed hemodynamic evidence of right heart failure. The authors paid special attention to the quantitative analysis of septal curvature. They found septal flattening both at end-diastole and end-systole in the acute phase of the disease and—although slightly less pronounced—3–5 days later. The shape of the interventricular septum returned to normal 2–3 weeks after the initial examination. The diastolic flattening of the interventricular septum could be explained by the inverted interventricular gradient caused by right ventricular failure and decreased left ventricular preload, both occurring inside a poorly distensible pericardium (Fig. 3). We could appreciate the role of pericardium

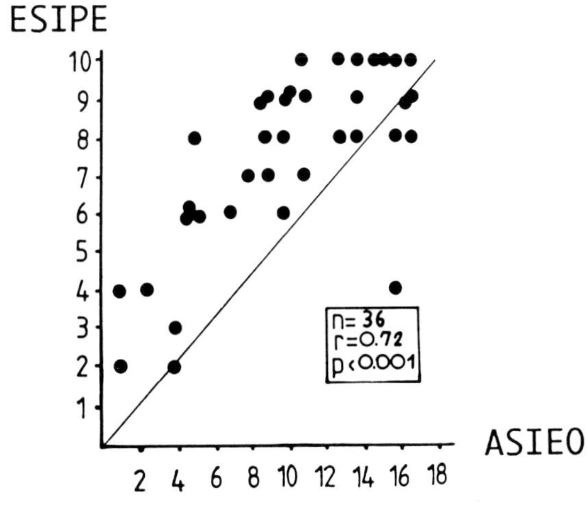

Figure 1 Correlation between echocardiographically determined severity index of pulmonary embolism (ESIPE) and angiographic severity index of embolic obstruction (ASIEO). (From Ref. 4, with permission.)

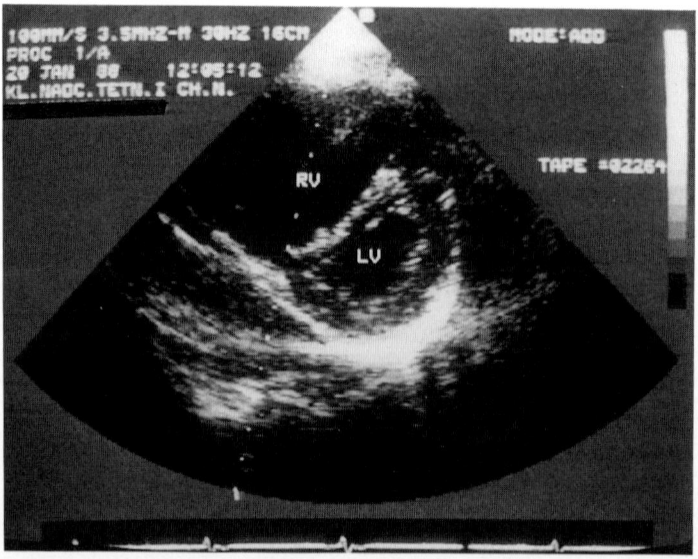

Figure 2 Echocardiographic image of enlarged right ventricle (RV) with diastolic bulging of the interventricular septum toward a small left ventricle (LV) seen in parasternal short axis view in a patient with acute massive pulmonary embolism. (From Ref. 69. Copyrighted and reprinted with the permission of Clinical Cardiology Publishing Co., Inc., and/or Foundation for Advances in Medicine and Science, P.O. Box 832, Mahwah, NJ 07430).

during acute pulmonary embolism by noting respiratory variations of the interventricular septal position and function similar to those described in pericardial tamponade or constriction. The mechanism of systolic septal flattening is less clear, because systolic right ventricular pressure in patients with acute pulmonary embolism is still well below left ventricular systolic pressure except for patients in shock. However, systolic septal flattening was observed by Come et al. (11) in four out of six patients with acute pulmonary embolism. After the treatment with rt-PA, the septal shape returned to normal. Diastolic changes of septal shape or function were not mentioned in their study, while other findings consisted of dilated and hypokinetic right ventricle and decreased left ventricular dimensions. Also, these changes resolved after thrombolytic treatment.

Considered together with similar findings reported by others (12–14), these observations suggest, that if acute burden is put on the right ventricle because of pulmonary embolus, its hemodynamic consequences can be quantified and monitored by the echocardiographic assessment of ventricular dimensions and of the interventricular septum.

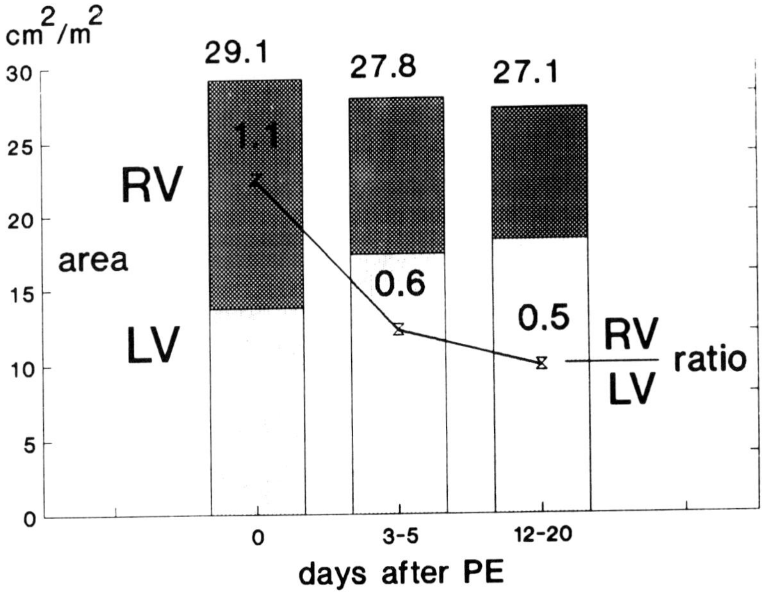

Figure 3 Average area of right (RV) and left ventricle (LV) as assessed from 4-chamber apical view in 14 patients with massive pulmonary embolism treated with heparin. Note relatively constant total bi-ventricular area limited by pericardium but progressive decrease of RV/LV area ratio at repeated follow-up. (Based on the data of Ref. 10.)

III. Doppler Echocardiography in the Differential Diagnosis of Right over Left Ventricular Domination

Dilatation of the right ventricle is not specific for pulmonary embolism. It may occur in right ventricular infarction or arrhythmogenic cardiomyopathy, in interventricular septal rupture or severe tricuspid regurgitation, and in a number of congenital cardiovascular defects. The domination of right over left ventricle is a rule in pretricuspid shunts, in isolated mitral stenosis, and in important chronic pulmonary hypertension regardless of the cause. Decompensation in the course of these diseases—if they were previously not diagnosed—may sometimes raise clinical suspicion of pulmonary embolism. Echocardiography provides clues for differential diagnosis in most of these cases.

A. Acquired and Congenital Heart Disease

Mitral stenosis, valvular or infundibular pulmonary arterial stenosis, and intracardiac shunts with right heart overload are reliably excluded with two-dimensional Doppler echocardiography. In case partial anomalous pulmonary venous return to the right atrium or sinus venosus type of atrial septal defect is suspected, transesophageal echocardiography with two-dimensional, color-coded Doppler and contrast might be useful for definite diagnosis.

B. Right Ventricular Afterload

Estimation of right ventricular systolic pressure is essential for understanding the cause of right ventricular dilatation found during echocardiographic examination in patients free from congenital cardiovascular abnormalities.

Measurement of peak velocity of the jet of tricuspid regurgitation with continuous wave Doppler echocardiography is the most reliable noninvasive method of the assessment of right ventricular systolic pressure. Although this method requires the presence of at least trivial tricuspid regurgitation (15,16), it occurs in the majority of patients' dilated right ventricles (17,18). The maximal velocity (V) of the tricuspid regurgitating jet is directly related to the maximal systolic pressure difference (ΔP) between the right ventricle and the right atrium. This relation is described by the simplified Bernoulli equation: $\Delta P = 4V^2$. However, in order to calculate noninvasively the right ventricular systolic pressure, an estimate of right atrial pressure should be added to the systolic pressure difference between right ventricle and right atrium calculated according to Doppler data. This is especially important in patients with right ventricular failure because their right atrial pressures may be severely elevated.

The diameter of the inferior vena cava measured with echocardiography in patients with chronic cardiovascular disorders was shown to correlate with their mean right atrial pressure ($r = 0.85$) (19). However, if one considers the limited compliance of the venous wall, this will probably not hold true for the acute increase in right atrial pressure expected in acute pulmonary embolism. Simonson and Shiller (20) described a method of estimation of the right atrial pressure based on the effect of loaded inspiration on the diameter of vena cava measured with echocardiography ($r = 0.87$, SEE 2.9 mm Hg). Theoretically, the method should work also in patients with acute right ventricular failure, but it requires multiple periods of sustained apnea and, therefore, may be difficult to apply in dyspnoeic patients with suspected pulmonary embolism.

Despite this limitation, tricuspid regurgitation peak jet velocity method is most useful to stratify the patients according to the level of right ventricular afterload. In patients in whom right ventricular dilatation/domination is not due to increased afterload peak velocity (V) of the tricuspid regurgitation jet is not elevated, i.e., does not exceed 2.5 m/s. According to the Bernoulli equation ($\Delta P = 4V^2$), this corresponds to the peak pressure difference (ΔP) between the contracting right ventricle and right atrium below 25 mm Hg. If right ventricular dilatation and hypokynesia is due to infarction or dysplasia resulting in its depressed function, the jet velocity may be even lower. This is due both to low systolic pressure inside the right ventricle and to elevated right atrial pressure.

In acute pulmonary embolism, right ventricular pressure rises to compensate for increased afterload, and, therefore, peak velocity of tricuspid regurgitant jet is higher—usually between 2.8 and 3.8 m/s. In fact—beside right over left ventricular domination—tricuspid jet velocity in this range is another important echocardiographic sign supporting the clinical suspicion of acute pulmonary embolism. With right ventricular dilatation, tricuspid insufficiency is almost universally found with continuous wave Doppler.

According to Metz et al. (8), peak jet velocity measurements of tricuspid insufficiency was possible in 52 out of 56 patients with pulmonary embolism, and it showed excellent correlation ($r = 0.91$) with directly measured pulmonary arterial systolic pressure. Interestingly, the linear correlation coefficient between Miller index of pulmonary vascular obstruction and tricuspid jet velocity was lower than that between Miller index and the ratio of diameters of right to left ventricle as measured with echocardiography ($r = 0.43$ and 0.68, respectively). A normal, nonhypertrophied right ventricle is unable to acutely generate systolic pressure exceeding 60 mm Hg. With severe acute embolic obstruction of the pulmonary arterial bed, right ventricular failure ensues resulting in right atrial pressure rise. Thus, with increasing hemodynamic severity of pulmonary embolism, one should indeed expect an inverted J-curve rather than progressive rise of tricuspid regurgitant jet velocity. This also implies that very high velocity of the jet of tricuspid regurgitation found with Doppler echocardiography in a patient with suspected pulmonary embolism cannot be explained by an isolated embolic episode, even if massive. Peak velocity of the jet of tricuspid regurgitation exceeding 3.8 m/s (corresponding to the systolic pressure difference between the right ventricle and right atrium of 58 mm Hg) can occur only with right ventricular hypertrophy, which may be due to chronic pulmonary hypertension of any origin.

C. Acute Versus Chronic Pulmonary Hypertension

Kasper et al. (21) listed echo/Doppler criteria that should be useful for the identification of patients with acute pulmonary hypertension. The velocity of tricuspid regurgitating jet between 2.8 m/s and 3.8 m/s complied with those criteria, while lower values suggested right ventricular infarction and higher ones suggested chronic pulmonary hypertension. Right ventricular hypokynesia, dilatation (defined as RVEDD >30 mm, or >16 mm/m^2 or RVEDD > LVEDD) together with a poorly collapsing inferior vena cava, suggested either acute pulmonary hypertension or right ventricular infarction. In the former case, paradoxical interventricular septal motion, dilated right pulmonary artery (RPA >12 mm/m^2), and short acceleration time of the flow velocity curve of the right ventricular ejection (AcT <90 msec) were expected.

Tricuspid Regurgitant Jet Velocity

As already discussed, hypertrophied right ventricle may generate much higher systolic pressures before it fails than those observed during acute pulmonary embolism. Systemic or near-systemic pressures are common in primary pulmonary hypertension or chronic unresolved pulmonary embolism, while a normal right ventricle faced with increased afterload is not supposed to generate pressure above 60 mm Hg. Thus, velocity of jet of tricuspid regurgitation exceeding 3.8 m/s suggests chronic pulmonary hypertension. However, it must be remembered that moderate to severe chronic pulmonary hypertension will result in elevation of tricuspid regurgitant jet velocity of the order encountered in acute pulmonary embolism, i.e., 2.8–3.8 m/s. Assessment of right ventricular hypertrophy, right atrial pressure, and flow velocity pattern of right ventricular ejection may sometimes help in echocardiographic differentiation between acute pulmonary embolism and moderate chronic pulmonary hypertension.

Right Ventricular Hypertrophy

Right ventricular free wall may be directly interrogated for signs of hypertrophy (22). While its normal thickness is below 5 mm, it can increase twofold and more in patients with chronic right ventricular pressure overload. This would not be expected in acute cor pulmonale: Acutely failing, distended ventricle will tend to be a thin-walled one. Unfortunately, the complex shape of the right ventricle does not allow for the calculation of its mass with echocardiography (23), and even if it did, heavy trabeculation and regional variations of the right ventricular free wall thickness would interfere with reproducibility of its echocardiographic measurements (23). Even so, if repeated M-mode echocardiographic measurements of right ventricular free wall from parasternal and/or subcostal windows exceed 5 mm in the presence of a prominent moderator band, right ventricular hypertrophy is most probably present.

Interventricular Septal Motion/Position

Although there is less constraint from the pericardium, abnormal septal motion as well as its leftward displacement found in acute pulmonary embolism occur also in chronic cor pulmonale (24,25). In chronic lung diseases, one can also sometimes appreciate the inspiration-related variations of the position of the interventricular septum. This is due to marked respiration-related pressure swings within the thorax and resulting large changes in the venous return to the right heart. In this case, observation of the inferior vena cava may be helpful: In chronic cor pulmonale, it usually collapses with inspiration by at least 40%, while in acute right ventricular failure, it remains dilated regardless of the respiratory phase (21).

Doppler Assessment of the Flow Velocity of Right Ventricular Ejection

No published data exist on the changes and diagnostic implications of flow velocity pattern during right ventricular ejection in patients with pulmonary embolism.

Acceleration time (AcT) of the flow velocity in the right ventricular outflow tract is a Doppler-derived systolic time interval. Since the report by Kitabatake et al. (26), the measurement of AcT was considered an important method of noninvasive estimation of pulmonary arterial pressure. Although AcT indeed tends to be shorter with increasing pressure, the relation between these two parameters does not seem direct (26,27). Probably, the characteristics of the early phase of right ventricular ejection, including AcT, have two major determinants: pulmonary arterial input impedance and right ventricular contractility (28–30). In cases with massive pulmonary embolism, we observed a rapid early ejection and a very short AcT, apparently shorter than could have been expected for the given level of pulmonary arterial pressure in the chronic setting. This was accompanied by an early systolic deceleration of flow in the right ventricular outflow tract, with forward flow returning rather gradually in the mid and late systole (Fig. 4). The deceleration of flow during right ventricular systole is a well-known sign of severe pulmonary hypertension, attributed to the increased velocity of the pressure wave reflected from the distal pulmonary arterial bed. Turkevich et al. (31) reported that the peak deceleration occurred earlier in systole with increasing pulmonary pressure. However, even with severe pulmonary hypertension, the deceleration was observed in the midsystole, while in our patients with massive pulmonary embolism, it occurred even earlier. Those observations could be explained by the increase in pulmonary arterial characteristic impedance caused by proximal massive acute embolization and/or by a very early return of the reflected pressure wave—both phenomena interfering with the initial phase of right ventricular ejection.

IV. Intraluminal Thrombi in Patients with Pulmonary Embolism

While echocardiographic signs of right ventricular pressure overload and failure indirectly support the clinical suspicion of pulmonary embolism, ultrasound methods provide sometimes direct visualization of a thromboembolus in the right atrium, right ventricle, or major pulmonary artery.

A. Thrombi Within Proximal Pulmonary Arteries

Transthoracic Echocardiography

Before the introduction of transesophageal probes, there were few reports on thrombi detected in the proximal pulmonary arteries with echocardiography (32–34). Only Kasper et al. (21) described pulmonary arterial thrombi in as many

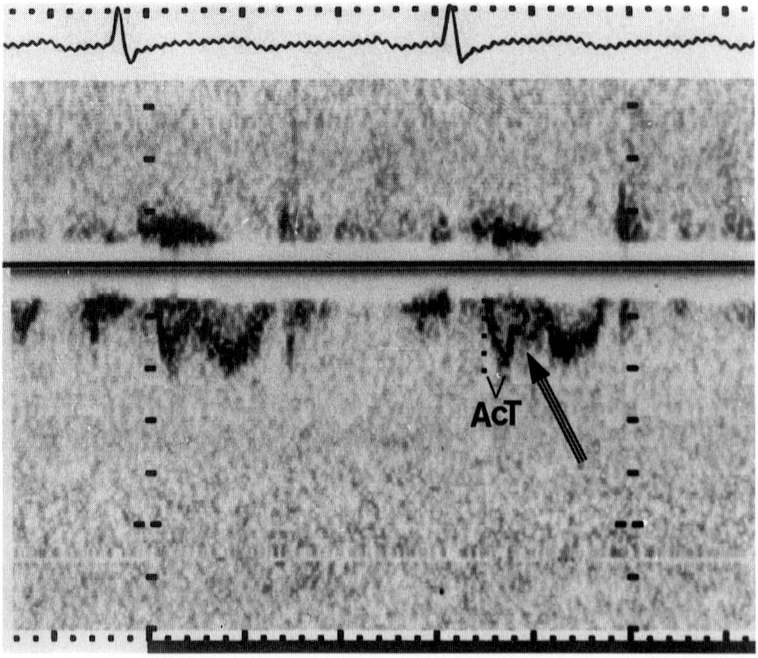

Figure 4 Flow velocity curve recorded with pulsed-wave Doppler in the right ventricular outflow tract in a patient with acute massive proximal pulmonary embolism: Very short acceleration time (AcT = 35 ms) and early systolic deceleration (arrow) despite only moderate elevation of pulmonary arterial systolic pressure (55 mm Hg). (From Ref. 69. Copyrighted and reprinted with the permission of Clinical Cardiology Publishing Co., Inc., and/or Foundation for Advances in Medicine and Science, P.O. Box 832, Mahwah, NJ 07430.)

as 20 out of 141 (14%) consecutive patients with confirmed acute or chronic pulmonary embolism. While suprasternal, subcostal, and parasternal approach were probably mostly used in their study, transesophageal echocardiography was also performed in an unspecified number of patients. No data regarding relative value of various acoustic windows were given. In three patients injections of echo-contrast were reported useful to confirm obstruction of the right pulmonary artery. Most of the thrombi described in the literature were found in the right pulmonary artery and in patients with echocardiographic signs of acute cor pulmonale. Recently, Gabrielsen et al. (35) reported on a large thrombus within the main pulmonary artery in a patient studied for left-sided valvular problems but free from signs of right ventricular overload. The patient died suddenly within a few minutes after the echocardiographic examination. Death was assigned by the authors to massive pulmonary embolism. Although no postmortem confirmation was available, the situation witnessed by Gabrielsen et al. might have corresponded to the last moments preceding an episode of the most dramatic clinical presentation of pulmonary embolism—sudden death.

Transesophageal Echocardiography

The first to report on transesophageal echocardiographic detection of right pulmonary artery thromboembolus were Nixdorf et al. (36). In some of the cases reported so far, the visualization of the clot in the main or right pulmonary artery was so suggestive that the authors decided to perform pulmonary embolectomy without angiographic confirmation (37,38). Transesophageal echocardiography was also found useful to document the disappearance of the previously observed pulmonary arterial thrombi after fibrinolytic therapy (39,40). So far, transesophageal echocardiographic visualization of pulmonary arterial thrombi was reported only in patients with massive pulmonary embolism (41). Most observations were confined to main and right pulmonary artery. In fact, proximal left pulmonary artery is shadowed by the left bronchus, which separates it from the esophagus (Fig. 5). However, with proper manipulation of the transesophageal probe, the distal part of the vessel can be identified and evaluated beyond its first branching in most of the patients in our laboratory (Fig. 6). Initially intravenous echocardiographic contrast injection was required to confirm the identification of the distal left pulmonary artery in each patient. At present, because of its characteristic pattern and position, the contrast is used only in case of doubts.

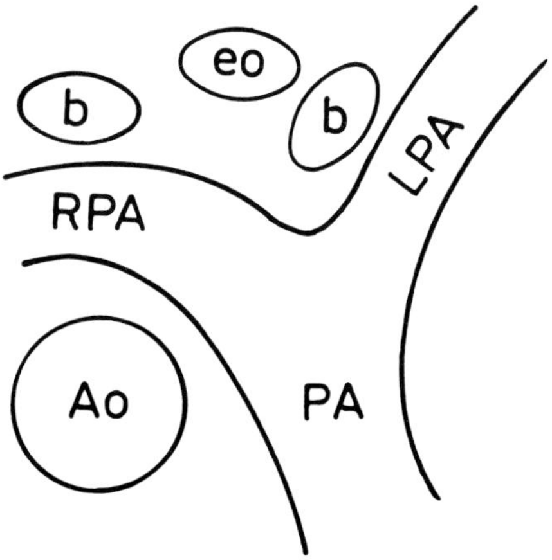

Figure 5 Main bronchi (b) do not allow for complete echocardiographic visualization of all segments of major pulmonary arteries from the esophagus (eo). Although topographic relations may vary between patients main (PA) and right pulmonary artery (RPA) as well as distal part of left pulmonary artery (LPA) can be usually assessed. Ao = ascending aorta.

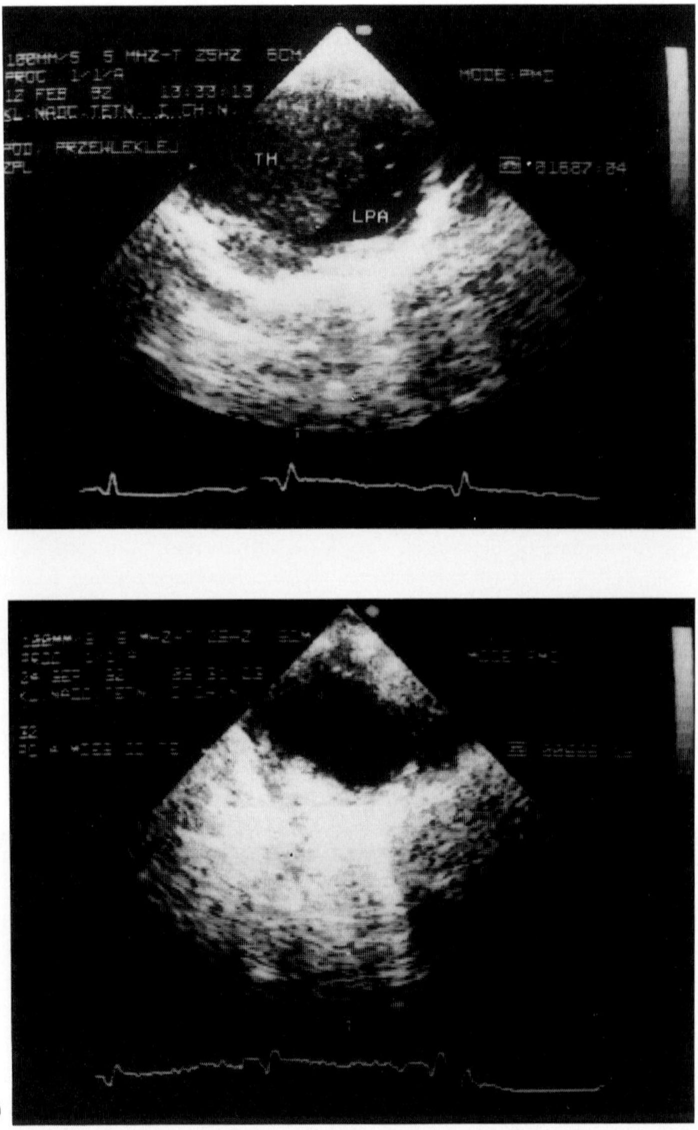

(A)

(B)

Figure 6 Transesophageal examination of the distal left pulmonary artery (LPA) near its first branching. (A) Large thrombus (TH) in a 33-year-old woman with severe chronic thromboembolic pulmonary hypertension. Three sparkling points in the vascular lumen represent microbubbles of echocardiographic contrast injected into a peripheral vein in order to confirm the identity of the vessel. (B) Irregular endothelial surface but no evidence of a thrombus on follow-up 6 weeks after successful thromboendarterectomy.

The possibility of assessment of the branching region of both left and right pulmonary arteries may increase the clinical value of transesophageal echocardiography. In fact, using this method, we recently observed pulmonary arterial thrombi not only in patients with massive proximal pulmonary embolism requiring surgery or fibrinolysis but also in hemodynamically stable patients with submassive pulmonary embolism, suitable for antithrombotic therapy (Fig. 7). Our experience is summarized in Table 1.

Intraluminal USG

Intracardiac and intravascular ultrasound studies were first reported by Cieszynski (42) in 1960. During his experiment, the ultrasonic catheter was introduced also to the main pulmonary artery of a dog, and the A-mode echoes of its walls were recorded. Modern intravascular ultrasound studies of normal pulmonary arteries in man were announced by Pandian et al. (43) in 1990. More recently, intravascular ultrasound proved useful in the diagnosis of experimental pulmonary embolism in dogs (44). Also, patients with acute (45) and chronic (46,47) pulmonary embolism were studied. Gorge et al. (46) found floating and/or adherent thrombi in all 10 patients with suspected acute pulmonary embolism. In five patients, wall adherent thrombi reducing vessel area less than 25% found at IVUS were missed by biplane pulmonary angiography. With 20-MHz transducers, vessels down to 3 mm diameter could be assessed, but pictures of the main pulmonary arteries were suboptimal. The authors concluded that IVUS may provide additional information in patients with mural pulmonary arterial

Table 1 Pulmonary Arterial Thrombi Detected with Transesophageal Echocardiography—Personal Experience

Age/sex	Pulmonary embolism type/confirmation/treatment	Right PA	Left PA
50/M	Chronic proximal/angio/surgery	Thrombus	
33/F	Chronic proximal/angio/surgery		Thrombus[a]
43/M	Chronic proximal/angio/surgery	Mural thrombus	No flow (occluding thrombus?)
75/F	Acute massive/scan/STK	Thrombus	
60/M	Acute submassive/angio/IVC filter		No flow[a] (occluding thrombus)
62/M	Acute submassive/scan/heparin	Thrombus[a]	Thrombus[a]
69/F	Acute submassive/scan/heparin	Thrombus[a]	Thrombus[a]
38/M	Chronic submassive/angio/acenocoumarol	Thrombus	

[a]Improvement after therapy confirmed by repeated TEE.

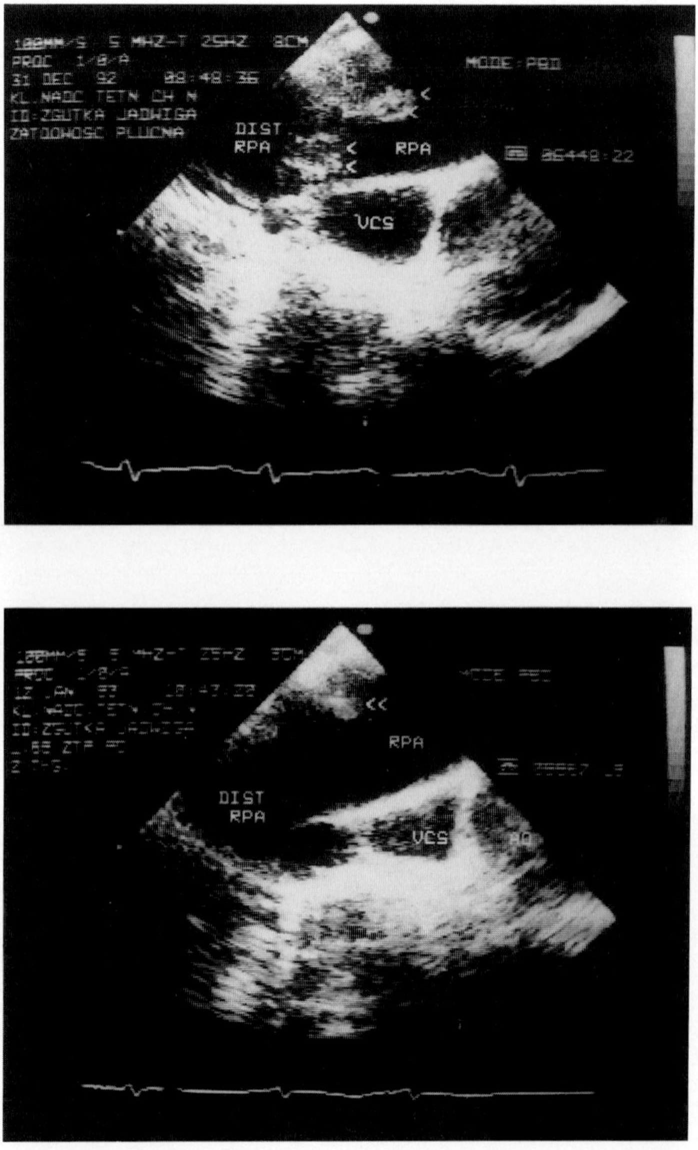

(A)

(B)

Figure 7 Transesophageal examination of the right pulmonary artery (RPA) in a 65-year-old woman with submassive pulmonary embolism: (A) Two large thrombi (arrowheads) partly occluding the vessel at the level of its passage behind vena cava superior (VCS). (B) Only a small remnant (arrowhead) of the previously extensive thrombi after 2 weeks of antithrombotic therapy (heparin followed by acenocoumarol).

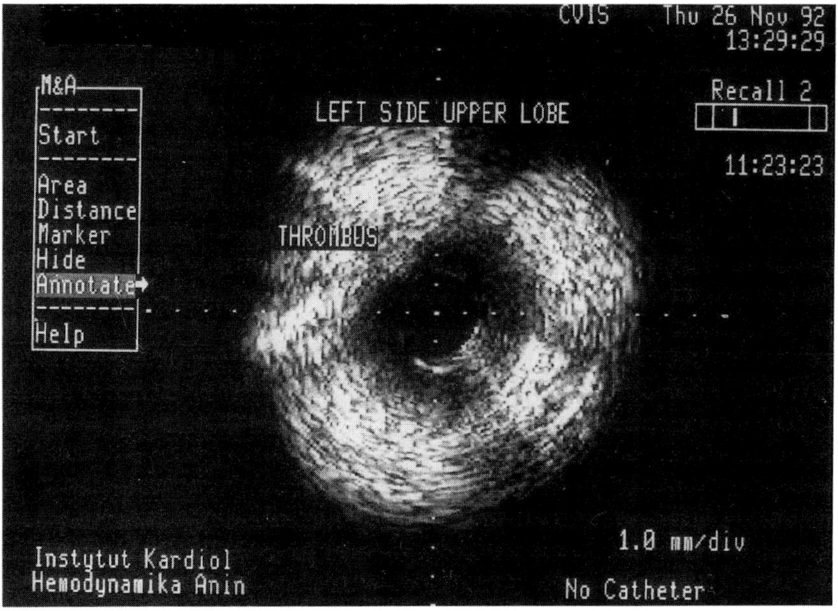

Figure 8 Intravascular ultrasound study of the left upper branch of the pulmonary artery in a 39-year-old patient with chronic pulmonary embolism. Organized mural thrombus disturbing the round shape of the arterial lumen was confirmed at surgery. (Courtesy of Dr J. Jodkowski and Dr. W. Ruzyllo, Institute of Cardiology, Warszawa.)

thrombi (Fig. 8). In their opinion, intravascular ultrasonic catheter remaining inside the pulmonary artery might prove useful in monitoring the effect of thrombolytic therapy.

Ricou et al. (47) were able to obtain intravascular ultrasound images of right pulmonary artery in 10 out of 11 patients with suspected chronic thromboembolic hypertension. Left pulmonary artery could be assessed in only three cases because of acute angulation at its origin from the main pulmonary artery. Among eight patients, changes were found in 10 vascular segments by ultrasound and in all cases confirmed at surgery. In one case a tumor (fibrous histiocytoma) was correctly suspected by intravascular ultrasound study. Among nine segments judged normal, one—within proximal right pulmonary artery—contained a clot at surgery. The authors stressed that after elimination of several technical problems, intravascular assessment of pulmonary arteries may be useful in defining surgical accessibility of chronic thromboemboli.

No complications caused by intravascular ultrasound examinations of pulmonary arteries were reported so far (42–47).

B. Right Atrial and Right Ventricular Thrombi

Right ventricular thrombi have been infrequently described (21). Typically they appeared with right ventricular infarction, in-dwelling catheters, pacemaker electrodes, etc. (Fig. 9). In a retrospective multicenter European registry (48), similar risk factors for local thrombogenesis were found in patients with right atrial thrombi that were oval, sessile, or mural and immobile. Such thrombi were often found incidentally, in the absence of clinical features suggestive of pulmonary embolism, and they responded well to thrombolytic treatment. Although 40% out of the 57 patients with right atrial thrombi of apparently intracardiac origin developed pulmonary emboli, there were no fatalities caused by pulmonary emboli in this subgroup irrespective of treatment (48). This was in sharp contrast with the outcome of patients whose right atrial thrombi had mobile and snakelike appearance (49) (Fig. 10). Out of 48 such patients, 47 (98%) had symptoms of pulmonary embolism during in-hospital observation, of which 13 were fatal (48). The 8-days' thrombus-related mortality in this group was 42% with 1/3 of the thromboembolic deaths occurring within 24 h from the echocardiographic diagnosis (Fig. 11). No local factors responsible for the in situ thrombus formation could usually be identified, while in many cases, signs of deep venous thrombosis have been noted. These observations led to the conclusion that mobile and snakelike thrombi were trapped in the right atrium on their way from the systemic veins to the pulmonary circulation (48,49). Patent foramen ovale, Chiari network, and Eustachian valve were considered as the site of entrapment, but free-floating, unattached thrombi were occasionally reported (50). Interestingly, when the outcome of patients with attached versus unattached right atrial thrombi was compared in a review, which used meta-analysis on cases reported in the literature between 1966 and 1989, no difference was found (51). It seemed that mobility, and not attachment, was of major importance for the outcome of a right atrial thrombus. Although cases of asymptomatic displacement of such thrombi to the pulmonary artery were witnessed by echocardiographers (48) (Morpurgo, personal communication), most authors point at high mortality from pulmonary embolism in the untreated patients with right atrial mobile thrombi. Farfel et al. (52) in their review found improvement of prognosis only with surgical treatment. Others, confirming relatively good results of surgery, pointed at the benefits of thrombolytic and/or anticoagulant therapy (48,49,51). Goldhaber (53) did not consider surgery among the therapeutic options at all, suggesting thrombolytic treatment. Thus, although approximately 400 cases of right atrial thrombi have been reported in the literature over last 10 years, the optimal treatment remains controversial. Despite these doubts, most authors agree that patients with mobile right atrial thrombi are at high risk of early fatal pulmonary embolism and should not be referred for pulmonary angiography but need immediate and aggressive treatment.

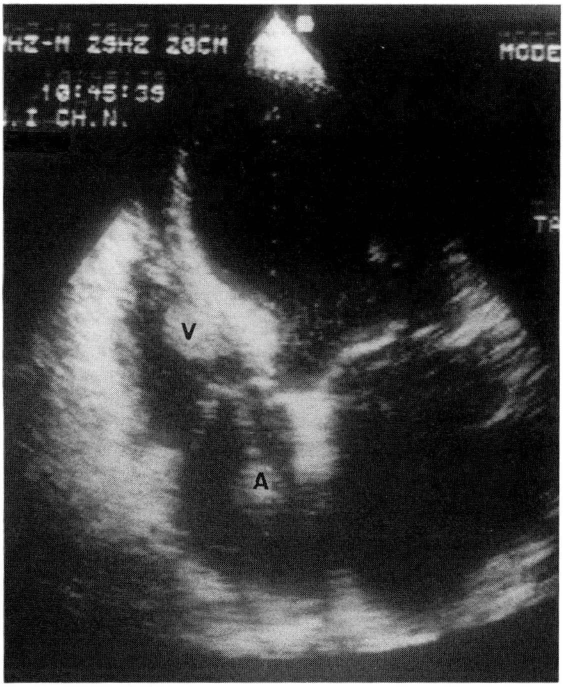

Figure 9 Right ventricular (V) and right atrial thrombus (A) along the pacing electrode in a 70-year-old patient with congestive heart failure.

While most of the cases of right heart thrombi were found with transthoracic echocardiography, Hunter et al. (54) reported on a case in which transesophageal echo showed right atrial mobile thrombus missed by standard approach. Transesophageal echocardiography was also used for real-time visualization of venous thromboemboli migrating across the right heart during orthopedic surgery (55).

V. Place of Echocardiography in Clinical Assessment of Suspected Pulmonary Embolism

A. Acute Pulmonary Embolism

Echocardiography may provide definitive diagnosis of pulmonary embolism or suggest an impending pulmonary embolism if thrombi inside major pulmonary arteries or in the right heart chambers are visualized. In the latter case,

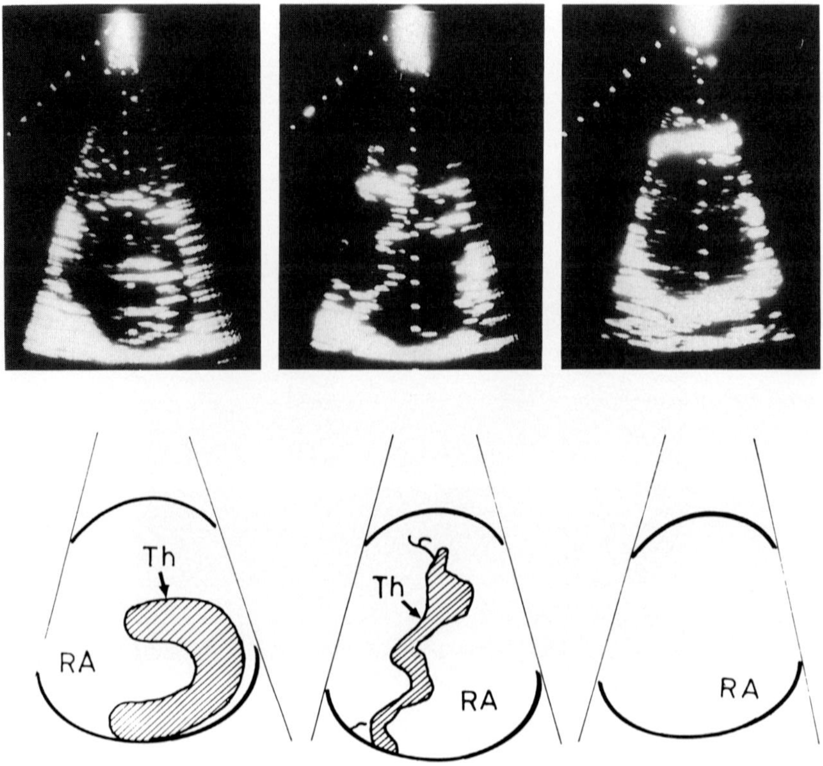

Figure 10 Highly mobile, snakelike right atrial thrombus in a 74-year-old patient with venous thromboembolism at the onset (left panel) and after 6 h of treatment with streptokinase (middle). At 24 h no trace of the thrombus could be found in the right atrium (right panel). (From Ref. 49, with permission.)

angiography is contraindicated because of risk of thrombus dislodgement; in the former case, it is not necessary. Thus, although no data are available regarding the prevalence of thrombi located within the reach of diagnostic ultrasound, transthoracic echo/Doppler followed by transesophageal echocardiographic may prove a reasonable choice in an unstable patient. This is especially so if immediate pulmonary angiography is not available or contraindicated, and thrombolytic treatment or embolectomy are considered. Even when thrombi in the pulmonary arteries are not visualized, signs of right ventricular pressure overload and failure with abnormal pulmonary arterial flow velocity pattern may reinforce the clinical suspicion. In a recent article, Bauer et al. (56) revealed that the decision to perform emergency pulmonary embolectomy was based on angiography in 15

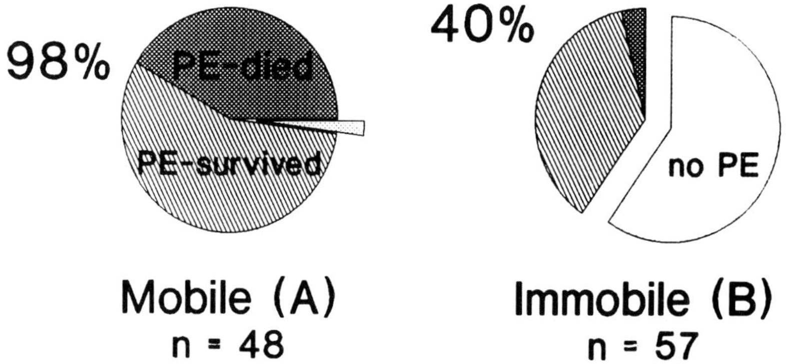

Figure 11 Prevalence of nonfatal pulmonary embolism (PE-survived) and embolism-related in-hospital mortality (PE-died) according to the mobility of right atrial thrombus as assessed by echocardiography. (Based on Multicenter European Study, Ref. 48, with permission.)

cases, on lung scan in 6, and on echocardiographic findings in 10 out of 44 patients treated with this method between 1978 and 1990 in their center. If thrombolytic therapy is considered without angiographic confirmation, echocardiography may be useful in excluding cardiac tamponade or aortic aneurysm and dissection. The latter was reported to cause unilateral compression of pulmonary artery resulting in acute cor pulmonale with false positive pulmonary angiogram for pulmonary embolism (57, 58) (M. Brochier, personal communication). Thus, transesophageal echocardiography might be useful before fibrinolysis is started in a patients with important risk factors for aortic dissection. Contrast echocardiography may provide information about the patency of foramen ovale in patients with acute pulmonary embolism. Recently Kasper et al. (59) reported on worse prognosis in this subgroup and higher prevalence of systemic emboli. Whether these patients may have higher prevalence of paradoxical subclinical cerebral emboli, increasing the risk of intracerebral bleeding during fibrinolytic treatment remains to be determined. If it was so, patients with pulmonary embolism and patent foramen ovale at contrast echocardiography should be treated preferably with heparin and/or evaluated for subclinical intracerebral lesions prior to fibrinolysis.

Echo/Doppler may provide data on cardiac output, useful in monitoring of patients with acute pulmonary embolism (60,61). However, topographic changes caused by the enlarged right ventricle may interfere with Doppler measurements of cardiac output at mitral or aortic valve level. The recording of the flow velocity in the ascending aorta with the probe in the suprasternal notch may sometimes prove useful. The abnormal pattern of right ventricular ejection together with dilatation of the right ventricular outflow tract resulting in low-flow velocities would probably increase the error in calculation of cardiac output at this level.

B. Chronic Pulmonary Embolism

Two types of chronic pulmonary embolism have been identified: the controversial small-vessel and the proximal-massive-unresolved (62). Both result in chronic pulmonary hypertension and ultimately in right ventricular failure. Echocardiography and Doppler provide clues for the diagnosis and quantification of the severity of pulmonary hypertension (63). Once pulmonary hypertension is diagnosed, echocardiography should help in excluding the possibility of postcapillary lesions and congenital heart disease. While severe malformations are usually obvious, sinus venosus defect or pulmonary venous abnormalities should always be thoroughly sought, including transesophageal echocardiographic evaluation if necessary. The diagnosis of chronic major-vessel thromboembolic pulmonary hypertension is of special importance because the patient can be cured definitely by thromboendarterectomy (62,64). Using transesophageal echocardiography and simultaneous direct pressure measurements, Dittrich et al. (65,66) showed that both right heart geometry and left ventricular filling improved immediately after the extraction of the obstructing thrombus and normalization of the right ventricular end diastolic pressure. Proximally located, organized thrombi can be sometimes seen with transthoracic and more readily with transesophageal echocardiography, while more distal thrombi are accessible with intravascular ultrasound. In both cases, proximal left pulmonary artery is more difficult to study than the right. Although pulmonary angiography is obligatory for the diagnosis of chronic thrombotic occlusion of proximal pulmonary arteries, it may be both false negative and dangerous in patients with severe pulmonary hypertension (67). Ultrasound methods may provide additional information especially in case of nonoccluding mural thrombi. Negative transesophageal and intravascular ultrasound studies for massive chronic proximal pulmonary embolism might in the future save the risks related to contrast injection in patients with primary pulmonary hypertension or recurrent small-vessel pulmonary emboli unsuitable for surgical treatment.

Primary sarcoma of the pulmonary artery may resemble chronic pulmonary embolism both clinically and angiographically. Although data on echocardiographic contribution to the differential diagnosis of this rare entity are limited to four cases studied with transthoracic echocardiography, transesophageal approach may be a promising method of visualization of this intravascular tumor usually located in the proximal right or left pulmonary arteries (68).

VI. Summary

Echocardiography with Doppler provides valuable information at the bedside of patients with suspected pulmonary embolism.

The most apparent M-mode and two-dimensional echocardiographic changes during pulmonary embolism consist of flattening or leftward bulging of the interventricular septum with right ventricular hypokinesis, dilatation, and domination over the left ventricle. These changes reflect increased right ventricular afterload and its subsequent failure. Pulmonary embolism may have such hemodynamic consequences when at least 40% of the pulmonary arterial bed is obliterated. Thus, echocardiography may be unrelevant in minor pulmonary embolism.

While intensity of echocardiographic changes correlate with the hemodynamic severity of major embolic episodes in patients free from preexisting cardiorespiratory disorders, the latter may sometimes result in similar M-mode and two-dimensional echocardiographic changes. Doppler echocardiographic methods of estimation of right ventricular afterload based on measurements of peak velocity of the jet of tricuspid regurgitation and on analysis of flow velocity curve in the right ventricular outflow tract may be of help: When Doppler measurement of tricuspid jet velocity indicates low to normal right ventricular systolic pressure, right ventricular dilatation should be attributed to its infarction or dysplasia/cardiomyopathy. Very high-peak velocity of the jet of tricuspid regurgitation is diagnostic for chronic pulmonary hypertension. Coexisting normal diameter and collapsibility of the inferior vena indicating normal right heart filling pressures make superimposed acute pulmonary embolic episode unlikely. Unfortunately, Doppler echocardiography does not permit excluding such an episode as a cause of decompensation of chronic cor pulmonale. On the other hand, acute increase of pulmonary arterial input impedance suggested by severely disturbed pattern of flow velocity curve in the right ventricular outflow tract in the presence of only moderate elevation of peak velocity of tricuspid regurgitation jet generated by a nonhypertrophied right ventricle suggests acute pulmonary embolism rather than chronic pulmonary hypertension, especially when accompanied by noncollapsing, distended inferior vena cava.

Direct echocardiographic visualization of intraluminal thrombi in patients with suspected pulmonary embolism is not frequent. However, echocardiographic diagnosis of a thrombus within major pulmonary arteries seems as reliable as it is in other vascular compartments and may be considered as definite confirmation of proximal pulmonary embolism. Transesophageal echocardiography and intravascular ultrasound may even prove superior to angiography in the diagnosis of flat mural chronic pulmonary arterial thrombi and in the differential diagnosis of tumor invasion of the pulmonary artery.

Echocardiography permits one to diagnose right ventricular and right atrial thrombi as well as may identify those trapped inside right heart chambers on their way from the peripheral veins to the pulmonary artery. Unlike thrombi of intracardiac origin, thrombi in transit are snakelike in appearence and highly mobile, and require prompt aggressive treatment without any further diagnostic evaluation because of a very high risk of early massive pulmonary embolism.

Even when echocardiography provides only indirect signs compatible with hemodynamic consequences of pulmonary embolism, it may be successfully used to search for and exclude most of the potential acute cardiovascular disorders that may mimic pulmonary embolism, including aortic dissection or hemopericardium. In an unstable patient requiring immediate treatment without the possibility of definite confirmation of pulmonary embolism, such information is of great importance.

Thus, although neither sensitive nor highly specific (except for cases of direct visualization of intraluminal thrombi), echocardiography with Doppler is still very helpful in the initial evaluation of a patient with suspected pulmonary embolism.

References

1. Conference de consensus. Diagnostic de l'embolie pulmonaire. Ann Cardiol Angeiol 1990; 39:357–62.
2. PIOPED Investigators. Value of the ventilation/perfusion scan in acute pulmonary embolism. JAMA 1990; 263:2753–9.
3. Copper TJ, Hayward MV, Hartog M. Survey on the use of pulmonary scintigraphy and angiography for suspected pulmonary thromboembolism in the UK. Clin Radiol 1991; 43:243–5.
4. Kasper W, Meinertz T, Henkel B, Eissner D, Hahn K, Hoffman T, Zeiher A, Just H. Echocardiographic findings in patients with proved pulmonary embolism. Am Heart J 1986; 112:1284–90.
5. Jardin F, Lacombe P, Dubourg O, Delorme G, Hardy A, Beauchet A. Echocardiographie bidimensionnelle quantitative au cours de l'embolie pulmonaire aigue. Presse Med 1991; 20:2085–9.
6. Jardin F. Letter to the editor. Presse Med 1992; 21:439.
7. Walsh PN, Greenspan RH, Simon M, Simon AL, Hyers TM, Woosley PC, Cole CM. An angiographic severity index for pulmonary embolism. Circulation 1973; 47(suppl II):101.
8. Metz D, Chapoutot L, Chabert JP, Laudinat JM, Doucet J, Bajolet A. Diagnostic value of echo Doppler in the assessment of the severity of acute pulmonary embolism. Eur Heart J 1990; 11:1860. Abstract.
9. Miller GAH, Sutton GC, Kerr IH, Gibson RV, Honey M. Comparison of streptokinase and heparin in treatment of isolated acute massive pulmonary embolism. Br Med J 1971; 2:681–4.

10. Jardin F, Dubourg O, Gueret P, Delorme G, Bourdarias J-P. Quantitative two-dimensional echocardiography in massive pulmonary embolism: emphasis on ventricular interdependence and leftward septal displacement. J Am Coll Cardiol 1987; 10:1201–6.
11. Come PC, Kim D, Parker A, Goldhaber S, Braunwald E, Markis JE. Early reversal of right ventricular dysfunction in patients with acute pulmonary embolism after treatment with intravenous tissue plasminogen activator. Am J Coll Cardiol 1987; 10:971–8.
12. Castillo-Fenoy A, Scheuble C, Benacerraf A, Brau J, Cereze P. Semeiologie echocardiographique de l'embolie pulmonaire aigue. Arch Mal Coeur 1980; 73:971–77.
13. Bouvier JL, Benichou M, Antar M, Elias A, LeCorff G, Vaillant A, Goudard A, Serradimigni A. Detection par echocardiographie de thrombus des cavites droites dans l'embolie pulmonaire aigue. Arch Mal Coeur 1987; 80:1441–6.
14. Vardan S, Mookherjee S, Smulyan HS, Obeid AI. Echocardiography in pulmonary embolism. 1983; 24:67–78.
15. Chan KL, Currie PJ, Seward JB, Hagler DJ, Mair DD, Tajik AJ. Comparison of three Doppler ultrasound methods in the prediction of pulmonary artery pressure. J Am Coll Cardiol 1987; 9:549–54.
16. Currie PJ, Seward JB, Chan KL, Fyfe DA, Hagler DJ, Mair DD, Reeder GS, Nishimura RA, Tajik JA. Continuous wave Doppler determination of right ventricular pressure: a simultaneous Doppler-catheterization study in 127 patients. J Am Coll Cardiol 1985; 6:750–6.
17. Berger M, Haimowitz A, Van Tosh A, Berdoff RL, Goldberg E. Quantitative assessment of pulmonary hypertension in patients with tricuspid regurgitation using continuous wave ultrasound. J Am Coll Cardiol 1985; 6:359–65.
18. Michelsen S, Hurlen M, Otterstad JE. Prevalence of tricuspid and pulmonary regurgitation diagnosed by Doppler in apparently healthy women. Possible influence on their physical performance? Eur Heart J 1988; 9:61–7.
19. Nakao S, Come PC, McKay R, Ransil BJ. Effects of positional changes on inferior vena caval size and dynamics and correlations with right-sided pressure. Am J Cardiol 1987; 59:125–32.
20. Simonson JS, Schiller NB. Sonospirometry: a new method for noninvasive estimation of mean right atrial pressure based on two-dimensional echographic measurements of the inferior vena cava during measured inspiration. J Am Coll Cardiol 1988; 11:557–64.
21. Kasper W, Geibel A, Tiede K, Hofmann T, Meinertz T, Just H. Die Echokardiographie in der Diagnostic der Lungembolie. Herz 1989; 14:82–101.
22. Prakash R, Matsukubo H. Usefulness of echocardiographic right ventricular measurements in estimating right ventricular hypertrophy and right ventricular pressure. Am J Cardiol 1983; 51:1036–40.
23. Foale R, Nihoyannopoulos P, McKenna W, Klienebenne A, Nadazdin A, Rowland E, Smith G. Echocardiographic measurement of the normal adult right ventricle. Br Heart J 1986; 56:33–44.
24. Tanaka H, Tei C, Nakao S, Tahaza M, Sakurai S, Kashima T, Kanehiso T. Diastolic bulging of the interventricular septum toward the left ventricle. An

echocardiographic manifestation of negative interventricular pressure gradient between left and right ventricle during diastole. Circulation 1980; 62:558–63.
25. Torbicki A, Hawrylkiewicz I, Zielinski J. Value of M-mode echocardiography in assessing pulmonary arterial pressure in patients with chronic lung disease. Bull Eur Physiopathol Respir 1987; 23:233–9.
26. Kitabatake A, Inoue M, Asao M, Masuyama T, Tanouchi J, Morita T, Mishima M, Uematsu M, Shimazu T, Hori M, Abe H. Non-invasive evaluation of pulmonary hypertension by a pulsed wave Doppler technique. Circulation 1983; 68:302–9.
27. Torbicki A, Tramarin R, Fracchia C, Mortara A, Ambrosino N, Pozzoli M, Rampulla C, Cobelli C. Reliability of pulsed wave Doppler monitoring of acute changes in pulmonary arterial pressure in patients with COPD. In: Widimsky J, Herget J, eds. Pulmonary Blood Vessels in Lung Disease. Progr. Resp. Res. Basel: Karger, 1990:26,133–41.
28. Matsuda M, Sekiguchi T, Sugishita Y, Kuwako K, Iida K, Ito I. Reliability of non-invasive estimates of pulmonary hypertension by pulsed Doppler echocardiography. Br Heart J; 1986; 56:158–64.
29. Mohiaddin R, Paz S, Theodoropoulos S, Longmore D, Yacoub M. Magnetic resonance flow measurement in the pulmonary arteries of patients with single lung transplantation. Eur Heart J 1990; 11:329. Abstract.
30. Vaska K, Sagar K, Wann LS. Pulmonary Doppler ultrasound depends on right ventricular inotropic state as well as pulmonary artery systolic pressure. Circulation 1988; 78(suppl II):402. Abstract.
31. Turkevich D, Groves BM, Micco A, Trapp JA. Early partial systolic closure of the pulmonic valve relates to severity of pulmonary hypertension. Am Heart J 1988; 115:409–18.
32. Busch U, Wirtzfeld A, Sebening H, von Bibra H, Petrik M. Pulmonary and intracardiac embolectomy based on echocardiographic findings. J Clin Ultrasound 1985; 13:949.
33. DiCarlo LA, Schiller NB, Herfkens RL, Brundage BJ, Lipton MJ. Noninvasive detection of proximal pulmonary artery thrombosis by two-dimensional echocardiography and computerized tomography. Am Heart J 1982; 104:879.
34. Erbel R, Schweizer P, Effert S. Direkter ein- und zweidimensionaler echokardiographischer Nachweis einer akuten Lungenarterienembolie. Dtsch Med Wschr 1981; 106:179.
35. Gabrielsen F, Schmidt A, Eggeling T, Hoeher M, Kochs M, Hombach V. Massive main pulmonary artery embolism diagnosed with two-dimensional Doppler echocardiography. Clin Cardiol 1992; 15:545–6.
36. Nixdorf U, Erbel R, Drexler M, Meyer J. Detection of thromboembolus of the right pulmonary artery by transesophageal two-dimensional echocardiography. Am J Cardiol 1988; 61:488.
37. Klein AL, Steward WC, Cosgrove DM, Mick MJ, Salcedo E. Visualization of acute pulmonary emboli by transesophageal echocardiography. J Am Soc Echocardiogr 1990; 3:412–5.
38. Deleuze P, Saada M, DePaulis R, Brochard L, Mazzucotelli JP, Rotman N, Loisance DY, Cachera JP. Intraoperative transesophageal echocardiography for

pulmonary embolectomy without cardiopulmonary by-pass. Ann Thorac Surg 1991; 52:137–8.
39. Dall'Aglio V, Nicolosi GL, Zanuttini D. Transthoracic and transesophageal echocardiographic documentation of disappearence of massive right atrial and pulmonary artery thromboemboli after fibrinolytic therapy and normalization of left ventricular dimensions and function. Eur Heart J 1990; 11:863–5.
40. Gelernt MD, Mogtader A, Hahn RT. Transesophageal echocardiography to diagnose and demonstrate resolution of an acute massive pulmonary embolus. Chest 1992; 102:297–9.
41. Popovic AD, Milanovic B, Nescovic AN, Pavlovski K, Putnikovic B, Hadzagic I. Detection of massive pulmonary embolism by transesophageal echocardiography. Cardiology 1992; 80:94–9.
42. Cieszynski T. Intracardiac method of ultrasonic heart structure investigation. Arch Imm Ter Dosw 1960; 8:551–7.
43. Pandian N, Weintraub A, Kreis A, Schwartz S, Konstam M, Salem D. Intracardiac, intravascular, high frequency ultrasound imaging of pulmonary artery and its branches in human and animals. Circulation 1990; 81:2007–12.
44. Tapson VF, Davidson CJ, Gurbel PA, Sheikh KH, Kisslo KB, Stack RS. Rapid and accurate diagnosis of pulmonary emboli in a canine model using intravascular ultrasound imaging. Chest 1991; 100:1410–3.
45. Gorge G, Erbel R, Schuster S, Ge J, Meyer J. Intravascular ultrasound in patients with acute pulmonary embolism: Comparison to angiography. J Am Coll Cardiol 1992; 19:314A.
46. Gorge G, Erbel R, Ge J, Schuster S, Wittlich N, Meyer J. Value of intravascular ultrasound for differential diagnosis of pulmonary hypertension. Abstracts 5th Mainz-Mayo Symposium "New Technologies in Cardiovascular Ultrasound," October 18–21, 1992, Mainz.
47. Ricou F, Nicod PH, Moser KM, Peterson KL. Catheter-based intravascular ultrasound imaging of chronic thromboembolic pulmonary disease. Am J Cardiol 1991; 67:749–52.
48. The European Working Group on Echocardiography. The European cooperative study on the clinical significance of right heart thrombi. Eur Heart J 1989; 10:1046–59.
49. Torbicki A, Pasierski T, Uchman B, Miskiewicz Z. Right atrial mobile thrombi: two dimensional echocardiographic diagnosis and clinical outcome. Cor Vasa 1987; 29:293–303.
50. Pasierski TJ, Alton ME, VanFossen DB, Pearson AC. Right atrial mobile thrombus: improved visualization by transesophageal echocardiography. Am Heart J 1992; 123:802–3.
51. Kinney EL, Wright RJ. Efficacy of treatment of patients with echocardiographically detected right sided thrombi: a meta-analysis. Am Heart J 1989; 110:569–73.
52. Farfel Z, Shechter M, Vered Z, Rath S, Goor D, Gafni J. Review on echocardiographically diagnosed right heart entrapment of pulmonary emboli-in-transit with emphasis on management. Am Heart J 1987; 113:171–8.

53. Goldhaber ZS. Optimal strategy for diagnosis and treatment of pulmonary embolism due to right atrial thrombus. Mayo Clin Proc 1988; 63:1261–4.
54. Hunter JJ, Johnson KR, Karagianes TG, Dittrich HC. Detection of massive pulmonary embolus-in-transit by transesophageal echocardiography. Chest 1991; 100:1210–14.
55. Mohanty N, Campbell D, McGrath B, Hsla J. Transesophageal echocardiographic visualization of pulmonary emboli during orthopedic surgery. Circulation 1992; 86(suppl I):193.
56. Bauer EP, Laske A, von Seggeser LK, Carrel T, Turina MI. Early and late results after surgery for massive pulmonary embolism. Thorac Cardiovasc Surg 1991; 39:353–6.
57. Heizel MV, Schindler G. A dissecting aortic aneurysm with unilateral compression of the pulmonary artery. Radiologe 1989; 29:282–4.
58. Taams MA, Gussenhoven WJ, Bos E, Roelandt J. Saccular aneurysm of the transverse thoracic aorta detected by transesophageal echocardiography. Chest 1988; 93:436–7.
59. Kasper W, Tiede N, Geibel A, Konstantinidis S, Just H. Clinical relevance of a patent forame ovale in patients with hemodynamic active pulmonary embolism. Circulation 1991; (suppl II):452.
60. Labovitz AJ, Williams GA. Doppler Echocardiography: The Quantitative Approach. Labovitz AJ, Williams GA, eds. Philadelphia: Lea & Febiger, 1988:85–95.
61. Torbicki A, Tramarin R, Fracchia C, Mortara A, Ambrosino A, Pozzoli M, Rampulla C, Cobelli C. Simultaneous Doppler and thermodilution assessment of pulmonary artery flow during acute interventions in patients with COPD. Cor Vasa 1990; 32:197–205.
62. Moser KM, Auger WR, Fedullo PF. Chronic major-vessel thromboembolic pulmonary hypertension. Circulation 1990; 81:1735–43.
63. Torbicki A, Tramarin R. Noninvasive assessment of pulmonary arterial pressure with ultrasound. CV World Report 1990; 3:84–90.
64. Rich S, Levitsky S, Brundage BH. Pulmonary hypertension from chronic pulmonary embolism. Ann Int Med 1988; 108:425–34.
65. Dittrich Hc, Nicod PH, Chow LC, Chappuis FP, Moser KM, Peterson KL. Early changes of right heart geometry after pulmonary thromboendarterectomy. J Am Coll Cardiol 1988; 11:937–43.
66. Dittrich Hc, Nicod PH, Thomas CT, Dembitsky WP, Moser KM. Acute intraoperative changes in cardiac geometry and left ventricular diastolic filling during surgical reduction of severe right ventricular pressure in man. J Am Coll Cardiol 1990; 15(suppl A):244. Abstract.
67. Brown KT, Bach AM. The paucity of angiographic findings despite extensive organized thrombus in chronic thromboembolic pulmonary hypertension. J Vasc Interv Radiology 1992; 3:99–102.
68. Kruger I, Borowski A, de Dievie ER, Theissen P, Gross-Fengels W. Symptoms, diagnosis and therapy of primary sarcomas of the pulmonary artery. Thorac Cardiovasc Surg 1990; 38:91–95.
69. Torbicki A, Tramarin R, Morpurgo M. Role of Echo/Doppler in the diagnosis of pulmonary embolism. Clin Cardiol 1992; 15:805–10.

14

Pulmonary Angiography in Pulmonary Embolism

MIREILLE L. BROCHIER

University of Tours
Tours, France

I. Introduction

Pulmonary angiography was until recently considered the "gold standard" for the diagnosis of pulmonary embolism despite the fact it is an invasive technique. This is due to the fact that neither standard chest radiology, hemodynamic data, nor radionuclear methods, alone or together, are specific enough for pulmonary embolism diagnosis. Pulmonary angiogram visualizes directly intrapulmonary thrombus or thrombi. As early as 1933, de Carvalho and Moniz (1), using in vivo angiography, detected intrapulmonary artery thrombi. Nonetheless, technical difficulties were responsible for the delay in developing pulmonary angiography. It was necessary to await development of new catheters; improved, more powerful X-ray generators and nonionic, well-tolerated dye products to use pulmonary arteriography routinely and safely in patients suspected for pulmonary embolism. The first large series of patients to be studied by pulmonary angiography because of suspected pulmonary embolism was reported by Williams and Wilcox (2) in 1963, followed by Sasahara et al. (3), who were the first to use selective pulmonary angiography. Pulmonary angiography has been until now considered highly desirable before any decision was made for major treatment such as thrombolysis or embolectomy.

II. Pulmonary Angiography as Reference Technique

The justification for pulmonary angiography as a referred technique for pulmonary embolism is mainly due to the low specificity of bedside clinical data and standard chest roentgenogram for clinically suspected pulmonary embolism. Ventilation-perfusion scanning mismatch in individual patients can increase the probability of acute embolism if segmental or larger perfusion defects are associated with normal ventilation scanning, but matching defects cannot be used to exclude the diagnosis of pulmonary embolism (4) (see Chap. 12).

Compared to perfusion lung scanning, the pulmonary angiography assesses both arterial obstruction and lobar or segmental perfusion defect, whereas lung scan assesses only perfusion defects and ignores intraarterial obstruction (Fig. 1A,B). Thus, lung scans usually underestimate pulmonary embolism severity (5). Moreover, a nonperfused deep area of 2 or 3 cm might be not detected by perfusion scanning. Also, a partial (<50%) arterial obstruction without reduction of blood flow does not impair lung perfusion. In the PIOPED study (6), interobserver variability was as much as 30% for classifying intermediate- and low-probability scan results. Therefore, pulmonary angiography was routinely done until now in most major multicenter trials for pulmonary embolism. Nevertheless, the practical issue for the clinician is the limited availability of pulmonary angiography, which requires special expertise and equipment not found in many hospitals. Further, the diagnostic accuracy of angiography in community practice is unknown compared with that in the major medical centers where most reported studies have been conducted (7). According to the patients with suspected pulmonary embolism admitted in some centers, a subset of 20% of patients might be unable to have pulmonary angiography because of life-threatening cardiac or respiratory illnesses (4). The only noninvasive technique able to confirm the presence of a clot in a large branch of pulmonary artery is echocardiography (see Chap. 13), especially transesophageal echo, but the percentage of positive echos for detection of intrapulmonary clots is low (15%–25%), whereas other abnormalities of echo are not specific.

A. Methods

Selective pulmonary angiography is the technique of choice to assess patients with suspected pulmonary embolism usually after chest X-ray and perfusion lung scanning as first screening tests, and more and more often after echocardiography.

Access may be through either a brachial or a femoral route. Brachial injection is easy, safe, and reduces local complications. Femoral route has the advantage to allow inferior vena cava angiography concomitantly. Arterial pressure measurements in right cavities and pulmonary artery are compulsory

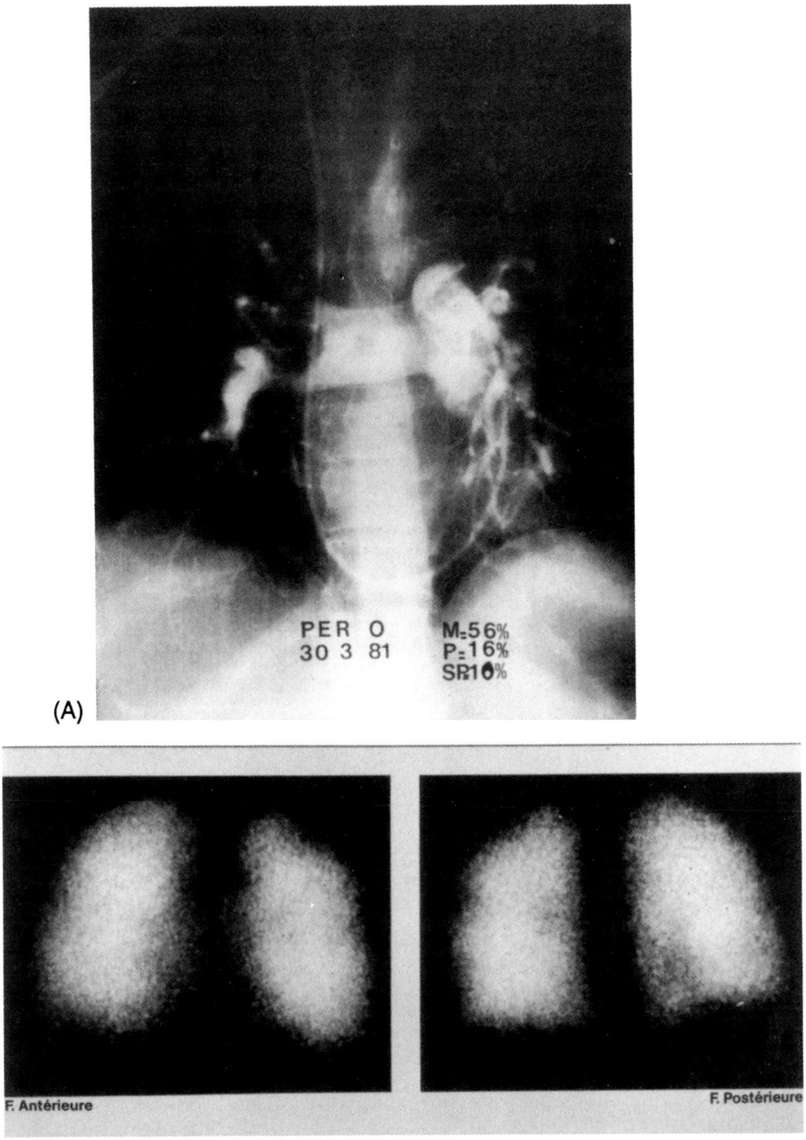

Figure 1 (A) Pulmonary angiogram showing large thrombus in the right proximal pulmonary artery (cut-off aspect), a constant filling defect into the main pulmonary trunk, and a partially obstructive thrombus in the left branch, whereas peripheral pulmonary vascularization is only reduced. Miller's index 56%, angiographic capillary flow 16%. (B) (Same patient as Fig. 1A.) Perfusion lung scan performed the same day showing a near normal pulmonary perfusion.

before dye-contrast injection especially in patients with previous pulmonary hypertension or chronic respiratory disease.

It is advisable to avoid injection in pulmonary trunk when end diastolic right ventricle pressure is >20 mm Hg and/or when main pulmonary artery pressure is >50 mm Hg. After collection of the usual serial hemodynamic data, the 6 or 7 French catheter is positioned in the main pulmonary artery. Contrast medium (usually a nonionic dye contrast) is injected with a powerful injector at a rate of 30–40 mL/s for a total dose of 1 mL/kg. All filming is made in the anteroposterior position with a serial film changer at a minimum rate of three to four films per second. Additional selective views are performed in case of doubtful identification of emboli, the choice to perform successive views being guided by previous lung scan abnormalities. Profile view is the best one to see the basal pyramid arteries. In order to obtain a good opacification of 6-order pulmonary branches and pulmonary parenchyma, the flow injection is about 20 mL/s for digital substraction angiography and 30–40 mL/s for conventional pulmonary angiography with a total dose <100mL.

B. Results of Pulmonary Angiography in Pulmonary Embolism

Among the four main angiographic abnormalities previously demonstrated in experimental pulmonary embolism studies are (a) intraarterial filling defects, (b) cutoffs of arteries, (c) areas of oligemia, and (d) asymmetry of flow; only the first and the second ones are specific for the diagnosis of pulmonary embolism (Fig. 1A). The third and the fourth abnormalities may occur in patients having chronic lung or congestive heart diseases without any pulmonary embolism. Oligemia is frequent in emphysematous patients, and asymmetry of flow is often seen in patients with left ventricular failure or in patients with mitral stenosis, whereas even in patients with chronic lung disease or congestive heart failure, constant filling defects and cutoffs of arteries occur only in patients with pulmonary embolism (8).

Therefore, constant intraarterial filling defects and cutoffs of arteries are considered as "direct" and specific, allowing confirmation of the partial or total arterial occlusion, whereas areas of oligemia and asymmetry of flow that reflect "indirect" disturbance of flow are not specific for pulmonary embolism and are even sometimes artifactual. The right lower lung is the most common site of embolism, followed closely by the left lower lung, then by the upper right lung (9).

III. Qualitative and Quantitative Assessment of Pulmonary Angiography

Qualitative assessment of severity is differently estimated according to the centers. Some authors consider that pulmonary embolism can be defined as "massive" with at least two lobar lacks of perfusion then lobar, segmental, or subsegmental defects (10), whereas for others, more than 50% of lung perfusion defects are required for "massive pulmonary embolism" qualitative assessment (5).

Quantitative assessment of severity is useful in order to provide guidelines for management and therapeutic strategy. Two scores have been proposed by Miller et al. (11) and by Walsh et al. (12), respectively:

Miller's Index (11)

Miller et al. proposed in 1971 a quantitative assessment of both artery obstruction and pulmonary filling defect (Fig. 2). Right pulmonary artery was considered as

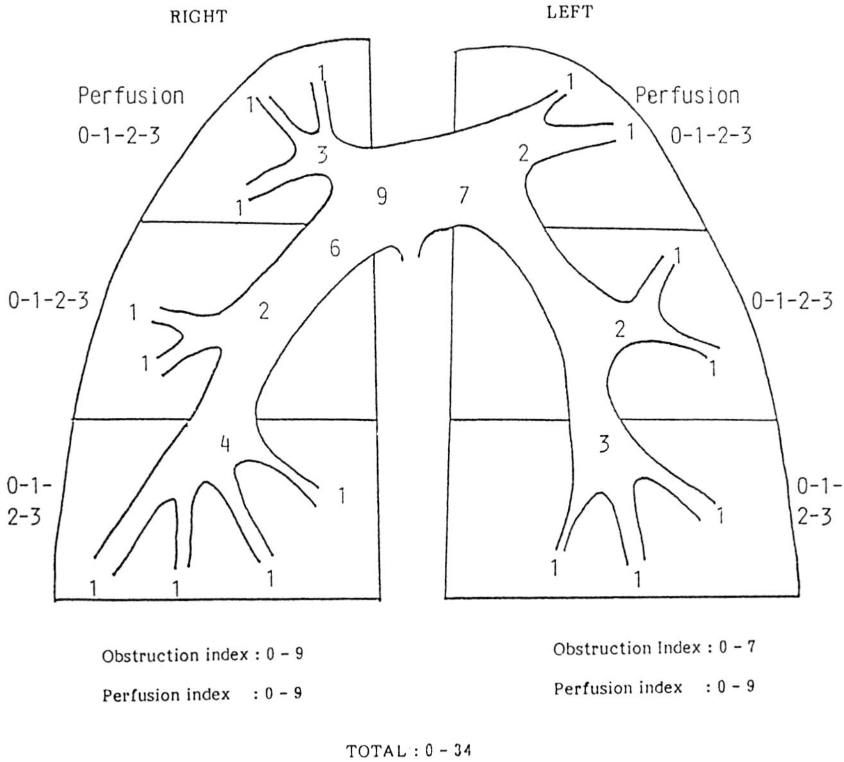

Figure 2 Miller's index scheme. Every thrombus visible in a branch of pulmonary artery whether obstructive or not is taken into account with a score depending upon the thrombus location (1–9). Pulmonary areas are divided in three zones for capillary flow with a score of 0 (normal) to 3 (total capillary filling defect).

nine segmental arteries (three for upper lobar artery, two for middle, and four for lower lobar artery). Left pulmonary artery was considered as seven segmental arteries (two for upper, two for lingula, three for lower lobar artery); thus, the maximum score for artery obstruction was 9 for the right lung and 7 for the left lung whereas for perfusion defect each lung area (up, middle, and low) had a normal score of 0 and an abnormal score of perfusion defect increasing from 1 to 3 with a maximum score of 9 for each lung. Thus, the global score was 34. This quantification, although open to criticism, allows to assess both the arterial obstruction and perfusion defect rate. The total score of 17/34 or more (>50%) characterizes massive pulmonary embolism. In the UKEP (13), the threshold given for submassive was 14/34 (41%) and for massive was 20/34 (60%).

Walsh's Index (12)

In order to express change of angiographic abnormalities objectively and quantitatively before and after therapy (thrombolytics or heparin therapy), Walsh et al. (12) developed an objective angiographic score for pulmonary embolism. Obstruction score depended upon the vessel involved (Table 1), and a perfusion defect received a score on the basis of anatomical location (Table 2). This score was used in the UPET trial (9) and was considered helpful to classify patients, predict prognosis, plan clinical studies, and assess treatment effects.

Interobserver agreement between experts has been estimated to be 80%–

Table 1 Walsh's Index—Obstruction Score

Vessel involved	Score for each obstruction
Main pulmonary artery	9
Intermediate artery	6
Lobar artery	
Upper	3
Middle (or lingular)	2
Lower	4
Segmental	1

Table 2 Walsh's Index—Filling Defect Score

Anatomical location	Score for a filling defect
Central region	3
Lobar or lingular	2
Segmental	1

95% (10,14). It is more related to the magnitude of thromboembolism than to the quality of the angiogram.

The initial vascularization defect judged on Miller's or Walsh's index allows classification of the severity before treatment and after treatment and to evaluate the therapeutic efficiency when compared to the postinfusion score. Usually the mean relative improvement 24 h after thrombolytics is about 25%–30%; therefore, additional or prolonged fibrinolytic infusion is often needed to clear residual intravascular thrombi (13). Fragmentation into lobar and segmental vessels occurs commonly, resulting in a disproportionate decrease in the number of large emboli on the postinfusion angiogram and a lesser decrease or even an increase in the number of small emboli in the segmental arteries (15). However, this is not frequent.

The objective quantitative analysis of the angiograms frequently demonstrates that patients with initial massive pulmonary embolism (≥50%) score defect show greater improvement than those with initial submassive pulmonary embolism (≥30% < 50%). In some patients in shock, the thrombolytic therapeutic effect may be impressive (Fig. 3A,B) (9). Such a beneficial therapeutic effect may be obtained after surgical endarterectomy until 3 months after failure of thrombolytics (Fig. 4A,B).

In USPET (15) as well as in UKEP (13) studies, there was no disagreement concerning the specificity of angiography in identifying thromboemboli. Angiogram measurements were obtained with little morbidity and no mortality, and they were the most sensitive indicator of clot resolution. The objective method for analyzing pulmonary angiograms developed by Miller et al. (11) and by Walsh et al. (12) allows a useful quantitative analysis and in UPET (9) confirmed the superiority of urokinase on heparin in dissolving thromboemboli.

IV. Other Advantages of Pulmonary Angiography

Pulmonary angiography offers other special diagnostic advantages: the opportunity to evaluate the hemodynamic status of the patient; the measurements of right atrial, ventricular, pulmonary arterial, and wedge pressures; total pulmonary resistance, and cardiac output—all information that may be vital for the assessment of massiveness and severity and for correcting therapeutic decisions.

Pulmonary angiography avoids some life-threatening differential diagnosis. We observed two patients with clinical and scanning high probability for massive pulmonary embolism who indeed had an ascendant aortic fissuration responsible for a major filling perfusion defect of the whole right lung. Pulmonary angiogram at the right arterial phase confirmed the near total absence of vascular filling because of an extrinsic compression of the proximal right pulmonary artery. Another exceptional personal case of high probability for a massive unilateral

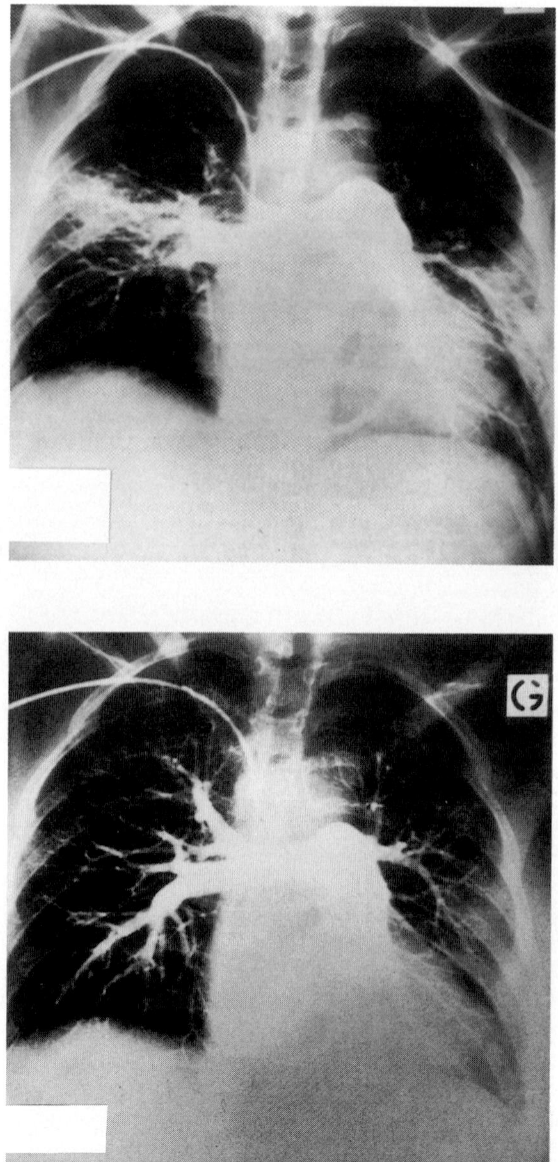

(A)

(B)

Figure 3 (A) Pulmonary angiogram before thrombolysis. Miller's index 53%. (B) Same patient immediately after a 24-h infusion of Urokinase (2.7 million units) associated with plasminogen loading dose. Miller's index 20%, showing an early excellent revascularization rate of 62%.

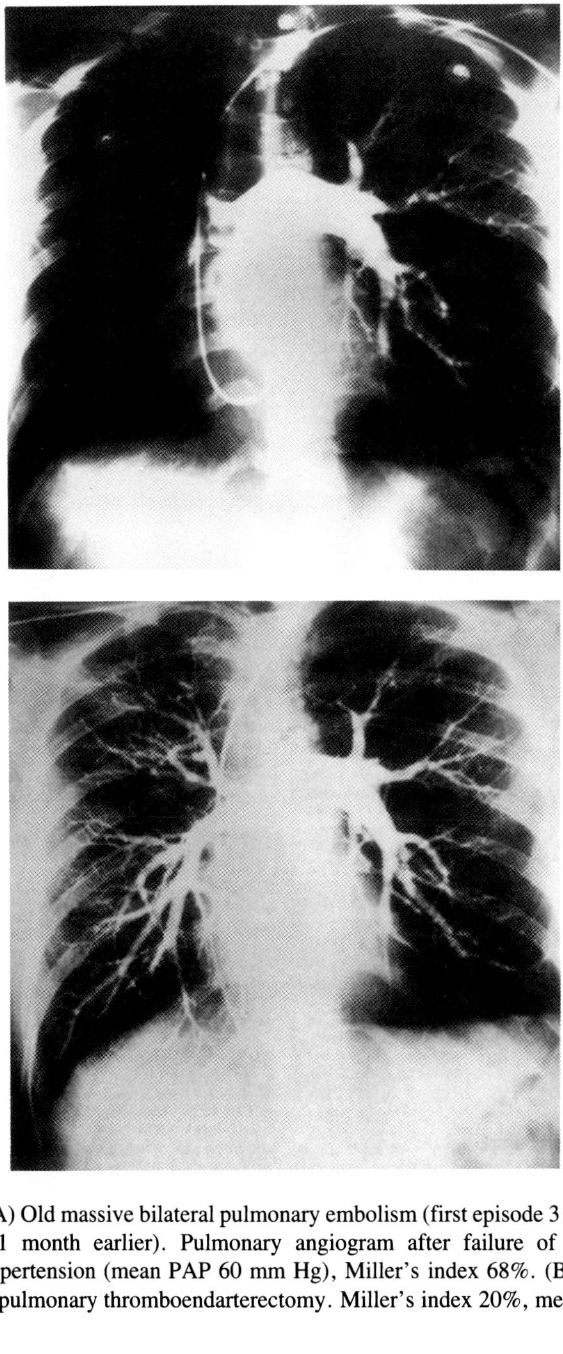

(A)

(B)

Figure 4 (A) Old massive bilateral pulmonary embolism (first episode 3 months earlier, last episode 1 month earlier). Pulmonary angiogram after failure of thrombolytics. Pulmonary hypertension (mean PAP 60 mm Hg), Miller's index 68%. (B) Same patient 3 weeks after pulmonary thromboendarterectomy. Miller's index 20%, mean PAP 15 mm Hg.

right pulmonary embolus was in fact a primary leiomyosarcoma of the right pulmonary artery, confirmed by scanner and surgery (16).

After pulmonary angiography has confirmed the diagnosis and the severity of pulmonary embolism, and after the proper therapy has been given, serial lung scans are generally sufficient to follow improvement or impairment of lung perfusion (see Chap. 12). However, in massive pulmonary embolism with major obstruction of the main or lobar pulmonary arteries that needed thrombolysis, pulmonary angiography that provides direct visualization of artery occlusion is the best technique to evaluate thrombolysis efficiency. Therefore, it is easier to repeat arteriography when the catheter remains in the main pulmonary artery for 24–48 h. Perfusion lung scanning only shows changes in pulmonary perfusion but does not allow detection of residual intraluminal thrombus, which is often responsible for local thrombosis extension or recurrence. Conversely, for the long-term follow-up, noninvasive technics such as perfusion lung scans in association with impedance plethysmography or duplex ultrasound for peripheral veins and echocardiography are currently used.

V. Intravenous Digital Subtraction Angiography

The precise role of intravenous digital subtraction angiography (DSA) in the diagnosis of pulmonary embolism was investigated in the 1980s and compared to selective pulmonary angiography, which was used as the "gold standard" (17–19). Emboli were detected in major and second-order branches and occasionally in third-order branches as well. Because of the limited spatial resolution of DSA, very small emboli were not visualized in the arterial phase of the intravenous study.

Improved spatial resolution has presently increased rates of image acquisition, large image intensifier fields, and biplane imaging. And intravenous DSA is now considered as an acceptable substitute for routine pulmonary angiography in most patients with suspected major pulmonary embolism. The technique is less expensive, safer, faster, and easier to perform than conventional pulmonary angiography (18).

Nevertheless, DSA images are frequently difficult to read, and Gutierrez et al. (17) found that motion artifacts can lead to serious image degradation. The appropriate breath holding may be extremely difficult to obtain for patients with major dyspnea (20).

In a recent prospective trial comparing diagnostic value of DSA and conventional angiography in acute pulmonary embolism, Musset et al. (21) concluded that DSA was technically unsatisfactory in 24% of cases in a series of 54 patients. The interpretable DSA had 81% sensitivity and 64% specificity. With DSA, one could not exclude the diagnosis of pulmonary embolism on the basis of normal angiograms (27% false-negative results). However, in medium to major pulmonary embolism, DSA showed a 94% sensitivity. Therefore, DSA may be the technique of choice in the screening of life-threatening major pulmonary embolism.

VI. Complementary Peripheral Veinography

Postmortem studies have shown that most patients with pulmonary embolism have deep vein thrombosis (DVT) of the legs (22–23). In the UKEP study (13), DVT was clinically present in 50% of pulmonary embolism patients, whereas phlebography detected DVT in 80% of patients. Despite impedance plethysmography can be done at bedside and is a noninvasive and safe technique; it is not able to detect floating thrombus in vena cava. Therefore, when pulmonary angiography is performed from a femoral vein approach, contrast material may be injected in the common iliac vein to detect or exclude iliac or caval thrombi. Although most patients with pulmonary embolism have previously had DVT, a negative venogram may be associated with documented pulmonary embolism in 20%–30% (4,10). In such cases, either the whole venous thrombus has migrated in the lungs, or pulmonary embolism may have derived from other sites (pelvic, renal veins, inferior vena cava, or right heart cavities). Therefore, a negative venogram does not exclude venous thromboembolism in patients with suspected or documented pulmonary embolism. Conversely, in patients with DVT, Moser and Lemoine (24) found that over 50% of patients with proximal DVT had lung scan suggestive of pulmonary embolism, sometimes despite the absence of cardiopulmonary symptoms (25).

VII. Side Effects

Pulmonary angiography is invasive, rather expensive, and requires specialized equipment and staff. In the 1970s, pulmonary angiography was considered to have a 10% risk of morbidity and 0.5% risk of mortality (26). The present utilization of pigtail catheter has considerably reduced complications like right ventricle perforation, intramyocardial effusion, pericardium effusion, and hemorrhage (27). Rhythm disturbances are limited to ventricular premature beats, whereas sustained ventricular tachycardia is exceptional. Nonetheless, the risk of complications is higher in patients with pulmonary hypertension >50 mm Hg (28).

In the UPET (9), 5 cases of ventricular tachycardia and 1 cardiac perforation occurred in 310 right heart catheterizations, all of which were successfully treated. In the literature, pulmonary angiographic morbidity is evaluated 3% and mortality rate 0.2%. From 1987 to 1992 in a personal series of 483 pulmonary embolisms (of which 38% were massive) and 427 pulmonary angiograms, the global in-hospital mortality rate was 5.4%. Only one death was related to the procedure (0.23%).

After rigorous selection and respect for contraindications, pulmonary angiography provides a simple, precise, and sensitive method of assessing quantitatively the resolution of pulmonary emboli and of evaluating treatment differences in clinical trials.

VIII. Conclusion

Pulmonary angiography and venography were often combined in the past for patients with suspected pulmonary embolism after initial isotopic screening in order to confirm the diagnosis, to establish the severity score, and to manage the therapy.

Selective pulmonary angiography in skilled hands is safe and remains the most suitable method for the diagnosis of pulmonary embolism and the precise evaluation of severity as well as therapeutic efficacy.

Nevertheless, the recent development of noninvasive techniques such as echocardiography and venous duplex echodoppler allows one to avoid the more aggressive explorations in a number of pulmonary embolisms.

Acknowledgment

The author is indebted to Viviane Poilpot for her help in the preparation of the manuscript.

References

1. de Carvalho L, Moniz E. Visibility of the pulmonary vessels (angiopneumography). Acta Radiol Lisbon 1933; 14:433–8.
2. Williams JR, Wilcox WC. Pulmonary embolism: roentgenographic and angiographic considerations. Am J Roentgen Rad Therapy Nucl Med 1963; 89:333–9.
3. Sasahara AA, Stein M, Simon M, et al. Pulmonary angiography in the diagnosis of thromboembolism disease. N Engl J Med 1964; 270:1075.
4. Hull RD, Hirsh J, Carter CJ, et al. Pulmonary angiography, ventilation lung scanning, and venography for clinically suspected pulmonary embolism with abnormal perfusion lung scan. Ann Intern Med 1983; 98:891–9.
5. Brochier M, Raynaud P, Fauchier JP, et al. Comparison between lung scans and pulmonary angiograms in the evaluation of the perfusion defect in massive and submassive pulmonary embolism. Prog Respir Res 1980; 13:120–6.
6. Pioped investigators. Value of the ventilation/perfusion scan in acute pulmonary

embolism. Results of the Prospective Investigation of Pulmonary Embolism Diagnosis (PIOPED). JAMA 1990; 263:2753–9.
7. Kelley MA, Carson JL, Palevsky HI, et al. Diagnosing pulmonary embolism: new facts and strategies. Ann Intern Med 1991; 114:300–6.
8. Dalen JE, Brooks HL, Johnson LW, et al. Pulmonary angiography in acute pulmonary embolism: indications, techniques and results in 367 patients. Am Heart J 1971; 31:175–85.
9. UPET. Urokinase Pulmonary Embolism Trial. Circulation 1973; vols. XLVII and XLVIII, no. 4 (suppl II): 47–8.
10. Quinn MF, Lundell CJ, Klotz TA, et al. Reliability of selective pulmonary arteriography in the diagnosis of pulmonary embolism. Am J Radiol 1987; 149:469–71.
11. Miller GAH, Sutton GC, Kerr IH, et al. Comparison of streptokinase and heparin in treatment of isolated acute massive pulmonary embolism. Br Med J 1971; 2:681–4.
12. Walsh PN, Greenspan RH, Simon M, et al. An angiographic severity index for pulmonary embolism. Circulation 1973; 47–48(suppl II):101–8.
13. The UKEP Study Research Group. The UKEP Study: multicentre clinical trial on two local regimens of urokinase in massive pulmonary embolism. Eur Heart J 1987; 8:2–10.
14. Sostman HD, Rapoport S, Gottschalk A, et al. Imaging of pulmonary embolism. Invest Radiol 1986; 21:443–54.
15. USPET. Urokinase Streptokinase Embolism Trial: Phase II. Results. JAMA 1974; 229:1606–13.
16. François G, Garnier LF, Charbonnier B, et al. Leimyosarcome primitif de l'artère pulmonaire. A propos d'un cas. Arch Mal Coeur 1987; 80:1417–21.
17. Gutierrez FR, Biello D, McKnight RC. Digital venous angiography in the diagnosis of pulmonary thromboembolism. Cathet Cardiovasc Diagn 1984; 10:343–8.
18. Reilley RF, Smith CW, Price RR, et al. Digital subtraction angiography. Limitations for the detection of pulmonary embolism. Radiology 1983; 149:379–82.
19. Pond GD, Ovitt TW, Capp M. Comparison of conventional pulmonary angiography with intravenous digital subtraction angiography for pulmonary embolic disease. Radiology 1983; 147:345–50.
20. Lacombe P, Bouchet D, Mouvier, et al. Angiographie pulmonaire numérique: technique et applications. In: Encycl Med Chir. Vol. 2. Paris: Poumons, 1987:1–6.
21. Musset D, Rosso J, Petitpretz, et al. Acute pulmonary embolism: diagnostic value of digital subtraction angiography. Radiology 1988; 166:455–9.
22. Sevitt S, Gallagher W. Venous thrombosis and pulmonary embolism. Br J Surg 1961; 48:475–89.
23. Havig GO. Source of pulmonary emboli. Acta Chir Scand 1977; 478(suppl):42–7.
24. Moser KM, Lemoine JR. Is embolic risk conditioned by location of deep venous thrombosis? Ann Intern Med 1981; 94:439–44.
25. Huisman MV, Buller HR, Ten cate JW, et al. Unexpected high prevalence of silent pulmonary embolism in patients with deep venous thrombosis. Chest 1989; 95:498–502.

26. Bell WR, Simon TL. A comparative analysis of pulmonary perfusion scans with pulmonary angiograms. Am Heart J 1976; 92:700–6.
27. Stein PD, Athanasoulis CH, Alavi A, et al. Complications and validity of pulmonary angiography in acute pulmonary embolism. Circulation 1992; 85:462–8.
28. Mills RS, Jackson DC, Older RA, et al. The incidences, etiologies, and avoidance of complications of pulmonary angiography in large series. Radiology 1980; 136:295–9.

Part Four

TREATMENT

15

ICU in the Management of Pulmonary Embolism

CLAUDE H. PERRET and FRANÇOIS FEIHL

Institute of Pathophysiology
University Hospital (CHUV)
Lausanne, Switzerland

I. Introduction

Pulmonary embolism (PE) justifies admission to an intensive care unit (ICU) when massive, i.e., when it is responsible for cardiocirculatory instability or severe respiratory failure. The purpose of this chapter is to define guidelines for the diagnosis, monitoring, and treatment of PE in an ICU setting.

II. Diagnostic Strategy

Patients with massive PE admitted to an ICU may present with one of the three following pictures: (a) acute right ventricular (RV) failure, (b) cardiorespiratory arrest (CRA), or (c) shock. In each of these settings, the diagnosis upon admission may be already established, only suspected, or not even evoked.

(a) For patients with suspected PE and acute RV failure without shock, the diagnostic work-up will proceed as usual, with lung scan first, followed by pulmonary angiography if necessary. To ascertain the diagnosis, angiography is required in the presence of an intermediate-probability scan or of a low-probability scan associated with a high clinical suspicion. If PE is strongly suspected, these procedures should be preceded by the administration of heparin (bolus of 5000 IU).

(b) The diagnosis of PE as a cause of CRA can be either extremely difficult or quick and simple as in patients known to have deep venous thrombosis and/or a previous episode of PE. It can be suspected on presence of evident risk factors (see Chap. 2) or a suggestive history (sudden asphyxia and cyanosis). The suspicion may also be raised by the development of physical signs of acute RV failure during or immediately after successful resuscitation. In such conditions of presumed diagnosis, emergency pulmonary embolectomy may be requested without further investigations. Otherwise, the diagnostic strategy will follow that of categories (a) or (c) according to circulatory conditions.

(c) The clinical picture of shock secondary to massive PE is highly suggestive of the diagnosis when typical signs of acute cor pulmonale including RV gallop (S3), loud pulmonary component of the second heart sound (P2), left parasternal lift, and distented neck veins are observed (see Chaps. 6 and 7). When these signs are not sufficiently demonstrative, screening tests are necessary in order to determine the cause of shock. The diagnostic value of the relevant tests is now briefly discussed.

A. Routine Tests

The chest X-ray, although nonspecific, is of primary importance (see Chap. 12). In order to be responsible for shock in patients without prior lung disease, PE is usually massive with the classical signs of elevated hemidiaphragm, oligemia, plumpness of the main pulmonary artery segment, and right heart enlargement (1,2). However, an apparently normal chest X-ray does not entirely exclude the diagnosis. In patients with chronic pulmonary disease, interpretation of chest X-ray is problematic.

Arterial blood gas analysis, contrary to a widespread opinion, is of poor diagnostic value (see Chap. 5). In patients with suspected PE, there is no significant difference between Pao_2 and $Paco_2$ values whether pulmonary angiography is positive or negative (3). Furthermore, normal Pao_2 values have been described in massive PE complicated with shock (4).

Electrocardiogram (ECG) is of little use because of lack of specificity and sensitivity (5,6). A normal ECG does not rule out massive PE because it is known that electric signs of RV strain may be transitory (7). However, when present in a patient known to have a recent normal ECG, they may be of value although nonspecific.

B. Blood Tests

A low plasma level of D-dimers (<500 μg/mL) appears to have a high negative predictive value when measured early after the onset of clinical signs (8) (see Chap. 8).

C. Investigation of the Deep Venous System

Demonstration of thrombosis of the iliofemoral axis by means of Doppler or impedance plethysmography is a strong argument for PE when associated with a high clinical suspicion.

D. Echocardiography

Two-dimensional echocardiography has three main advantages: (a) it is noninvasive and easily available; (b) it can exclude other causes of cardiogenic shock such as extensive or complicated left ventricular (LV) myocardial infarction, pericardial tamponade, or dissecting aortic aneurysm; and (c) it allows one to estimate pulmonary arterial pressure, thus providing an additional clue to the severity of pulmonary artery (PA) obstruction (9) (see Chap. 13). Most of the echocardiographic signs of massive pulmonary embolism are not specific; they reflect the response of the right heart to acute pulmonary arterial hypertension. They consist in distension of the pulmonary arterial trunk (a good index of the average pulmonary artery pressure [PAP] [10]), RV dilatation and hypokinesis, a reduced LV size, an increased RV/LV diameter ratio, diastolic and systolic flattening of the interventricular septum with paradoxical systolic motion, and less frequently a bulging of the interatrial wall into the left atrium (11–14). Such a pattern is not specific and may be entirely mimicked by an extensive RV infarction (15–17) especially when associated with LV dysfunction and secondary pulmonary hypertension. Actually, echocardiography is able to ascertain the diagnosis of PA in only one rare condition: the visualization of thromboemboli in the right ventricle (14,18,19).

Unfortunately, the information given by echocardiography is frequently limited by technical difficulties and largely dependent on the expertise of the operator. In the ICU, it is notoriously difficult or at times impossible to obtain satisfactory echocardiographic images with the transthoracic approach. In such conditions, transoesophageal echocardiography (TEE) is a valuable tool, providing high-quality data in almost every patient (20). With this technique, direct visualization of thrombi in the right or main pulmonary artery may be possible (21,22). Transoesophageal echocardiography is a semiinvasive procedure and has been associated with complications such as worsening hypoxemia, arterial hypotension, or cardiac arrythmias. Fortunately, these last two complications occur rarely even in hemodynamically unstable ICU patients (20,23). Nevertheless, TEE should be performed under close monitoring of ECG, arterial blood pressure, and oxygen saturation ($Sa{O_2}$ or $S\bar{v}{O_2}$).

E. Bedside Hemodynamic Investigation

In presence of shock of undetermined origin, bedside hemodynamic investigation is of primary interest in providing essential clues regarding the cause of circulatory failure. In patients without prior cardiopulmonary disease, the following hemodynamic profile is highly suggestive of massive PE: cardiac and stroke indices are severely depressed, mean pulmonary artery pressure (PAP) is moderately elevated (<40 mm Hg), and total pulmonary vascular resistances (PVR) are significantly increased (>400 dynes/s/cm^{-5}) (13,24,25) (see Chap. 7). Pulmonary artery occlusion pressure (PAOP), although usually normal, is sometimes elevated. This may be the consequence of either a reduced LV compliance caused by ventricular interdependence or of a defective equilibration of PAOP with left atrial pressure. The latter phenomenon is explained either by increased critical closing pressures in the pulmonary micro circulation (26) or by total embolic obstruction downstream from the inflated balloon (27). Right atrial pressure (RAP) may surprisingly be within normal limits (25), which may be explained by the relatively high compliance of the normal RV.

One additional clue to the hemodynamic diagnosis of massive PE is worth noting: The obstruction of PA trunk or of proximal pulmonary arteries alters the morphology of PA pulse pressure, which becomes somewhat similar to the RV pressure waveform with a rapid end systolic drop and the absence of the dicrotic notch (Fig. 1). This unusual morphology attests to profound changes in pulmo-

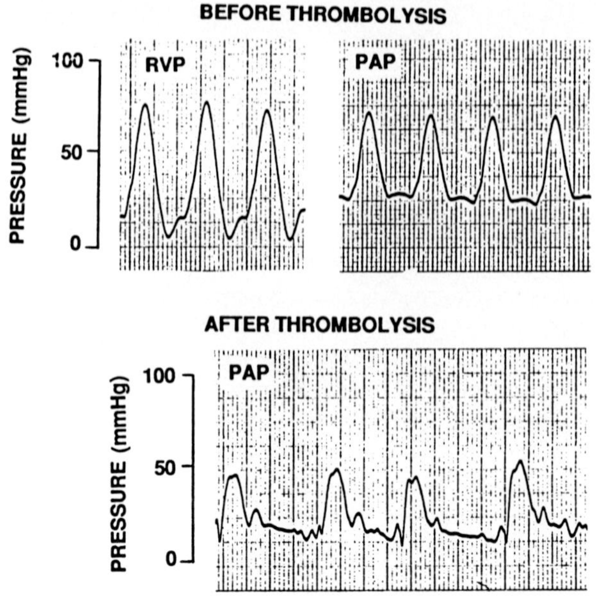

Figure 1 Pulmonary arterial pressure (PAP) waveforms recorded before and after thrombolysis in one patient with massive pulmonary embolism. Before thrombolysis, note the similar morphologies of the PAP and right ventricular pressure (RVP) waveforms.

nary arterial impedance essentially related to reduced compliance of the dilated arterial bed and increased amplitude of reflected pressure waves (28,29).

In patients with concomitant pulmonary disease, the diagnostic value of bedside hemodynamic investigation is quite limited because of the nonspecificity of increased PVR (30). In fact, a highly increased PAP (>50 mm Hg) attests in principle to the existence of preexisting cardiopulmonary disease (25,31). Depending on the particular clinical circumstances, this may lead to reconsideration of diagnosis of PE as the sole cause of cardiocirculatory failure.

Experience shows that correct placement of balloon-tipped catheters is often difficult in presence of massive proximal PA obstruction, most likely because of the dilated right heart cavities and the resulting tricuspid regurgitation. Exceptionally, the clot may impinge on the catheter tip, leading to either a sudden artifactual increase or a loss of the pressure signal recorded from the distal lumen; in addition, the measurement of thermodilution cardiac output may become impossible. Such incidents in the course of PA catheterization are not specific but suggestive of PE (32).

Because of the major risk of bleeding, Swan-Ganz catheterization should be avoided when thrombolysis is considered, except when a percutaneous antecubital insertion is possible.

F. Lung Scan

In the absence of shock, ventilation-perfusion scan has been shown of great value in the diagnostic work-up of suspected PE, provided the state of the art procedures are strictly adhered to (33,34) (see Chap. 12). However, in shock patients, this technique may be misleading and should be avoided if angiography is immediately available (35): First, the ventilation scan is difficult to obtain in uncooperative subjects; and second, the perfusion scan may be markedly altered by an uneven pulmonary blood-flow distribution induced by shock (36–38). This may conceivably lead to intermediate probability scan, or even worse, to a false positive diagnosis. Third, there are documented instances of massive central PE with normal lung scans (Fig. 2) (39,41).

G. Pulmonary Angiography

Pulmonary angiography is the only specific diagnostic test (see Chap. 14). It is a prerequisite to thrombolytic therapy or surgery, except in the emergency situation of a life-threatening, rapidly progressive circulatory collapse when the clinical and echocardiographic data strongly support the diagnosis of PE. Even in such catastrophic conditions, skilled cardiosurgical teams might be able to put the patient on partial extracorporeal circulatory support, thus providing acceptable hemodynamic conditions for performing angiography (42). It is surprising to note that pulmonary angiography still has a bad reputation, and clinicians fail to use

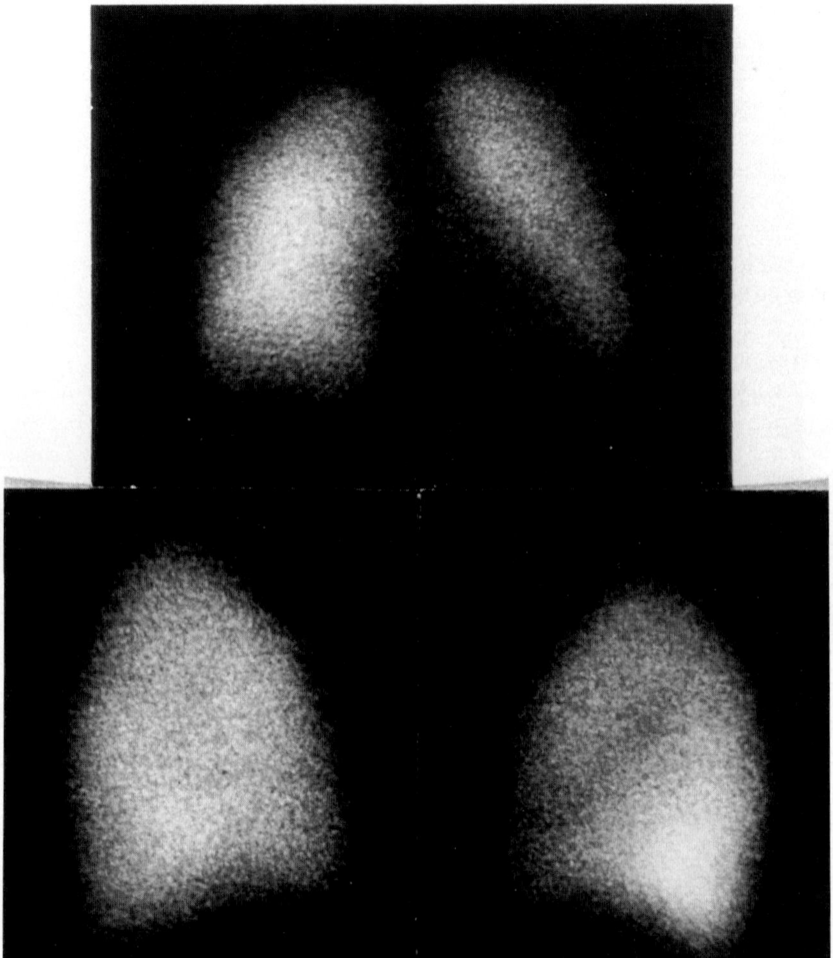

Figure 2 Perfusion scan obtained in a 37-year-old woman admitted in shock with clinically highly suggestive signs of pulmonary embolism. The patient died 1 h later in spite of aggressive medical support. Autopsy demonstrated massive obstruction of both pulmonary arteries by a saddle embolus.

it sufficiently (43), although several large series report a low morbidity and an extremely low fatality rate (0%–0.5%) (44–48). Although mortality increases in presence of RV failure secondary to severe pulmonary hypertension, it remains low (3%–5%) even in such conditions (44,45,48). Death is almost exclusively related to refractory low output and systemic hypotension caused by the injected contrast material. In that respect, nonionic agents appear significantly safer than ionic agents (49,50)

Various technical points have been developed to maximize the safety of pulmonary angiography in patients to be treated with thrombolytics (51). They include a percutaneous femoral (or superficial antecubital) approach and the use of a pigtail catheter (52) to avoid inadvertent perforation of the RV, which could lead to tamponade when thrombolytics are administered.

Patients with preexisting left bundle branch block may develop a complete atrioventricular block during the procedure. In such conditions, the preventive placement of a pacing catheter, or preferably of an external pacemaker, is recommended (51).

H. Newer Imaging Techniques

There is presently no data demonstrating the interest of computed tomography and nuclear magnetic resonance imaging in the diagnostic strategy (53). Furthermore, these techniques are not feasible in unstable patients.

I. Diagnosis of Acute Pulmonary Embolism in Patients with Chronic Obstructive Pulmonary Disease

As already mentioned, functional abnormalities in pulmonary embolism are not specific and have been described in a number of cardiac or pulmonary diseases. In such conditions, routine tests such as chest X-ray, ECG, and blood gas analysis—including the alveolar-arterial O_2 gradient—are of poor diagnostic value (54). In chronic obstructive pulmonary disease (COPD) patients, the same is true for intermediate probability scans that have been described in the absence of pulmonary embolism, demonstrating the need for further investigations (55). The positive predictive value of a high-probability image still seems close to 100% (54).

Echocardiography contributes little diagnostically in COPD patients. Because of pulmonary hyperinflation and breathlessness, these patients are usually difficult to investigate. Furthermore, the demonstration of pulmonary hypertension or RV dilatation does not allow one to discriminate between acute and chronic cor pulmonale (see Chap. 13). The same is true for hemodynamic investigation so that whenever the diagnosis has to be confirmed, pulmonary angiography must be considered.

III. Patient Monitoring

In the absence of circulatory failure, routine monitoring is sufficient. In patients with shock, invasive monitoring with a pulmonary artery catheter provides an effective means to evaluate cardiocirculatory balance and an extremely useful guide for estimating response to therapy. Continuous monitoring of mixed venous O_2 saturation ($S\bar{v}O_2$) might be of interest to detect recurrences or progressive hemodynamic deterioration.

When invasive monitoring is not available, indirect estimation of PAP with Doppler-echocardiography may be useful, in particular to follow the response to thrombolytic therapy (12).

At least a central venous line should be inserted to permit repeated measurements of central venous pressure and the administration of drugs. When thrombolytic therapy is considered, the antecubital route should be preferred and insertion of arterial lines avoided.

IV. Therapy

The aim of therapy is fivefold: to improve pulmonary gas exchange, to manage circulatory imbalance, to obtain pulmonary vascular tree desobstruction, to inhibit thrombus extension, and to prevent recurrences.

A. Respiratory Support

Hypoxemia is a frequent but not mandatory manifestation of massive PE (Chap. 9). There is no tight relationship between the extent of pulmonary vascular obstruction and the severity of hypoxemia (4,24,56,57). As a rule, oxygenotherapy (FIO_2: 0.40–0.60, Venturi mask) is quite effective in correcting hypoxemia, which is mainly due to $\dot{V}A/\dot{Q}$ maldistribution (58,59). The latter is related to an incomplete adaptation of regional ventilation to the abnormal pulmonary blood flow distribution induced by PE. When refractory, hypoxemia is dependent on a right to left shunt (60), which may be intracardiac (through a patent foramen ovale) (61) or intrapulmonary (pulmonary atelectasis) (62) or, rarely, a pulmonary edema in nonobstructed areas exposed to high vascular pressures (62,63). In such conditions, when hypoxemia is severe, intubation and mechanical ventilation may be necessary, but the risk exists to further deteriorate cardiocirculatory conditions by impeding venous return, thus reducing RV preload with positive airway pressure. Indeed, improving cardiac output is more effective by increasing the O_2 content of mixed venous blood and thus reducing the effect of right to left shunt (58,64), even if $\dot{Q}S/\dot{Q}T$ increases with increased flow (57). Still more important is to obtain rapid deobstruction of the pulmonary vascular bed.

B. Cardiocirculatory Support

This subject has been recently and carefully reviewed (32,65). In patients who are admitted in cardiorespiratory arrest, cardiopulmonary resuscitation (CPR) must be performed according to usual guidelines (66). Because of the increased risks of bleeding related to the large incidence of traumatic complications of CPR (rib fractures, hemothorax, lung contusion, laceration of the liver and spleen), it is recommended to avoid thrombolysis and to prefer embolectomy for those patients who do not recover promptly.

In patients with shock, there is no demonstrated benefit of volume expansion in patients with massive PE (67). Experimental data (68–70) and an isolated case report (71) even suggest that volume loading may cause further hemodynamic deterioration by enhancing RV distension and ventricular interference, thus worsening RV myocardial oxygen imbalance. The only exception concerns the worsening of circulatory imbalance induced by positive pressure mechanical ventilation. In such conditions, volume expansion appears to be useful (57,72) provided it is accomplished under close hemodynamic monitoring in order to prevent progressive equalization of filling pressures.

Attempts to reduce RV afterload by vasodilators in patients with shock are likely to be dangerous. Experimental results imply that the concomitant reduction in systemic vascular resistances may induce or worsen RV myocardial ischemia by decreasing coronary perfusion pressure (73,74). In the absence of shock, however, data obtained from animal models of massive PE suggest that, under strict hemodynamic monitoring, cautious administration of pulmonary vasodilators such as isoproterenol (75) or hydralazine (76) may be of benefit by improving cardiac output and reducing pulmonary hypertension. There is one favorable case report on the use of hydralazine in clinical PE (77), but others mention deleterious effects of this drug in patients with chronic pulmonary hypertension (78). Indeed, it must be noted that the actual role in humans of an increased pulmonary vascular tone in the development of acute pulmonary hypertension following massive PE is still uncertain.

In the setting of low cardiac output with severe systemic hypotension, the failure of preload and afterload manipulations limits the possible interventions to stimulating inotropism. In massive pulmonary embolism, a high RV myocardial oxygen demand (increased wall stress and tachycardia) is associated with a reduced coronary perfusion pressure. This may lead to isolated RV myocardial ischemia and loss of contractility (73,74). Experimental data have clearly demonstrated that combining α and β_1 adrenergic stimulation (norepinephrine) may dramatically improve RV performance, while pure β_2 stimulation produces a rapidly fatal course (74). In the present state of knowledge, norepinephrine appears to be an effective drug for short-term cardiorcirculatory support. A continuous intravenous infusion should be started at 0.1 μg/kg/min and titrated according to the observed response of arterial blood pressure. There is no present data concerning the upper limit of dosis; however, it can be expected that too high doses (>1 μg/kg/min) may be harmful by favoring the development of arrythmia or by producing excessive peripheral or coronary vasoconstriction with further anoxia or right ventricular ischemia. As a rule, blood pressure should not be raised to more than normotensive levels.

In the setting of low cardiac output with relatively maintained arterial blood pressure, RV ischemia is unlikely, and α adrenergic stimulation is of no benefit (79). In such conditions, dobutamine (5–15 μg/kg/min) has been shown to be clinically effective (80). In our experience and that of others (81), this is also true for dopamine (8–12 μg/kg/min) (see Chap. 16).

C. Thrombolysis

The use of thrombolytic agents represents a logical approach to alleviate the effects of an impeded RV ejection. Controlled studies with urokinase (UK) and streptokinase (SK) have clearly shown a beneficial effect of these drugs on the rate of thrombotic material resolution and improvement in hemodynamics when compared to conventional heparin therapy (56,82–84). But they failed to demonstrate a significant reduction in mortality rate, a fact that might be related to the potentially large type II error related to the small size of the series. Long-term benefit on diffusing capacity and pulmonary capillary blood volume has been shown (85,86), but the clinical significance of these findings is still unknown.

Thrombolysis appears as a treatment of choice in patients with massive PE associated with signs of acute RV failure. It is true that the bleeding hazards are considerably limited if invasive procedures are strictly controlled and contraindications followed. But most of the published series mention a definite, although low, incidence of intracranial bleeding with potentially important neurologic sequelae (87,88). Such complications are presently not predictable. On the other hand, thrombolytic agents have not been shown to result in clinically significant long-term benefits. For these reasons, it seems cautious to restrict thrombolysis to patients with life-threatening cardio-circulatory imbalance who do not respond to symptomatic treatment. In such patients, thrombolysis might reduce the indications for surgery. Experimental data and clinical studies suggest that marked and rapid hemodynamic improvement may be obtained with any of the three FDA-approved regimen (89,90), i.e., (a) streptokinase 250,000 IU as a loading dose over 30 min, followed by 100,000 IU/h for 24 h; (b) urokinase 4400 IU/kg as a loading dose over 10 min, followed by 4400 IU/kg/h for 12–24 h; or (c) recombinant tissue plasminogen activator (rt-PA) 100 mg over 2 h. Present trends seem to favor the use of more concentrated and shorter regimens (88), based on experimental (91,92) and clinical evidence (93,94) suggesting faster clot lysis and improved safety. In particular, the bolus injection of a weight-adjusted dose of rt-PA received some very recent attention (94,95) (see Chap. 16).

In the present state of knowledge, many issues remain to be resolved including the agent of choice, the optimal dosing regimen, and the choice between clot lysis and surgical clot extraction. In the meantime, the recommendations of the Consensus Development Panel from the NIH (96) are still valid. Before considering thrombolytic therapy, the following conditions have to be followed:

The diagnosis is established.
The severity of the clinical problem exceeds the risk of bleeding associated with a major contraindication.
Proper care is taken in the handling of the patients and in avoiding all but absolutely essential invasive procedures.
There is a clear understanding of the details of therapy, including monitoring, management of bleeding complications, and the control of subsequent anticoagulation.

D. Embolectomy

Most patients with massive PE and shock respond to maximal medical treatment, including thombolysis. For those who fail to improve or deteriorate, pulmonary embolectomy represents the last-resort treatment that has to be performed within the hours of unsuccessful therapy (see also Chap. 17). Angiography is mandatory to assess the diagnosis and precise the extent of obstruction (97). It usually requires circulatory support with partial cardiopulmonary bypass in order to improve hemodynamic conditions and to prevent further strain on the RV.

Pulmonary embolectomy is also indicated in patients with refractory RV failure who need prompt reduction in RV afterload and in which thrombolytics are contraindicated. Recent studies on emergency pulmonary embolectomy under cardiopulmonary bypass report an operative mortality rate of 20%–44% (42, 98,99).

Indications to surgery largely depend on local surgical facilities, including the training and availability of the cardio-thoracic surgical team. When emergency cardiopulmonary bypass is not available, the normothermic inflow occlusion technique can be used (100). This technique is surgically simple but entails a very high mortality (74%) in patients who had to be resuscitated preoperatively.

E. Catheter Embolectomy

Favorable results have been recently reported in massive PE with a new approach: the percutaneous retrieval of the embolus using suction exercised by means of a special 10F catheter (101).

F. Heparin Therapy

Heparin therapy in acute pulmonary embolism is well established (see Chap. 16). As soon as the diagnosis is suspected, heparin administration is recommended: intravenous bolus of 5000 U followed by the continuous IV infusion (1000–1200 U/h). The dose should be adjusted to maintain the partial thromboplastin time (PTT) at 1.5–2 times normal. In presence of underlying diseases favoring bleeding, monitoring should be particularly close, especially in patients with recent cerebrovascular accident or a history of previous bleeding. Frequent controls of platelet count should be performed.

The option to administer heparin in patients who were successfully resuscitated must be considered after an individual evaluation of the risks: benefits ratio.

G. Inferior Vena Caval Interruption

Filter devices (53, 87,102) are classically used for the treatment and prophylaxis in patients in whom anticoagulants are contraindicated or ineffective, and, as a routine procedure, after pulmonary embolectomy. They are also proposed as adjunct therapy to thrombolysis in high-risk patients who are hemodynamically compromised and for whom it is expected that a recurrent pulmonary embolism would be fatal. Actually, thrombolysis does not completely eliminate the risk of early recurrence (56,103), especially in presence of dangerous floating femoral or ilio-caval large clots. When the conditions that led to pulmonary embolism are unlikely to recur (postpartum, posttraumatic, following immobilization) implantation of a retrievable vena cava filter is appropriate (104). Because of the well-known increased incidence of hemorrhagic complications associated with thrombolysis therapy, it is mandatory to use a proper device that spares the vessel wall from any damage. Such filters are now available and seem as effective as older devices (104) (see Chap. 20). Further experience is needed to clarify the role of filter devices in acute massive pulmonary embolism.

V. Conclusions

Massive PE represents a life-threatening condition. It justifies close monitoring, most easily achieved in an ICU, which guarantees state of the art management in patients with acute RV dysfunction, shock, or acute respiratory failure. The proximity of an ICU is an asset even for patients with nonmassive PE, who may abruptly deteriorate following a new embolic event; this usually happens within 24 h following the beginning of therapy.

Massive PE may represent a unique diagnostic challenge, because of the low specificity of clinical signs as well as most available diagnostic methods. Because of the important risks associated with present aggressive therapy, the diagnosis must not be presumptive but ascertained. Angiography represents the only specific diagnostic test and appears safe in experienced hands. When angiography is not available, diagnosis rests upon suggestive findings from PA catheterization, echocardiography, and lung scan.

Symptomatic treatment aims at restoring acceptable cardiorespiratory conditions. Rapid deobstruction may be obtained with thrombolytic agents. Pulmonary embolectomy is indicated when thrombolysis fails or is contraindicated. The place of catheter pulmonary embolectomy, a recent development, remains to be defined.

References

1. Fleischner FG. Observations on the radiologic changes in pulmonary embolism. In: Sasahara AA, Stein M, eds. Pulmonary Embolic Disease. New York: Grune & Stratton, 1965:206–13.
2. Kerr IH, Simon G, Sutton GC. The value of the plain radiograph in acute massive pulmonary embolism. Br J Radiol 1971; 44:751–7.
3. Menzoian JO, Williams LF. Is pulmonary angiography essential for the diagnosis of acute pulmonary embolism? Am J Surg 1979; 137:543–8.
4. Jardin F, Bardet J, Sanchez A, Blanchet F, Bourdarias JP, Margairaz A. Massive pulmonary embolism without arterial hypoxaemia. Pathophysiology in two cases. Intens Care Med 1977; 3:77–80.
5. Miller GAH, Sutton GC. Acute massive pulmonary embolism. Clinical and haemodynamic findings in 23 patients studied by cardiac catheterization and pulmonary arteriography. Br Heart J 1970; 32:518–23.
6. McIntyre KM, Sasahara AA, Littmann D. Relation of the electrocardiogram to hemodynamic alterations in pulmonary embolism. Am J Cardiol 1972; 30:205–10.
7. Chou TC. Electrocardiography in clinical practice. 2nd ed. Orlando: Grune & Stratton, 1986:312–5.
8. Bounameaux H, Cirafici P, De Moerloose, P, Schneider PA, Slosman D, Reber G, Unger PF. Measurement of D-dimer in plasma as diagnostic aid in suspected pulmonary embolism. Lancet 1991; 337:196–200.
9. Stevenson JG. Comparison of several noninvasive methods for estimation of pulmonary artery pressure. J Am Soc Echocardiogr 1989; 2:157–171.
10. Kasper W., Meinertz T, Kersting F, Löllgen H, Limbourg, P, Just H. Echocardiography in assessing acute pulmonary hypertension due to pulmonary embolism. Am J Cardiol 1980; 45:567–72.
11. Come PC. Echocardiographic evaluation of pulmonary embolism and its response to therapeutic interventions. Chest 1992; 101(suppl):151S–162S.
12. Come PC, Kim D, Parker A, Goldhaber SZ, Braunwald E, Markis JE, and participating investigators. Early reversal of right ventricular dysfunction in patients with acute pulmonary embolism after treatment with intravenous tissue plasminogen activator. J Am Coll Cardiol 1987; 10:971–8.
13. Jardin F, Dubourg O, Guéret P, Delorme G, Bourdarias JP. Quantitative two-dimensional echocardiography in massive pulmonary embolism: emphasis on ventricular interdependence and leftward septal displacement. J Am Coll Cardiol 1987; 10:1201–6.

14. Kasper W, Meinertz T, Henkel B, Eissner D, Hahn K, Hofmann T, Zeiher A, Just H. Echocardiographic findings in patients with proved pulmonary embolism. Am Heart J 1986; 112:1284–90.
15. Goldstein JA, Tweddell JS, Barzilai B, Yagi Y, Jaffe AS, Cox JL. Importance of left ventricular function and systolic ventricular interaction to right ventricular performance during acute right heart ischemia. J Am Coll Cardiol 1992; 19:704–11.
16. Jugdutt BI, Sussex BA, Sivaram CA, Rossall RE. Right ventricular infarction: two-dimensional echocardiographic evaluation. Am Heart J 1984; 107:505–18.
17. D'Arcy B, Nanda NC. Two-dimensional echocardiographic features of right ventricular infarction. Circulation 1982; 65:167–73.
18. Farfel Z, Shechter M, Vered Z, Rath S, Goor D, Gafni J. Review of echocardiographically diagnosed right heart entrapment of pulmonary emboli-in-transit with emphasis on management. Am Heart J 1987; 113:171–8.
19. Saner HE, Asinger RW, Daniel JA, Elsperger KJ. Two-dimendional echocardiographic detection of right-sided cardiac intracavitary thromboembolus with pulmonary embolism. J Am Coll Cardiol 1984; 4:1294–1301.
20. Oh JK, Seward JB, Khandheria BK, Gersh GJ, McGregor CGA, Freeman WK, Sinak LJ, Tajik AJ. Transesophageal echocardiography in critically ill patients. Am J Cardiol 1990; 66:1492–5.
21. Deleuze Ph, Saada M, De Paulis R, Brochard L, Mazzucotelli JP, Rotman N, Loisance DY, Cachera JP. Intraoperative transesophageal echocardiography for pulmonary embolectomy without cardiopulmonary bypass. Ann Thorac Surg 1991; 52:137–8.
22. Nixdorff U, Erbel R, Drexler M, Meyer J. Detection of thromboembolus of the right pulmonary artery by transesophageal two-dimensional echocardiography. Am J Cardiol 1988; 61:488–9.
23. Oh JK, Sinak LJ, Freeman WK, Seward JB, Khandheria BK, Tajik AJ. Transesophageal echocardiography in patients with shock syndrome. Circulation 1991; 84(supp II):II–127.
24. McIntyre KM, Sasahara AA. The hemodynamic response to pulmonary embolism in patients without prior cardiopulmonary disease. Am J Cardiol 1971; 28:288–94.
25. Sharma GVRK, McIntyre KM, Sharma S, Sasahara AA. Clinical and hemodynamic correlates in pulmonary embolism. Clin Chest Med 1984; 5:421–37.
26. Butler BD, Drake RE, Hills BA. Effect of bronchial blood flow on pulmonary artery wedge pressure with pulmonary embolism. Crit Care Med 1986; 14:495–8.
27. Quintana E, Sanchez JM, Serra C, Net A. Erroneous interpretation of pulmonary capillary wedge pressure in massive pulmonary embolism. Crit Care Med 1983; 11:933–5.
28. Duroux P, Simonneau G, Petitpretz P, Herve P. Therapeutic approach to acute pulmonary embolism. Intens Care Med 1984; 10:99–102.
29. Fitzpatrick JM, Grant BJB. Effects of pulmonary vascular obstruction on right ventricular afterload. Am Rev Respir Dis 1990; 141:944–52.
30. McIntyre KM, Sasahara AA. Determinants of right ventricular function and hemodynamics after pulmonary embolism. Chest 1974; 65:534–43.
31. West JW. Pulmonary embolism. Med Clin North Am 1986; 70:877–94.

32. Dehring DJ, Arens JF. Pulmonary thromboembolism: disease recognition and patient management. Anesthesiology 1990; 73:146–64.
33. Hull RD, Hirsh J, Carter CJ, Raskob GE, Gill GJ, Jay RM, Leclerc JR, David M, Coates G. Diagnostic value of ventilation-perfusion lung scanning in patients with suspected pulmonary embolism. Chest 1985; 88:819–28.
34. The PIOPED Investigators. Value of the ventilation/perfusion scan in acute pulmonary embolism. JAMA 1990; 263:2753–9.
35. Benotti JR, Dalen JE, Alpert JS. Pulmonary embolism. In: Rippe JM, Irwin RS, Alpert JS, Fink MP, eds. Intensive Care Medicine. 2nd ed. Boston: Little, Brown and Company, 1991:308–16.
36. Ohlsson, J, Middaugh M, Hlastala MP. Reduction of lung perfusion increases VA/Q heterogeneity. J Appl Physiol 1989; 66:2423–30.
37. Fortune JB, Mazzone RW, Wagner PD. Ventilation-perfusion relationships during hemorrhagic hypotension and reinfusion in the dog. J Appl Physiol 1983; 54:1071–82.
38. Tiefenbrun J, Shoemaker WC. Sequential changes in pulmonary blood flow distribution in hemorrhagic shock. Ann Surg 1971; 174:727–33.
39. Brandstetter RD, Naccarato E, Sperber RJ, Ozick H, Novich I, Neglia W, Levitt A. Normal lung perfusion scan with extensive thromboembolic disease. Chest 1987; 92:565–7.
40. Ceraldi CM, Schabel SI, Waxman K. Normal ventilation/perfusion lung scan in a patient with proven pulmonary embolus. Crit Care Med 1990; 18:577–8.
41. Hackbarth R, Kuhns L, Sarnaik A. Central pulmonary embolism with normal ventilation/perfusion scan-Diagnosis by nuclear pulmonary artery flow studies. Ann Emerg Med 1991; 20:95–8.
42. Meyer G, Tamisier D, Sors H, Stern M, Vouhé P, Makowski S, Neveux JY, Leca F, Even P. Pulmonary embolectomy: a 20-year experience at one center. Ann Thorac Surg 1991; 51:232–6.
43. Millward SF, Peterson RA. UK survey on pulmonary scintigraphy and angiography: the underuse of angiography. Clin Radiol 1991; 44:287–8.
44. Perlmutt LM, Braun SD, Newman GE, Oke EJ, Dunnick NR. Pulmonary arteriography in the high-risk patient. Radiology 1987; 162:187–9.
45. Mills SR, Jackson DC, Older RA, Heaston DK, Moore AV. The incidence, etiologies, and avoidance of complications of pulmonary angiography in a large series. Radiology 1980; 136:295–9.
46. Dalen JE, Brooks HL, Johnson LW, Meister SG, Szucs MM, Dexter L. Pulmonary angiography in acute pulmonary embolism: indications, techniques, and results in 367 patients. Am Heart J 1971; 81:175–85.
47. Goodman PC. Pulmonary angiography. Clin Chest Med 1984; 5:465–77.
48. Stein PD, Athanasoulis C, Alavi A, Greenspan RH, Hales CA, Saltzman HA, Breim CE, Terrin ML, Weg JG. Complications and validity of pulmonary angiography in acute pulmonary embolism. Circulation 1992; 85:462–8.
49. Rees CR, Palmaz JC, Garcia O, Alvarado R, Siegle RL. The hemodynamic effects of the administration of ionic and nonionic contrast matherials into the pulmonary arteries of a canine model of acute pulmonary hypertension. Invest Radiol 1988; 23:184–9.

50. Tajima H, Kumazaki T, Tajima N, Ebata K. Effect of iohexol and diatrizoate on pulmonary arterial pressure following pulmonary angiography. Acta Radiologica 1988; 29:487–90.
51. Meyerovitz MF. How to maximize the safety of coronary and pulmonary angiography in patients receiving thrombolytic therapy. Chest 1990; 97(suppl): 132S–135S.
52. Grollman JH, Renner JW. Transfemoral pulmonary angiography: update on technique. AJR 1981; 136:624–6.
53. Goldhaber SZ, Braunwald E. Pulmonary embolism. In: Braunwald E, ed. Heart Disease: a Textbook of Cardiovascular Medicine. 4th ed. Philadelphia: WB Saunders Co, 1992:1558–80.
54. Lesser BA, Leeper KV, Stein PD, Saltzman HA, Chen J, Thompson T, Hales CA, Popovich J, Greenspan RH, Weg JG. The diagnosis of acute pulmonary embolism in patients with chronic obstructive pulmonary disease. Chest 1992; 102:17–22.
55. Stein PD, Coleman RE, Gottschalk A, Saltzman HA, Terrin ML, Weg JG. Diagnostic utility of ventilation/perfusion lung scans in acute pulmonary embolism is not diminished by pre-existing cardiac or pulmonary disease. Chest 1991; 100:604–6.
56. National Cooperative Study. The urokinase pulmonary embolism trial. Circulation 1973; 47:II1–II108.
57. Jardin F, Gurdjian F, Desponds P, Fouilladieu JL, Margairaz A. Hemodynamic factors influencing arterial hypoxemia in massive pulmonary embolism with circulatory failure. Circulation 1979; 59:909–12.
58. Manier G, Castaing Y, Guenard H. Determinants of hypoxemia during the acute phase of pulmonary embolism in humans. Am Rev Respir Dis 1985; 132:332–8.
59. Huet Y, Lemaire F, Brun-Buisson C, Knaus WA. Teisseire B, Payen DI, Mathieu D. Hypoxemia in acute pulmonary embolism. Chest 1985; 88:829–36.
60. D'Alonzo GE, Bower JS, De Hart P, Dantzker DR. The mechanisms of abnormal gas exchange in acute massive pulmonary embolism. Am Rev Respir Dis 1983; 128:170–2.
61. Hervé Ph, Petitpretz P, Simonneau G, Salmeron S, Laine JF, Duroux P. The mechanisms of abnormal gas exchange in acute massive pulmonary embolism. Am Rev Respir Dis 1983; 128:1101.
62. Johnson A, Malik AB. Effect of different-size microemboli on lung fluid and protein exchange. J Appl Physiol 1981; 51:461–4.
63. Manier G, Mora B, Castaing Y, Guénard H. Oedème pulmonaire au cours d'une embolie pulmonaire. Bull Eur Physiopathol Resp 1984; 20:55–60.
64. Dantzker DR. The influence of cardiovascular function on gas exchange. Clin Chest Med 1983; 4:149–59.
65. Prewitt RM. Hemodynamic management in pulmonary embolism and acute hypoxemic respiratory failure. Crit Care Med 1990; 18:S61–S69.
66. Emergency Cardiac Care Committee and Subcommittees, American Heart Association. Guidelines for cardiopulmonary resuscitation and emergency cardiac care. JAMA 1992; 268:2171–2298.

67. Ozier Y, Dubourg O, Farcot JC, Bazin M, Jardin F, Margairaz A. Circulatory failure in acute pulmonary embolism. Intens Care Med 1984; 10:91–7.
68. Paetkau D, Kettner J, Girling L, Slykerman K, Prewitt RM. What is the appropriate therapy to maintain cardiac output as pulmonary vascular resistance increases? Anesthesiology 1982; 57(suppl):A56.
69. Ghignone M, Girling L, Prewitt RM. Volume expansion versus norepinephrine in treatment of a low cardiac output complicating an acute increase in right ventricular afterload in dogs. Anesthesiology 1984; 60:132–5.
70. Belenkie I, Dani R, Smith ER, Tyberg JV. Effects of volume loading during experimental acute pulmonary embolism. Circulation 1989; 80:178–88.
71. Prewitt RM, Matthay MA, Ghignone M. Hemodynamic management in the adult respiratory distress syndrome. Clin Chest Med 1983; 4:251–68.
72. Hauser CJ, Shoemaker WC. Volume loading in massive acute pulmonary embolus. Crit Care Med 1979; 7:304–6.
73. Vlahakes GJ, Turley K, Hoffman JIE. The pathophysiology of failure in acute right ventricular hypertension: hemodynamic and biochemical correlations. Circulation 1981; 63:87–95.
74. Molloy WD, Lee KY, Girling L, Schick U, Prewitt RM. Treatment of shock in a canine model of pulmonary embolism. Am Rev Respir Dis 1984; 130:870–4.
75. Mathru M, Venus B, Smith RA, Shirakawa Y, Sugiura A. Treatment of low cardiac output complicating acute pulmonary hypertension in normovolemic goats. Crit Care Med 1986; 14:120–4.
76. Priebe HJ. Efficacy of vasodilator therapy in canine model of acute pulmonary hypertension. Am J Physiol 1988; 255:H1232–H1239.
77. Bates ER, Crevey BJ, Sprague FR, Pitt B. Oral hydralazine therapy for acute pulmonary embolism and low output state. Arch Intern Med 1981; 141: 1537–8.
78. Packer M, Greenberg B, Massie B, Dash H. Deleterious effects of hydralazine in patients with pulmonary hypertension. N Engl J Med 1982; 306:1326–31.
79. Molloy DW, Lee KY, Jones D, Penner B, Prewitt RM. Effects of noradrenaline and isoproterenol on cardiopulmonary function in a canine model of acute pulmonary hypertension. Chest 1985; 88:432–5.
80. Jardin F, Genevray B, Brun-Ney D, Margairaz A. Dobutamine: a hemodynamic evaluation in pulmonary embolism shock. Crit Care Med 1985; 13:1009–12.
81. Bourdarias JP, Dubourg O, Gueret P, Ferrier A, Bardet J. Inotropic agents in the treatment of cardiogenic shock. Pharmacol Ther 1983; 22:53–79.
82. Tibbutt DA, Davies JA, Anderson JA, Fletcher EWL, Hamill J, Holt JM, Thomas ML, Lee G de J, Miller GAH, Sharp AA, Sutton GC. Comparison by controlled clinical trial of streptokinase and heparin in treatment of life-threatening pulmonary embolism. Br Med J 1974; 2:343–7.
83. Ly B, Arnesen B, Eie H, Hol R. A controlled clinical trial of streptokinase and heparin in the treatment of major pulmonary embolism. Acta Med Scand 1978; 203:465–70.
84. Dalla-Volta S, Palla A, Santolicandro A, Giuntini C, Pengo, V, Visioli O, Zonzin

P, Zanuttini D, Barbaresi F, Agnelli G, Morpurgo M, Marini MG, Visani L. PAIMS 2: alteplase combined with heparin versus heparin in the treatment of acute pulmonary embolism. J Am Coll Cardiol 1992; 20:520–6.
85. Sharma GVRK, Burleson VA, Sasahara AA. Effect of thrombolytic therapy on pulmonary-capillary blood volume in patients with pulmonary embolism. N Eng J Med 1980; 303:842–5.
86. Sharma GVRK, Folland ED, McIntyre KM, Sasahara AA. Longterm hemodynamic benefit of thrombolytic therapy in pulmonary disease. J Am Coll Cardiol 1990; 15:65A.
87. Goldhaber SZ, Grassi CJ. Management of pulmonary embolism. In: Sabiston DS, ed. Textbook of Surgery. Update 8. 14th ed. Philadelphia: WB Saunders Co, 1990:115–27.
88. Goldhaber SZ, Kessler CM, Heit JA, Elliott CG, Friedenberg WE, Heiselman DE, Wilson DB, Parker JA, Bennett D, Feldstein ML, Selwyn AP, Kim D, Sharma GVRK, Nagel J, Meyerovitz MF. Recombinant tissue-type plasminogen activator versus a novel dosing regimen of urokinase in acute pulmonary embolism: a randomized controlled multicenter trial. J Am Coll Cardiol 1992; 20:24–30.
89. Goldhaber SZ. Thrombolysis for pulmonary embolism. Prog Cardiovasc Dis 1991; 34:113–34.
90. Goldhaber SZ. Evolving concepts in thrombolytic therapy for pulmonary embolism. Chest 1992; 101(suppl):183S–185S.
91. Shiffmann F, Ducas J, Hollett P, Israels E, Greenberg D, Cook R, Prewitt RM. Treatment of canine embolic pulmonary hypertension with recombinant tissue plasminogen activator. Circulation 1988; 78:214–20.
92. Prewitt RM, Shiffman F, Greenberg D, Cook R, Ducas J. Recombinant tissue-type plasminogen activator in canine embolic pulmonary hypertension. Circulation 1989; 79:929–38.
93. Goldhaber SZ, Heit J, Sharma GVRK, Nagel JS, Kim D, Parker JA, Drum D, Reagan K, Anderson J, Kessler CM, Markis J, Dawley D, Meyerovitz M, Vaughan DE, Tumeh SS, Loscalzo J, Selwyn AP, Braunwald E. Randomised controlled trial of recombinant tissue plasminogen activator versus urokinase in the treatment of acute pulmonary embolism. Lancet 1988; 2:293–8.
94. Levine M, Hirsh J, Weitz J, Cruickshank M, Neemeh J, Turpie AG, Gent M. A randomized trial of a single volume dosage regimen of recombinant tissue plasminogen activator in patients with acute pulmonary embolism. Chest 1990; 98:1473–9.
95. Diehl JL, Meyer G, Igual J, Collignon MA, Giselbrecht M, Even P, Sors H. Effectiveness and safety of bolus administration of alteplase in massive pulmonary embolism. Am J Cardiol 1992; 70:1477–80.
96. Symposium at the National Institutes of Health. Thrombolytic therapy in thrombosis: a national institutes of health consensus development conference. Ann Intern Med 1980; 93:141–4.
97. Gray HH, Miller GAH, Paneth M. Pulmonary embolectomy: its place in the management of pulmonary embolism. Lancet 1988; 1:1441–5.

98. Schmid C, Zietlow S, Wagner TOF, Laas J, Borst HG. Fulminant pulmonary embolism: symptoms, diagnostics, operative technique, and results. Ann Thorac Surg 1991; 52:1102–7.
99. Bauer EP, Laske A, Von Segesser LK, Carrel T, Turina MI. Early and late results after surgery for massive pulmonary embolism. Thorac Cardiovasc Surg 1991; 39:353–6.

16

Thrombolytic Treatment of Pulmonary Embolism

MARC VERSTRAETE

Center for Molecular and Vascular Biology
University of Leuven
Leuven, Belgium

I. Medical Treatment of Pulmonary Embolism

On the basis of pure clinical findings, pulmonary emboli may be schematically represented in four different types: massive pulmonary embolism, often immediately fatal, coming on unexpectedly; massive pulmonary embolism developing rapidly in hemodynamically unstable patients; pulmonary embolism obvious from clinical signs without major hemodynamic disturbances; and minor forms involving multiple small pulmonary emboli but causing dyspnoea, pulmonary hypertension, and eventually right heart failure (1,2).

A. Massive Pulmonary Embolism, Acute and Often Immediately Fatal

A massive pulmonary embolus arises suddenly like a thunderbolt in a clear sky; the patient sits up in his bed, lets out a loud cry, loses consciousness, and generally dies within a few minutes from cardiac and respiratory arrest. In this case the embolus is found astride the bifurcation of the pulmonary artery, or else it obliterates one or two parts of the pulmonary vascular systems.

Acute pulmonary hypertension is due not only to obliteration of the affected pulmonary artery but also to intense reflex vasoconstriction in other parts of the pulmonary vascular system.

The hemodynamic effect is a purely mechanical obstruction of the right ventricular outflow, which is unable to overcome the resistance affected by the embolus; consequently, it dilates, and the picture of right-sided heart failure develops. When cardiac function has been compromised by previous cardiopulmonary illness, relatively smaller emboli obstructing only one or two pulmonary segments can already exert a similar hemodynamic effect.

In about half of the cases caused by acute massive pulmonary embolism, death occurs within a period of 15 min, and about two thirds of the patients die in less than 2 h in a state of acute cardiogenic shock. The time factor is by itself decisive for success no matter what form of treatment is given. The prevention of massive pulmonary embolism is therefore essential if these patients are to be saved.

In a few cases, acute massive pulmonary emboli permit respite from death for an hour or more. If the unconscious cyanotic patient is in cardiac arrest, heart massage and artificial respiration may possibly save the patient; if the patient is in hospital at the time of the acute complication, immediate thrombolytic therapy with a bolus of 30,000 IU urokinase/kg, 3,000,000 U of streptokinase, or 50 mg alteplase administered in a peripheral vein should be instituted while the patient is urgently taken to the operating theater (3–5). The clinical response may be rapid and dramatically advantageous to the patient. Pressors such as epinephrine should be given simultaneously in case of persistent hypotension. If the cardiovascular situation did not improve by the time an experienced surgeon becomes available, closed heart pulmonary embolectomy (modified Trendelenburg operation with clamping the venae cavae) can be tried if there is no time to prepare the heart-lung machine.

It is, however, such that surgery is not always available in an emergency, and it often fails to restore circulation in small arteries. The in-hospital mortality was 37% in 96 consecutive patients with acute massive pulmonary embolism who underwent pulmonary embolectomy with total cardiopulmonary bypass under normothermia and without aortic cross-clamping (6). Mortality following pulmonary embolectomy performed with extracorporeal circulation is in most reports between 30% and 50% and depends, among other things, on the interval that elapses from the onset of the pulmonary embolism to operation; prognosis is much more favorable the longer the interval is, because the most severe cases die as time goes on: the operative mortality is about 80% if operation is carried out within 1 h, but it is 20% if the patient is not operated until 7 h after the pulmonary embolism (7).

B. Rapidly Evolving Major Pulmonary Embolism of Hemodynamic Importance

In these patients, a considerable part of the pulmonary circulation is interrupted, and right ventricular afterload increases when the pulmonary obstruction reduces the pulmonary vascular bed by 50% or more. To compensate, right ventricular and pulmonary artery pressures rise. As right ventricular afterload increases acutely, this chamber dilates and becomes hypokinetic, leading to tricuspid regurgitation. As the right ventricle fails, right atrial pressure rises, and cardiogenic shock ensues. Right ventricular hypertension can displace the interventricular septum toward the left ventricle, resulting in a decreased left ventricular diastolic filling and end diastolic volume (8–10). Thus, acute major pulmonary embolism is characterized by high pulmonary vascular resistance and low systemic blood pressure in combination with a decreased cardiac output.

The clinical results of major pulmonary embolism cannot be explained solely by the sudden occlusion of a large pulmonary artery; during unilateral occlusion of a pulmonary artery at the time of pneumectomy, the features of massive pulmonary embolism do not appear. There are, undoubtedly, also nervous and humoral reflexes that cause both vasoconstriction and severe bronchoconstriction.

Chronologically, the steps of right ventricular support are provision of adequate filling volume as indicated by central venous pressure, maintenance of adequate coronary perfusion pressure, use of vasoactive drugs to control the capacitance bed, and application of inotropic support for direct impact on ventricular contractility. Immediate action consists of treating this constriction and pulmonary hypertension with isoprenalin (10 mg dissolved in 250 mL and beginning with 2 μg/kg/min). Ketanserin (10 mg bolus followed by 4 mg/h) has also been used to reverse the abnormal vascular impedance (11). This substance stimulates adrenergic beta-receptors and causes bronchodilatation, increases the pulmonary arterial output, improves atrioventricular conduction, and constricts the veins. Isoprenalin has the disadvantage of possibly lowering the blood pressure through peripheral vasodilatation. It may be preferable to use dopamine, which in low doses (2–10 μg/kg/min) stimulates the adrenergic beta-receptors and renal delta receptors and does not decrease peripheral vascular resistance (12). In high doses (10–20 μg/kg/min), dopamine stimulates the adrenergic alpha-receptors.

If there is no hypercapnia, oxygen in high concentration serves to combat the hypoxia and the secondary collapse. Hydrocortisone hemisuccinate (50–100 mg intravenously) helps to break the vicious circle caused by peripheral collapse of the precapillaries. To alleviate pain, morphine is indicated (in milligram dosage up to a total of 5–10 mg). Slow infusion of 500 mL dextran increases cardiac output and inhibits the aggregation of platelets. For cases of heart failure, lanotoside C may be injected intravenously. Heparin (a bolus of 10,000–15,000 IU intravenously followed by a maintenance intravenous infusion of 1000–1500 U/h) prevents enlargement of the thrombus and recurrence of new emboli. It should be noted that patients with pulmonary embolism have a higher heparin requirement than those who have only deep vein thrombosis. Among patients with pulmonary embolism, the half-life of heparin is shorter, and the clearance of heparin is greater compared with patients having only deep vein thrombosis (13). Heparin administration should be started without delay.

Most patients with rapidly evolving major pulmonary embolism can be treated successfully with intensive heparin therapy. In some patients, however, acute pulmonary embolism severely compromises cardiorespiratory function, and, in these, thrombolytic therapy may be life-saving. There are three thrombolytic regimens approved by the Food and Drug Administration (FDA) and in most European countries (Table 1). The traditional 12–24-h regimens of streptokinase and urokinase are not optimal because of their logistic complexity and associated hemorrhagic complications (14).

The first reported case of treatment with alteplase of massive pulmonary embolism was in a 63-year-old man who had undergone renal transplantation 5 weeks before the acute pulmonary event (15). Further favorable experience was soon gained from the intravenous infusion of 50 mg alteplase administered over 2 h followed, if necessary, by an additional 4-h infusion of 40 mg in 30 patients with acute major pulmonary embolism (16). The quantitative angiographic score improved 21% by 2 h and 46% by 6 h.

The first trial with alteplase of the European Cooperative Study Group for Pulmonary Embolism was a pilot study in 34 patients with massive pulmonary embolism. This study indicated that an infusion in the pulmonary artery of alteplase does not offer a significant benefit over the systemic intravenous route (random allocation) and that a prolonged infusion of alteplase over 7 h (100 mg) is superior to a single infusion of 50 mg over 2 h (17).

Twelve European centers participated in a second trial (18). This was a double-blind study in which 63 patients with angiographically documented acute massive pulmonary embolism were randomly assigned to treatment with either urokinase (UK, 4400 IU/kg as a bolus, then 4400 IU/kg/h over 12 h), or to alteplase (10 mg as a bolus, then 90 mg over 2 h) followed by heparin. The primary objective was to compare the resolution of pulmonary emboli as judged by the change in total pulmonary resistance over the initial 2 h. Further objectives were to evaluate the changes in total pulmonary resistance over the next 10 h

Table 1 FDA-Approved Thrombolytic Regimens for Acute Massive Pulmonary Embolism

Streptokinase: 250,000 IU as a loading dose over 30 min, followed by 100,000 U/h for 24 h
Urokinase: 2000 IU/lb as a loading dose over 10 min, followed by 2000 IU/lb/h for 12–24 h
Alteplase: 100 mg as a continuous peripheral intravenous infusion administered over 2 h.

and the degree of angiographic resolution at 12–18 h. At 2 h, total pulmonary resistance decreased by 18 ± 22% in the urokinase group and by 36 ± 17% in the alteplase group (P = 0.0009). Continuous monitoring of pulmonary artery mean pressure, cardiac index, and total pulmonary resistance revealed that these variables improved faster in the alteplase group with consistently significant intergroup differences from 30 min up to 3–4 h. After 12 h, the decrease in total pulmonary resistance was 53 ± 19% in the urokinase group compared with 48 ± 17% in the alteplase group, and the reduction of the angiographic severity score was 30 ± 25% compared with 24 ± 18%, respectively, with no significant intergroup differences. Bleeding was equally frequent in the two treatment groups, except that more urokinase-treated patients experienced hematomas at puncture sites. This European experience with alteplase is in full agreement with the angiographic results of a similar U.S. randomized trial comparing alteplase and urokinase used at the same dose as in the European trial; however, total pulmonary resistance was not measured in the latter trial (19). To determine the effects of a more concentrated urokinase dose administered over a shorter time course, 90 patients with acute pulmonary embolism were randomized to receive either 100 mg alteplase over 2 h or 3 million IU urokinase over 2 h (the initial 1 million units were given as a bolus injection over 10 min), both drugs being delivered through a peripheral vein (20). The results indicated a statistically nonsignificant trend favoring alteplase over urokinase at quantitative angiographic assessment at 2 h and identical angiographic improvement at 24 h. The mean change in perfusion lung scans between baseline and 24 h was similar for both treatment groups.

The concept of bolus thrombolytic treatment was introduced by Dickie et al. (21). With 15,000 IU/kg of urokinase over 10 min, there was 34% decrease in vascular obstruction within 12 h after treatment (22). In addition to anatomic improvement, there was a 20%–30% decrease of pulmonary artery mean pressure and in total pulmonary resistance within the first 3 h after the injection of urokinase. This is an important point because a prompt decrease of right ventricular strain may be of critical value to unstable patients. It has been shown that the relationship between total pulmonary resistance and the level of pulmonary vascular obstruction is hyperbolic, and a sharp increase of total peripheral resistance occurs when the pulmonary vascular obstruction exceeds 60% (23). Therefore, even a small early revascularization could result in a marked decrease in total pulmonary resistance. This latter finding also emphasizes the lack of sensitivity of the pulmonary angiography to assess the early effects of thrombolytic agents.

Recently, Levine et al. (24) and Levine (25) published a clinical study of pulmonary embolism that suggests that weight-adjusted bolus alteplase can achieve a reasonable comparable efficacy (assessed by pulmonary reperfusion on pre- and posttreatment perfusion lung scans) when compared to the efficacy achieved with alteplase infusion (17–20) and to the pulmonary reperfusion observed in the historical landmark Urokinase Pulmonary Embolism Trial (14). Fifty-eight patients with subacute pulmonary embolism were randomized either to alteplase (0.6 mg/kg ideal body weight) as a bolus over 2 min or to placebo. Continuous intravenous heparin therapy was given in the two groups and interrupted only for the duration of the study drug infusion. At 24 h, the mean relative improvement in the baseline perfusion lung scan defect was 37% in alteplase-treated patients compared with 18.8% in the placebo group ($P = 0.017$). There were no major bleeds in either group. For patients who received alteplase, there was an approximate one-third decrease from the baseline fibrinogen level at 30 min.

Thus, a bolus of alteplase appears to be a promising treatment strategy for patients with pulmonary emboli. However, its safety and efficacy have not been tested in a randomized controlled trial against a standard FDA-approved regimen for thrombolytic treatment of pulmonary embolism. Furthermore, use of bolus alteplase does not confer a guarantee of protection against major bleeding complications. Nevertheless, bolus thrombolysis warrants intensive investigation with randomized clinical trials.

Interruption of vena cava flow should be reserved for patients who develop emboli while receiving anticoagulant drugs or in whom anticoagulation is contraindicated or who had serious bleeding notwithstanding a therapeutic INR level (26,27). In most circumstances, the filter is placed percutaneously, but occasionally a surgical venotomy is preferred. The presence of a nonadherent large vena caval thrombi will help in the decision making. Early techniques required major operations and resulted in a high incidence of extensive distal thrombosis, peripheral edema, and postphlebitic change. Modern equipment such as the Greenfield and Günther filters do not have these disadvantages because they permit continued caval flow and may be inserted through the jugular vein with the patient under local anesthesia (28).

A well-coordinated team consisting of a vascular surgeon, an interventional radiologist, and a cardiologist or angiologist, all comprehensively and specifically trained, is the most effective way to secure the best possible results for patients with acute major pulmonary embolism. Two thirds of the patients with acute massive pulmonary embolism die in less than 2 h in acute cardiogenic shock. In those reaching the hospital alive and being properly treated, the mortality is presently 2.5%, but clinically apparent pulmonary embolism recurred in 8.3%, of whom 45% died during the 1-year follow-up (29).

C. Intermediate Forms of Pulmonary Embolism of Moderate to Minor Hemodynamic Importance

In hemodynamically uncomplicated pulmonary embolism, the National Institutes of Health (NIH)-sponsored Urokinase Pulmonary Embolism Trial (UPET) (14) provided evidence that the incidence of pulmonary vascular reperfusion was quite identical whether the patients had been treated with heparin or with urokinase. More recently, a U.S. trial comparing alteplase usually in conjunction with heparin versus heparin alone has been started in patients with symptoms of pulmonary embolism within 7 days of the qualifying angiogram (30). This study was discontinued after 13 patients because of slow recruitment. The same drug comparison was investigated in 36 patients pertaining to a multicenter Italian trial (31). Alteplase (100 mg over 2 h followed by 1750 IU heparin per hour for 7–10 days) resulted in a greater and faster improvement of the angiographic variables and of the pulmonary artery pressure compared with heparin alone (1750 IU heparin per hour for 7–10 days). A larger U.S. study in 99 hemodynamically stable patients with symptoms or signs of pulmonary embolism up to 14 days compared the effect of alteplase (100 mg over 2 h followed by heparin) and heparin alone (32). In 39% of alteplase-treated patients but in only 17% of heparin alone patients, right ventricular wall motion at 24 h had improved from baseline, and in 2% and 17%, respectively, it worsened. Alteplase patients also had a significant decrease in right ventricular and end diastolic area during the 24 h after randomization and a significant absolute improvement in pulmonary perfusion. However, still a larger trial is required to correlate these findings with clinically meaningful end points such as death, recurrent pulmonary embolism, and pulmonary function over a long follow-up period.

In the meantime, anticoagulation is usually preferred to thrombolysis in intermediate forms of pulmonary embolism. The main objective in treating venous thromboembolism with heparin is to reduce the risk of further pulmonary emboli, while natural endogenous fibrinolysis is lysing the thrombi in the pulmonary circulation.

Treatment should begin with intravenous injection of 10,000–15,000 IU of unfractionated (standard) heparin in a bolus dose, followed by intravenous infusion of 1000–1500 IU hourly. It is well known that patients with pulmonary embolism require much higher doses to obtain satisfactory anticoagulant protection than patients with only deep venous thrombosis (13). The target-activated partial thromboplastin time (aPTT) is 1.5–2 times the upper limit of the control value; the aPTT is to be checked every 4–6 h until the target aPTT range is obtained. When the aPTT is less than 1.5 times the control, the continuous heparin infusion dose should be increased rapidly by an increase of at least 25%. Conversely, if an aPTT level exceeds three times the control value, a reduction in the infusion rate of no more than 25% of the dose should be made (33). After circa 1 week, it is possible to transfer to oral anticoagulants, which are maintained for 3–6 months at moderate anticoagulation (INR 2.0–2.5) (33–36).

D. Minor Forms of Pulmonary Embolism

For the most part, this involves a large number of small emboli, obliterating only some peripheral branches of the pulmonary artery. It is likely that these multiple pulmonary microemboli occur much more often than is suspected because they are usually asymptomatic. These emboli do not cause infarcts because enough anastomoses open up between the small branches of the pulmonary and bronchial arteries. Recurrent small pulmonary emboli (miliary emboli) cause increasing dyspnea, right heart failure, and may insidiously lead to pulmonary hypertension) (12).

II. Summary

Thrombolytic therapy with streptokinase, urokinase, or alteplase should be reserved for patients with acute massive pulmonary embolism particularly if, notwithstanding intravenous heparin and further medical treatment, there is rapid further impairment of the cardiovascular status. Thrombolysis is most effective when the thrombus is reasonably fresh and only partly occlusive, and may salvage deep vein valves—thus reducing the incidence of postphlebitic changes. The administration of these agents is simple but requires careful medical supervision because thrombolytic treatment carries a greater risk of bleeding than simple anticoagulant drugs.

References

1. Meyer G, Charbonnier B, Stern M, Brochier ML, Sors S. Thrombolysis in pulmonary embolism. In: Julian DG, Kübler W, Norris RM, Swan HJ, Collen D, Verstraete M, eds. Thrombolysis in Cardiovascular Disease. New York: Marcel Dekker 1989:337–60.
2. Verstraete M, Vermylen J. Thrombosis. Oxford: Pergamon Press, 1984:312–24.
3. Previtt RM. Principles of thrombolysis in pulmonary embolism. Chest 1991; 99(suppl 4):157S–164S.
4. Ozbek C, Sen S, Frank S, Dyckmans J, Schieffer H. Rapid high dose streptokinase in severe pulmonary embolism. Lancet 1989; ii:229–30.
5. Mitchell JP, Trulock EP. Tissue-plasminogen activator for pulmonary embolism resulting in shock: two case reports and discussion of the literature. Am J Med 1991; 90:255–60.
6. Meyer G, Tamisier D, Sors H, Stern M, Vouhé P, Makowski S, Neveux JY, Leca F, Even P. Pulmonary embolectomy: a 20-year experience at one center. Ann Thorac Surg 1991; 51:232–6.
7. Dorfman GS. Percutaneous inferior vena caval filters. Radiology 1990; 174:987–92.
8. Elert O, Satter P. Diagnose der Lungenarterienembolie und Ihre Chirurgische Behandlung. Med Welt 1981; 32:1317–21.
9. Jardin F, Dubourg O, Gueret P, Delorme G, Bourdarias P. Quantitative two-dimensional echocardiography in massive pulmonary embolism: emphasis on ven-

tricular interdependence and leftward septal displacement. J Am Coll Cardiol 1987; 10:1201–6.

10. Visner MC, Arentzen CE, O'Connor M, Larson EV, Anderson RW. Alterations in left ventricular three-dimensional dynamic geometry and systolic function during acute right ventricular hypertension in the conscious dog. Circulation 1983; 67:353–65.
11. Huet Y, Brun-Buisson C, Lemaire F, Teisseire B, Lhoste F, Rapin M. Cardiopulmonary effects of ketanserin infusion in human pulmonary embolism. Am Rev Resp Dis 1987; 135:114–7.
12. D'Orio Y, Mendes P, Saad G, Marcelle R. Pathogenesis and management of acute pulmonary embolism. Acta Clin Belg 1989; 44:396–408.
13. Hirsh J, van Aken WG, Gallus AS, Dollery CT, Cade JF, Yung WL. Heparin kinetics in venous thrombosis and pulmonary embolism. Circulation 1976; 53:691–5.
14. The Urokinase Pulmonary Embolism Trial. A national cooperative study. Circulation 1973; 47(suppl 2):1–108.
15. Bounameaux H, Vermylen J, Collen D. Thrombolytic treatment with recombinant tissue-type plasminogen activator in a patient with massive pulmonary embolism. Ann Int Med 1985; 103:64–5.
16. Goldhaber SZ, Vaughan DE, Markis JE, Selwyn AP, Meyerovitz MF, Loscalzo J, Kim DS, Kessler CM, Dawley DL, Sharma GVRK, Sasahara A, Grossbard EB, Braunwald E. Acute pulmonary embolism treated with tissue plasminogen activator. Lancet 1986; ii:886–9.
17. Verstraete M, Miller GAH, Bounameaux H, Charbonnier B, Colle JP, Lecorf G. Marbet GA, Mombaerts P, Olsson CG. Intravenous and intrapulmonary recombinant tissue-type plasminogen activator in the treatment of acute massive pulmonary embolism. Circulation 1988; 77:353–60.
18. Meyer G, Sors H, Charbonnier B, Kasper W, Bassand P, Kerr IH, Lesaffre E, Vanhove P, Verstraete M. The effect of intravenous urokinase versus alteplase on total pulmonary resistance in acute massive pulmonary embolism. A European multicenter double-blind trial. J Am Coll Cardiol 1992; 19:239–45.
19. Goldhaber SZ, Kessler CM, Heit A, Markis J, Sharma GVRK, Dawley D, Nagel JS, Meyerovitz M, Kim D, Vaughan DE, Parker JA, Tumeh SS, Drum D, Loscalzo J, Reagan K, Selwyn AP, Anderson J, Braunwald E. Randomised controlled trial of recombinant tissue plasminogen activator versus urokinase in the treatment of acute pulmonary embolism. Lancet 1988; ii:293–8.
20. Goldhaber SZ, Kessler CM, Heit A, Elliott CG, Friedenberg WR, Heiselman DE, Wilson DB, Parker JA, Bennett D, Feldstein ML, Selwyn AP, Kim D, Sharma GVRK, Nagel JS, Meyerovitz MF. Recombinant tissue-type plasminogen activator versus a novel dosing regimen of urokinase in acute pulmonary embolism: a randomized controlled multicenter trial. J Am Coll Cardiol 1992; 20:24–30.
21. Dickie KJ, de Groot WJ, Cooley RN, Bond TP, Guest MM. Hemodynamic effects of bolus infusion of urokinase in pulmonary thromboembolism. Am Rev Respir Dis 1974; 109:48–56.
22. Petitpretz P, Simmoneau G, Cerrina J, Musset D, Dreyfus M, Vandenbroek MD, Duroux P. Effects of a single bolus of urokinase in patients with life-threatening pulmonary emboli: a descriptive trial. Circulation 1984; 70:861–6.

23. Safran D, Raynaud P, Dennewald G, Sors H, Even P. Hémodynamique et échanges gazeux dans l'embolie pulmonaire. A propos de 150 cas. In Goulon M, Rapin M, eds. Réanimation et Médecine d'Urgence. Paris: Expansion Scientifique Française, 1981:195–204.
24. Levine MN, Hirsh J, Weitz J, Cruickshank M, Neemen J, Turpie AG, Gent M. A randomized trial of a single bolus dosage regimen of recombinant tissue plasminogen activator in patients with acute pulmonary embolism. Chest 1990; 98:1473–9.
25. Levine MN. Bolus, front-loaded, and accelerated thrombolytic infusions for myocardial infarction and pulmonary embolism. Chest 1991; 99(suppl):128–34.
26. Grassi CJ, Goldhaber SZ. Interruption of the inferior vena cava for the prevention of pulmonary embolism: transvenous filter devices. Herz 1989; 14:182–91.
27. Meyer G, Raynaud P, Even P, Penaud D, Sors M. L'interruption de la veine cave inférieure et pathologie thrombo-embolique. Presse Méd 1990; 19:1347–48.
28. Hopkins NFG, Wolfe JHN. ABC of Vascular Diseases, Thrombosis and pulmonary embolism. Br Med J 1991; 303:1260–2.
29. Carson JL, Kelley MA, Duff A, Weg JG, Fulkerson WJ, Palevsky HI, Schwartz JS, Thompson BT, Popovich Jr, Hobbins TE, Spera MA, Alavi A, Terrin ML. The clinical course of pulmonary embolism. N Engl J Med 1992; 326:1240–45.
30. A Collaborative Study by the PIOPED Investigators. Tissue plasminogen activator for the treatment of acute pulmonary embolism. Chest 1990; 97:528–33.
31. Dalla-Volta S, Palla A, Santolicondro A, Giuntini C, Pengo V, Visioli O, Zonzin P, Zanuttini D, Barbaresi F, Agnelli G, Morpurgo M, Marini MG, Visani L. PAIMS 2: alteplase combined with heparin versus heparin in the treatment of acute pulmonary embolism. Plasminogen Activator Italian Multicenter Study 2. J Am Coll Cardiol 1992; 20:520–6.
32. Goldhaber S, Haire WD, Feldstein ML, Miller M, Toltzis R, Smith JL, Taveira DA, da Silva AM, Come PC, Lee RT, Parker JA, Mostader A, McDonough TJ, Braunwald E. Alteplase versus heparin in acute pulmonary embolism: randomised trial assessing right-ventricular function and pulmonary perfusion. Lancet 1993; 341:507–11.
33. Hirsh J. Optimal therapeutic ranges for unfractionated heparin and low molecular weight heparins. In: Fuster V, Verstraete M, eds. Thrombosis in Cardiovascular Disorders. Philadelphia: WB Saunders Co, 1992:147–60.
34. Research Committee of the British Thoracic Society. Optimum duration of anticoagulation for deep-vein thrombosis and pulmonary embolism. Lancet 1992; 340:873–6.
35. Hull R, Hirsh J, Jay R, Carter C, England CRN, Gent M, Turpie AGG, McLoughlin D, Dodd P, Thomas M, Raskob G, Ockelford P. Different intensities of oral anticoagulant therapy in the treatment of proximal-vein thrombosis. N Engl J Med 1982; 307:1676–81.
36. Hull RD, Raskob GE, Rosenbloom D, Panju AA, Brill-Edwards P, Ginsberg JS, Hirsh J, Martin GJ, Green D. Heparin for 5 days as compared with 10 days in the initial treatment of proximal venous thrombosis. N Engl J Med 1990; 322:1260–4.

17

Surgical Management of Pulmonary Embolism

PETER F. FEDULLO, WILLIAM R. AUGER, RICHARD N. CHANNICK, KENNETH M. MOSER, and STUART W. JAMIESON

School of Medicine
University of California, San Diego
and UCSD Medical Center
San Diego, California

I. Introduction

Surgical intervention plays a limited role in the management of patients with pulmonary embolism. Although pulmonary embolism remains a major and often unexpected cause of death in hospitalized patients, death from pulmonary embolism is more commonly the result of diagnostic error than therapeutic failure (1–3). A recent multicenter study, in which patient treatment decisions were left to the discretion of the attending physicians, demonstrated that only 10 of 399 patients (2.5%) with clinically apparent pulmonary embolism died from that disease (4). The overwhelming majority of pulmonary embolic events that result in death, therefore, can be characterized as sudden and unexpected, or as recurrent and unsuspected.

Over the last 30 years, considerable progress has been made in the prevention, diagnosis, and therapy of venous thromboembolism. The epidemiology of the disease has been investigated, defining patient groups at risk. Safe and effective methods of venous thrombosis prophylaxis have been evaluated in a wide range of patient populations, and recommendations for their application have been widely disseminated. Noninvasive techniques for the diagnosis of venous thrombosis and pulmonary embolism have been developed, and their capabilities and limitations have been defined. Guidelines for existing therapy have been refined, and new therapeutic agents have been introduced into clinical practice.

Despite these important advances in the prevention, diagnosis, and management of pulmonary embolism, two situations exist in which surgical intervention may be indicated. In the first, pulmonary thromboendarterectomy for chronic thromboembolic pulmonary hypertension, the indications for surgical intervention and the optimal surgical technique have been well defined (5,6). In the second, pulmonary embolectomy for acute, hemodynamically massive pulmonary embolism, controversy continues to be generated regarding indications for the procedure and the optimal surgical approach (7–10). It is important to note that the two procedures differ substantially in technique. In chronic thromboembolic pulmonary hypertension, restoration of pulmonary arterial patency involves a true *endarterectomy* of organized, recanalized and endothelialized thrombus. In this circumstance, performing a pulmonary embolectomy will not reduce pulmonary vascular resistance if the distal obstruction is not alleviated. Given the differences in patient population, indications for surgery and surgical techniques, it is important that each entity be considered individually.

II. Thromboendarterectomy for Chronic Thromboembolic Pulmonary Hypertension

A pulmonary thromboendarterectomy represents a distinct surgical procedure designed to remove occlusive, or partially occlusive, organized thrombotic material from main, lobar, or segmental pulmonary arteries of patients with chronic thromboembolic pulmonary hypertension. A successful therapeutic approach to patients with this disease entity requires not only an understanding of the surgical procedure itself but also an appreciation of the natural history of the disease, the diagnostic difficulties encountered in the evaluation of these patients, and the unique perioperative problems that may arise following the procedure.

Discussions of the natural history of pulmonary thromboembolism, whether the event is hemodynamically massive or submassive, have focused primarily on the clinical, hemodynamic, and gas exchange consequences of the acute embolic event. The natural history of most emboli is to undergo total resolution, or resolution leaving minimal residua with restoration of normal pulmonary hemodynamics. This course has now been amply documented in a number of studies (11–16) (see Chap. 10). Considerably less emphasis has been placed on potential long-term consequences. During the past decade, however, an alternate natural history has been identified in a minority of embolic survivors. In these patients, an embolic event, which is commonly not diagnosed or treated during its acute phase, results in organized, recanalized residua that obstruct or significantly narrow major pulmonary arteries. Depending on the extent and duration of the residual pulmonary vascular obstruction, a spectrum of clinical presentations may be encountered, from those patients with virtually no symptoms to those with severe pulmonary hypertension and right-heart failure.

Limited data are available regarding the hemodynamic evolution of chronic thromboembolic pulmonary hypertension because clinical recognition often occurs in the later stages of the disease. The symptomatic history, however, does follow a predictable course. Although a significant number of these patients do not have a *documented* history of venous thrombosis or pulmonary embolism, a careful history can often elicit a remote episode consistent with an acute venous thromboembolic event. In the case of venous thrombosis, the event may have been diagnosed as a muscle strain or as cellulitis; in the case of pulmonary embolism, the event may have been considered viral pleurisy or atypical pneumonia. This lack of a documented history likely reflects the often subtle clinical presentation of venous thromboembolism and the frequency with which the diagnosis is overlooked in the population at large (17–19). After a variable period of time, which may range from months to years, the patient has increasing dyspnea and varying degrees of right ventricular hypertrophy or overt right ventricular failure. For those with only modest degrees of pulmonary hypertension at rest, striking increases in pulmonary artery pressure can be elicited with minimal exercise (20).

The exact basis for this asymptomatic period and subsequent decline remain uncertain. Although certain patients may suffer from recurrent thromboembolic events, the majority of those with sequential perfusion scans available for review do not. Alternatively, retrograde extension of embolic obstruction proximal to a partially obstructing lesion may occur within the pulmonary arteries as a result of turbulent and/or sluggish flow (see Chap. 5). Finally, in certain patients it appears increasingly likely that small vessel changes, indistinguishable from those seen in primary pulmonary hypertension, develop in the unobstructed pulmonary vascular bed as a result of high flows and pressures, or the effects of an unidentified mediator (21). These changes in the small pulmonary arteries further increase pulmonary vascular resistance and place an increased demand on the right ventricle. Whatever the mechanisms of hemodynamic decline in a given patient, the historical facts are clear. The patient begins to complain of increasing exertional dyspnea, and over time slowly demonstrates all of the other features of right ventricular dysfunction.

Diagnostic delay occurs commonly, particularly in the absence of an acute history of venous thromboembolism. The progressive dyspnea and exercise intolerance that motivate these patients to seek medical advice are often attributed to coronary artery disease, interstitial lung disease, asthma, deconditioning, or psychogenic dyspnea. Abnormalities of the pulmonary vascular bed as a basis for the patient's dyspnea are often not considered because the findings of pulmonary hypertension in its early stages are subtle and easily overlooked. In time, obvious findings such as jugular venous distention, a right ventricular impulse, wide or fixed splitting of the second heart sound, a prominent pulmonary component of the second heart sound, hepatomegaly, ascites, or peripheral edema may develop. One unique physical finding, not described in small-vessel or other secondary forms of pulmonary hypertension, is the presence of flow murmurs over the lung fields, a result of turbulent flow through partially obstructing or recanalized thrombi (22). These often subtle murmurs are high-pitched and blowing in quality, accentuated during inspiration, and frequently heard only during periods of breath holding.

Initial laboratory studies are usually unremarkable. Approximately 20% of patients demonstrate a mild to moderate restrictive defect on pulmonary function testing, which may, in part, be related to scarring from areas of infarction (23). Although the majority of patients do have a reduction in the single breath diffusing capacity for carbon monoxide, a normal value does not exclude the diagnosis. Virtually all patients, even those normoxic at rest, have a decline in the arterial Po_2 and a rise in the alveolar-arterial gradient with exercise. Dead space ventilation (VD/VT) is increased at rest and worsens with exercise, accounting for part of the exertional dyspnea experienced by these patients. The blood count is normal until late in the course, when hypoxemia induces an increase in the hematocrit and hemoglobin. Blood chemistry studies are normal until right ventricular failure induces hepatic and/or renal abnormalities. The chest radiograph may demonstrate assymetry in the size of the central pulmonary arteries, zones of avascularity, or pleural-based densities consistent with prior areas of infarction. Early in the course of the disease, the electrocardiogram is often quite normal. Later in the course, classical evidence of right ventricular hypertrophy and strain will develop.

Two noninvasive studies, echocardiography and ventilation-perfusion scanning, commonly provide the initial objective evidence that pulmonary hypertension is present and that it might be related to chronic thromboembolic obstruction. Echocardiographic findings include right atrial and right ventricular enlargement, flattening or paradoxic motion of the interventricular septum, tricuspid regurgitation, and elevated pulmonary artery pressure by Doppler interrogation (24) (see Chap. 13). Once the presence of pulmonary hypertension has been established, ventilation-perfusion scanning provides an excellent noninvasive method of distinguishing between potentially operable, major-vessel thromboembolic pulmonary hypertension and obliterative, small-vessel pulmonary hypertension (25). In chronic, major-vessel thromboembolic disease, at least one (and more commonly, several) mismatched segmental defects are present. In contrast, the perfusion scan is either normal or demonstrates patchy subsegmental abnormalities in primary pulmonary hypertension. It is important to recognize, however, that the ventilation-perfusion scan does not define the proximal extent of the chronic thromboembolic obstruction, a critical determinant of operability, and that it often dramatically underestimates the actual extent of pulmonary vascular obstruction (26). Patients may have extensive, central pulmonary artery thrombotic obstruction with quite modest perfusion scan defects.

Right-heart catheterization and pulmonary angiography, therefore, are essential to quantitate the degree of pulmonary hypertension (at rest and, if indicated, with exercise), to exclude competing diagnoses, and to define the proximal extent and surgical accessibility of the obstructing thrombotic lesions. Despite concerns regarding the safe performance of pulmonary angiography in patients with severe pulmonary hypertension, the procedure can be performed safely by a rigorously followed technique, which includes: (a) catheterization via arm or neck, thereby avoiding the femoral veins and the possible induction or dislodgement of lower extremity, iliac or inferior vena caval thrombi; (b) a single injection of nonionic contrast media into the right and left main pulmonary arteries; (c) avoidance of repeated, selective injections; and (d) administration of oxygen and careful rhythm, hemodynamic and gas exchange monitoring during the procedure (27).

Interpretive difficulties exist in assessing the angiographic findings in chronic thromboembolic pulmonary hypertension. A distinction must be made between the sharply defined, intraluminal defects diagnostic of acute pulmonary embolism and the variable angiographic appearance of organized and recanalized chronic thromboemboli (28). Characteristic abnormalities that indicate the presence of chronic thromboembolic pulmonary artery obstruction, one or several of which may be present in the same patient, include arterial "webs" and "bands," intimal irregularities, complete arterial obstruction at the main, lobar or segmental level, and abrupt narrowing of major vessels rather than the usual gradual tapering of vessel size.

Uncertainty about the cause of the angiographic findings or about the surgical accessibility of the obstructing thrombi may still exist after angiography has been performed. Congenital stenotic lesions of the pulmonary arteries and a certain form of large vessel arteritis (Takayasu arteritis) may present a similar angiographic appearance. Total obstruction of major pulmonary arteries occurs in a number of other disorders including carcinoma (vascular or primary lung), extrinsic compression from mediastinal lymphadenopathy, fibrosing mediastinitis, and pulmonary artery agenesis (28). The absence of a main pulmonary vessel at angiography should not be considered to indicate pulmonary artery agenesis. Moser et al. (29) reported six patients initially considered to have congenitally absent pulmonary arteries who were demonstrated to have chronic thromboembolic obstruction. Careful examination of the contralateral pulmonary vascular pattern and a meticulous review of historic and prior radiographic and perfusion scan data may help assist in this distinction. Other ancillary procedures such as computerized tomography to define mediastinal anatomy and arch aortography may be required to exclude possible competing diagnoses.

Pulmonary angioscopy has been found to be useful in establishing a thromboembolic basis for the angiographic findings and in defining the proximal extent of the chronic thromboembolic obstruction (30). The angioscope is a transvenous fiberoptic device with flexion and extension capabilities. At the distal end of the device is a balloon that can be inflated through the angioscope's single channel. Under fluoroscopic guidance, the angioscope is introduced into the pulmonary arteries by way of an internal jugular sheath or a brachial venotomy. Once the angioscope is in place, the balloon is inflated with CO_2 and touched against the walls of the pulmonary artery, thereby displacing blood and allowing direct visualization of the vessel wall. Classic angioscopic signs of chronic thromboemboli include distinct vessel wall irregularities such as pits and ridges, intraluminal webs, and recanalized organized thrombus.

Although pulmonary angiography and/or pulmonary angioscopy usually completes the diagnostic evaluation, adjunctive studies are indicated in selective patients. Coronary angiography is routinely performed on patients above 35 years of age and occasionally in younger patients who have significant coronary risk factors. Noninvasive carotid studies are performed in patients with a history of transient ischemic attacks and/or cerebrovascular accidents and in those with carotid bruits. Prior to thromboendarterectomy, an inferior vena caval filter is placed by way of a percutaneous, transfemoral approach if possible. Every effort is made to protect the patient from additional embolic events, both in the high-risk, early postoperative period when full anticoagulation is contraindicated, and over the long term.

The decision to proceed to pulmonary thromboendarterectomy is based on several objective factors and a willingness by the patient to accept an estimation of the mortal and morbid risks of the procedure that are individualized and based on prior experience. Objective factors, carefully defined during the preoperative evaluation, include (a) the surgical accessibility of the chronic thromboemboli (originating at the main, lobar, or segmental level) as determined by pulmonary angiography and/or angioscopy, and (b) the degree of hemodynamic or ventilatory impairment resulting from the vascular obstruction. Although the overwhelming majority of operated patients have a pulmonary vascular resistance in excess of 300 dyne/s/cm^{-5} at rest or with exercise, occasional patients, especially those with involvement of one main pulmonary artery, have a marked increase in dead space ventilation and significant exercise impairment caused by high minute ventilation demands without substantially altered pulmonary hemodynamics. (c) Also, the presence of co-morbid conditions such as severe parenchymal lung disease might limit the efficacy of the procedure or make the risk of the procedure unacceptable. Age in itself is not a contraindication to the procedure. Patients up to 80 years of age who are otherwise fit have successfully undergone a pulmonary thromboendarterectomy.

Pulmonary thromboendarterectomy is carried out through a median sternotomy incision that provides access to both main pulmonary arteries (5,31–33). Approach by way of a thoracotomy is contraindicated because of the risk of traversing pleural adhesions and bronchial artery collateral vessels and by the need for cardiopulmonary bypass with periods of circulatory arrest to avoid bronchial artery backflow. Furthermore, a thoracotomy approach allows access to only one element of a disease that is almost always bilateral in nature. Cardiopulmonary bypass is instituted with ascending aortic cannulation and two caval cannulae. Hypothermia is initiated on bypass. A temporary pulmonary artery vent is inserted and, when the heart fibrillates, a left ventricular vent is placed through the right upper lobe pulmonary vein.

The patient is cooled to 20° C. During the period of cooling (which takes approximately 45 min), the superior vena cava is thoroughly mobilized as far as the innominate vein with care being taken to avoid injury to the phrenic nerve. The azygos vein is not divided, but the reflection of the right atrium and left atrium to the right pulmonary artery is mobilized to allow the superior vena cava to be lifted from the pulmonary artery. The right pulmonary artery is mobilized intrapericardially and freed as far as the hilum. An incision is made in the right pulmonary artery from the level of the aorta beneath the superior vena cava to enter the lower lobe artery just past the origin of the right middle lobe artery. Separate incisions are not found to be necessary to gain adequate exposure of the upper lobe and middle lobe arteries. Any loose thrombus is removed. Although it is difficult to proceed with the operation prior to full circulatory arrest because of bronchial arterial backflow, an endarterectomy plane often can be raised during the cooling period.

The aorta is cross-clamped when the patient's temperature reaches 20° C and 1000 cc of cold cardioplegic solution is inserted into the aortic root. Additional myocardial protection is obtained throughout the cross-clamp period by the use of a special cooling jacket. Topical cold saline is not used because it obscures the operative site and may induce phrenic nerve injury when combined with profound hypothermia and circulatory arrest. An endarterectomy plane is raised posteriorly, after which each lobe and then the segmental and subsegmental vessels are endarterectomized. For a successful thromboendarterectomy, it is necessary to mobilize the thrombus in each branch circumferentially. Progressive advancement of the endarterectomy specimen is then obtained while it is being freed from the vessel wall so that a cast of the involved pulmonary arteries is obtained. When the endarterectomy is complete on the right side, the left side is then endarterectomized. Again, only one incision is necessary. Bilateral endarterectomy is always performed because unilateral disease is extremely rare in the pulmonary hypertensive patient.

When bronchial arterial back-bleeding impairs optimal visualization, circulatory arrest is imperative. Each period of hypothermic arrest is limited to a maximum of 20 min with resumption of flow between each interruption. With increased experience, the total arrest times have been considerably reduced, and an endarterectomy usually can be performed within a single arrest period on each side (32).

It should be emphasized that restoration of pulmonary arterial patency involves a true endarterectomy of organized, recanalized, and endothelialized thrombus. Considerable surgical experience and an awareness of the angiographic and/or angioscopic findings are essential to differentiate the neointima from the native intima. A pulmonary embolectomy alone of any loose thrombus within the pulmonary artery will not reduce pulmonary vascular resistance if the distal obstruction is not alleviated. Adequate definition of the endarterectomy plane is critical to the success of the procedure. Although it is possible to raise a plane at many levels, only one plane will strip adequately from the underlying media without leaving the vessel wall too thin or with residual intimal thickening.

At the completion of the thromboendarterectomy, circulation is recommenced and the patient rewarmed. The right atrium is always explored for a persistent foramen ovale or atrial septal defect, which occurs in approximately 25% of cases. If additional procedures such as valve replacement or coronary bypass surgery are required, they are conveniently performed during the period of rewarming. Although tricuspid valve repair was carried out in the past in patients with severe preoperative tricuspid regurgitation, this has proven unnecessary. With adequate resolution of pulmonary arterial hypertension, right ventricular dilatation resolves with subsequent reestablishment of tricuspid competence (34).

Careful postoperative management is vital to a successful outcome in these patients. Although most patients have an immediate improvement in postoperative pulmonary hemodynamics, their postoperative management can be complex. In addition to complications common to other forms of cardiac surgery (arrhythmias, atelectasis, wound infections, delirium), patients undergoing pulmonary thromboendarterectomy have two unique complications that may adversely affect early postoperative gas exchange: reperfusion edema and pulmonary artery "steal" (35,36).

Reperfusion pulmonary edema, in its severe form, is now seen in a minority of patients. Reperfusion edema is limited to those areas of the lung from which proximal obstructions have been removed, may appear up to 72 h after surgery and is highly variable in severity, ranging from a mild form of edema to an acute, hemorrhagic, and fatal complication. Less severe forms that result in postoperative hypoxemia are common. Because the areas of alveolar edema involve those segments of lung being preferentially perfused, meticulous ventilatory management is often required until the edema resolves. Based on the relative distribution of ventilation and perfusion, patients may also be dramatically position sensitive with respect to their hypoxemia.

Pulmonary artery steal represents a postoperative redistribution of pulmonary arterial flow caused by the establishment of differential pulmonary vascular resistances within the pulmonary vascular bed: a low-resistance circuit in the endarterectomized bed and a high-resistance circuit in the previously "open" bed. Whether this phenomenon represents a consequence of abnormal vasoregulation in the newly opened pulmonary vascular bed, secondary pulmonary hypertensive changes in the previously open pulmonary vascular bed, or a combination of the two is unknown. Whatever its etiology, the steal phenomenon commonly improves over time (37).

The operative and perioperative mortality rate in the 400 patients who have undergone pulmonary thromboendarterectomy at UCSD Medical Center has been 10.5%. During the development of and early experience with this procedure, mortality was related to many causes including myocardial infarction from unsuspected coronary artery disease, bilateral phrenic nerve paralysis, pulmonary hemorrhage, and sepsis. Over the last 200 cases, the mortality rate has been 6.5%, the majority related either to the presence of thrombi too distal to allow removal or to the development of overwhelming reperfusion edema (Table 1).

Among survivors of the procedure, the immediate postoperative hemodynamic results have been excellent (Table 2). Long-term hemodynamic and functional improvement have also been excellent. Of the first 150 patients, hemodynamic results obtained in 47 who returned for follow-up catheterization at 6–24 months after surgery are demonstrated in Table 3. New York Heart Association functional classification of 117 patients in this same group who were evaluated at 1 year following surgery is demonstrated in Table 4.

Chronic, major vessel thromboembolic pulmonary hypertension, although an uncommon outcome in patients who suffer an acute thromboembolic event, is amenable to surgical correction at an acceptable risk. Compared to transplan-

Table 1 Causes of Death in 13 of the Last 200 Patients Undergoing Pulmonary Thromboendarterectomy at UCSD Medical Center

No.	Cause
6	Inadequate thromboendarterectomy/RV failure
3	Reperfusion pulmonary edema
1	Intraoperative arrest
1	Arrhythmia (presumed)
1	Mediastinal hemorrhage
1	Aortic dissection

Table 2 Pulmonary Hemodynamics in 128 of 150 Patients in Whom Postoperative Values Were Obtained 48–72 h After Intensive Care Unit Admission, Off All Vasoactive Drugs

	Preoperative	Postoperative
PA mean pressure (mm Hg)	46 ± 12	28 ± 9[a]
PA systolic (mm Hg)	76 ± 21	47 ± 16[a]
Cardiac output (L/min)	3.7 ± 1.1	5.7 ± 1.2[a]
PVR (dyne/sec/cm^{-5})	901 ± 467	261 ± 163[a]

Abbreviations: PA, pulmonary artery; PVR, pulmonary vascular resistance.
[a]$P < 0.001$ versus preoperative value.

Table 3 Pulmonary Hemodynamics Obtained in 47 of the First 150 Patients Who Returned for Follow-Up Catheterization at 6–24 Months After Surgery

	Preoperative	Postoperative	Follow-up
PA mean pressure	48 ± 12	27 ± 8[a]	24 ± 10
PA systolic pressure	80 ± 21	44 ± 15[a]	39 ± 17[b]
Cardiac output (L/min)	3.7 ± 1.2	6.0 ± 1.1[a]	4.8 ± 1.0[c]
PVR (dynes/sec/cm^{-5})	971 ± 551	232 ± 111[a]	282 ± 251

Abbreviations: see Table 2 footnotes.
[a]$P < 0.001$ vs preoperative value.
[b]$P < 0.0015$ versus postoperative value.
[c]$P < 0.0001$ versus postoperative value.

Table 4 New York Heart Association Functional Classification of 117 Patients of the First 150 Who Were Evaluated at 1 Year Following Surgery

Class	Preoperative	Follow-up
IV	63	0
III	49	6
II	5	26
I	0	85
Total	117	117

tation, its only therapeutic alternative, pulmonary thromboendarterectomy has much to recommend it in terms of its lower acute and long-term mortality and the absence of need for long-term immunosuppressive therapy. Future initiatives aimed at more exactly defining surgical accessibility; in preventing or ameliorating reperfusion pulmonary edema; in noninvasively identifying patients who have developed irreversible, secondary pulmonary hypertensive changes in their "open" pulmonary vascular bed; and in achieving recognition earlier in the patient's course will further lower this mortality. Although optimal evaluation, operation, and postoperative management require considerable time, skill, and experience, substantial hemodynamic and functional improvement can be achieved in most patients with the majority being able to resume normal functional status.

III. Acute Pulmonary Embolectomy for Massive Pulmonary Embolism

Unlike the now established role of pulmonary thromboendarterectomy for chronic thromboembolic pulmonary hypertension, the role of pulmonary embolectomy in acute massive pulmonary embolism remains controversial. There are those who believe that pulmonary embolectomy is rarely if ever indicated in massive pulmonary embolism (7). Others have suggested that surgical intervention should be considered more often (8–10,38–41). Part of the controversy involves details of operative technique and the necessary extent of preoperative evaluation; the major component, however, is generated by questions regarding the indications for the procedure. Although the overwhelming majority of patients with pulmonary embolism have a favorable outcome with conventional therapy, it is apparent that a subset of patients afflicted with pulmonary embolism have a prognosis that justifies more aggressive therapy. Whether this approach should at times involve surgical intervention or be limited to aggressive medical and thrombolytic therapy cannot be resolved based on current data. However, as stated by Gray et al. (9), the difficulty in defining the group of patients for whom pulmonary embolectomy is appropriate does not necessarily deny the existence of such patients.

The significant mortality associated with acute massive pulmonary embolism justifies a separate consideration of the diagnostic and therapeutic approach to this problem than that of submassive embolism. The hemodynamic response to acute pulmonary thromboembolism is a function of embolic size and, therefore, the degree of pulmonary vascular obstruction, as well as to the preexisting status of the cardiopulmonary system (42–44) (see Chap. 7). Obstruction of the pulmonary vascular bed by embolism acutely increases right ventricular afterload. In patients without preexisting cardiopulmonary disease, obstruction of less than

20% of the pulmonary vascular bed results in a number of compensatory events that minimize adverse hemodynamic consequences. Pulmonary artery mean pressure and pulmonary vascular resistance may remain unchanged as recruitment and distension of pulmonary vessels occur; cardiac output is maintained by increases in right ventricular stroke volume and increases in heart rate. As the degree of pulmonary vascular obstruction exceeds 30%–40%, increases in pulmonary artery mean pressure occur followed by modest increases in right atrial pressure. As end-diastolic pressure increases, Frank-Starling mechanisms maintain right ventricular stroke work and cardiac output. Finally, as the degree of pulmonary obstruction exceeds 50%–60%, compensatory mechanisms are overcome, cardiac output begins to fall, and right atrial pressure increases dramatically. At this point, acute right ventricular failure occurs, accompanied by systemic hypotension. In patients without prior cardiopulmonary disease, a pulmonary artery mean pressure of 30–40 mm Hg represents severe pulmonary hypertension because this is the maximum mean pressure a previously normal right ventricle can generate before it fails. The hemodynamic response to pulmonary thromboembolism in patients with preexisting cardiopulmonary disease is considerably different. In contrast to patients without prior cardiopulmonary disease, in whom there is a general relationship between the degree of pulmonary artery obstruction and level of pulmonary artery mean pressure, patients with prior cardiopulmonary disease demonstrate degrees of pulmonary hypertension that are disproportionate to the degree of embolic obstruction.

Although the traditional definition of massive embolism had been purely anatomic, outcome analysis clearly suggests that a hemodynamic definition is more appropriate clinically (48). This impression is supported by mortality statistics from the urokinase trials and others, which demonstrated that the best predictors of outcome are hemodynamic rather than anatomical (45–48). Although it is true that anatomically massive emboli have a greater likelihood of being associated with hemodynamic compromise, not all anatomically massive emboli necessarily lead to that end. For example, of the 160 patients entered into the Urokinase-Pulmonary Embolism Trial, 90 patients (63%) had anatomically massive emboli, defined as obstruction equivalent to two or more lobar arteries (45). Of these, only 11 patients (12%) were hemodynamically compromised, defined as a documented systolic blood pressure less than 80 mm Hg for at least 10 min with clinical evidence of circulatory insufficiency and resulting organ dysfunction. Three additional patients with anatomically submassive pulmonary emboli had evidence of hemodynamic compromise. Mortality in patients with anatomically massive embolism without evidence of hemodynamic compromise was 6.3%. Mortality in patients with hemodynamic compromise, whether or not the pulmonary embolic event was anatomically massive, was 36%. It is this latter group of patients in whom a more aggressive therapeutic approach is warranted and that is often used as justification for a more widespread application of acute embolectomy. It must be remembered, however, that the number of patients in whom embolectomy might even by considered is small. The majority of patients who die of massive pulmonary embolism either do so suddenly or within 2 h of the acute event, before a diagnosis can be firmly established and before effective therapy can be instituted (49,50). Further, a significant number of patients who do not succumb during those critical early hours will survive without surgery if they receive intensive medical therapy (51). Spontaneous improvement often occurs as fragmentation and distal migration of the obstructing emboli occur.

Given the inability to define precisely the indications for acute embolectomy, it is useful to define those patients who are clearly not candidates. Based on the previously noted mortality statistics, patients with anatomically submassive or massive emboli who are not hemodynamically compromised are not candidates for the procedure. Patients with anatomically submassive or massive emboli who are hemodynamically compromised, who have not had a cardiac arrest, and who do not have an absolute contraindication to thrombolytic therapy should be managed initially with aggressive medical therapy. Although a definite improvement in survival has not been demonstrated with thrombolytic therapy, a conclusion that might reflect sample size limitation, the early anatomical and hemodynamic benefits of thrombolytic therapy have been confirmed (48,52). Because the central goal of therapy in hemodynamically massive pulmonary embolism is to relieve pulmonary vascular obstruction, utilization of agents that might increase the rate of thrombolysis seems warranted. Basic care of a critically ill patient should not be overlooked while specific diagnostic and therapeutic considerations are being implemented (see Chap. 15). Oxygen should be administered to alleviate the hypoxic pulmonary vasoconstriction that might be contributing to the pulmonary hypertension. Intubation and mechanical ventilatory support might be required to improve oxygenation and to decrease metabolic demands. Careful attention should be paid to the patient's volume status. The judicious use of vasopressors and inotropic support can also prove useful in increasing blood pressure and supporting right ventricular function. Although there is a tendency to utilize central hemodynamic monitoring in critically ill, hypotensive patients, this intervention should be considered carefully in the patient with massive pulmonary embolism. A femoral approach poses the risk of dislodging residual ileofemoral thrombus. Furthermore, balloon flotation poses the risk of dislodging embolic material that might be trapped within the right atrium or ventricle.

As noted by Sautter et al. (51), the *only* indication for pulmonary embolectomy is to prevent death. Unfortunately, it is impossible to identify accurately and consistently patients with pulmonary embolism who will die without embolectomy. It is this conundrum that poses the most difficult dilemma for physicians. Under most circumstances, an embolectomy is most feasible and will be most successful in patients who ultimately might not have required it. Yet to delay definitive surgical intervention in a critically ill patient until a cardiac arrest occurs dramatically worsens the potential outcome of those who might have required it. However, based on current data, the only patients in whom acute embolectomy might be considered are those with hemodynamically massive pulmonary embolism who have an absolute contraindication to anticoagulant or thrombolytic therapy, those who have suffered a cardiac arrest, and those in whom aggressive medical therapy, including the use of thrombolytics, has proven ineffective in restoring hemodynamic integrity. Of course, the availability, experience, and expertise of the surgical team should be important considerations in whether an embolectomy should be attempted. *Every* possible attempt should be made to confirm the diagnosis before an embolectomy is considered, even if this requires partial cardiopulmonary bypass while definitive diagnostic procedures are being performed. Mortality in patients referred for pulmonary embolectomy with an incorrect diagnosis approaches 100%.

The surgical approach to pulmonary embolectomy has evolved considerably since Trendelenburg's original description of the procedure using pulmonary artery and aortic outflow occlusion in 1908 (53,54). Currently, the most commonly utilized procedure involves normothermic cardiopulmonary bypass with or without aortic cross-clamping (6–10,38–40). Longitudinal incisions are made in the pulmonary arteries and the emboli extracted using standard forceps or sucking devices. Partial bypass (femoral vein to femoral artery) is often instituted prior to the sternotomy to maintain circulatory integrity and to allow time for definitive diagnostic studies. Others have reported acceptable results utilizing temporary inflow occlusion without cardiopulmonary bypass (40,41). During a short period of circulatory arrest (3 min), the occluding emboli are removed using a common bile duct forceps followed by a sucker to remove smaller, more distal clots.

Perioperative mortality rates for pulmonary embolectomy range from 23% to 80%, a figure obviously influenced by the patient population to which the procedure is applied and the operative technique (7,40). It has been clearly demonstrated that outcome in patients who have not suffered a cardiac arrest is dramatically different than those who have. Gray et al. (8) reported a 29% mortality in 71 patients undergoing pulmonary embolectomy, 11% in those who had not sustained a cardiac arrest, and 64% in those who had. Similar results have been reported recently by Clarke and Abrams (41) and by Meyer et al. (10).

Because the primary purpose of pulmonary embolectomy in massive pulmonary embolism is to relieve the degree of pulmonary vascular obstruction, the concept of doing so with a percutaneous catheter device has been an appealing one. In 1971, Greenfield et al. (55) reported the successful management of acute massive pulmonary embolism in two patients using an embolectomy catheter device. In 1984, Greenfield and Langham (56) reported significant clot extraction in 23 out of 26 patients with an in-hospital mortality rate of 27%. More recently, Timsit et al. (57) reported their results in 18 patients. Although hemodynamic data in the report are limited, thrombus extraction was successful in 11 patients (61%). Overall mortality was 28%, 11% in whom thrombus extraction was successful, and 43% in those in whom it was not. An alternative to catheter embolectomy, a procedure that poses considerable technical challenges, is the application of devices designed to fragment centrally occluding emboli and to disperse them distally, thereby diminishing the absolute extent of pulmonary vascular obstruction. Brady et al. (58) reported dramatic improvement in pulmonary hemodynamics in three patients in whom catheter fragmentation was accomplished using standard cardiac catheters. In an experimental model of pulmonary embolism, Stein et al. (59) were able to fragment occluding emboli with a rotating tip catheter in 6 of 11 animals.

It is unlikely that a randomized trial will ever be performed comparing aggressive medical therapy to surgical therapy in massive pulmonary embolism. As a result, the decision whether or not to refer a critically ill patient for embolectomy will remain one of the most difficult in medicine. Such a decision will continue to be made on a case-by-case basis, guided by a thorough understanding of the natural history of the disease, the results of nonrandomized trials in which these alternative methods of therapy were utilized, and the experience, judgment, and facilities available to the referring physician. Hopefully, the widespread application of venous thrombosis prophylaxis, improved methods of clinical detection and noninvasive diagnosis of venous thromboembolism, and the optimal application of existing therapeutic modalities will assure that this complex and difficult decision is one physicians rarely have to consider.

References

1. Rao MG, Rangwala AF. Diagnostic yield from 231 autopsies in a community hospital. Am J Clin Pathol 1990; 93:486–90.
2. Gross JS, et al. Autopsy study of the elderly institutionalized patient. Review of 234 autopsies. Arch Intern Med 1988; 148:173–6.
3. Berqvist D, Lindblad B. A 30-year survey of pulmonary embolism verified at autopsy: an analysis of 1274 surgical patients. Br J Surg 1985; 72:105–8.
4. Carson JL, et al. The clinical course of pulmonary embolism. N Engl J Med 1992; 326:1240–5.
5. Moser KM, Auger WR, Fedullo PF. Chronic major-vessel thromboembolic pulmonary hypertension. Circulation 1990; 81:1735–43.
6. Moser KM, Auger WR, Fedullo PF, Jamieson SW. Chronic thromboembolic pulmonary hypertension: clinical picture and surgical treatment. Eur Respir J 1992; 5:334–42.

7. Sautter RD, Myers WO, Ray JF III, Wenzel FJ. Pulmonary embolectomy: review and current status. Prog Cardiovasc Dis 1975; 17:371–89.
8. Gr / HH, Morgan JM, Paneth M, Miller GAH. Pulmonary embolectomy for acute massive pulmonary embolism: an analysis of 71 cases. Br Heart J 1988; 60:196–200.
9. Gray HH, Miller GAH, Paneth M. Pulmonary embolectomy: its place in the management of pulmonary embolism. Lancet 1988; i:1441–5.
10. Meyer G, Tamisier D, Herve-Sors, et al. Pulmonary embolectomy: a 20-year experience at one center. Ann Thorac Surg 1991; 51:232–6.
11. Benotti JR, Dalen JE. The natural history of pulmonary embolism. Clin Chest Med 1984; 5:403–10.
12. DeSoyza NDB, Murphy ML. Persistent post-embolic pulmonary hypertension. Chest 1972; 62:665–8.
13. Fred HL, Axelrad MA, Lewis JM, Alexander JK. Rapid resolution of pulmonary thromboemboli in man: an angiographic study. JAMA 1966; 196:121–3.
14. Hall RJC, Sutton GC, Kerr H. Long-term prognosis of treated, acute massive pulmonary embolism. Br Heart J 1977; 39:1128–34.
15. Paraskos JA, Adelstein SJ, Smith RE, et al. Late prognosis of acute pulmonary embolism. N Engl J Med 1973; 289:55–8.
16. Dalen JE, Banas JS, Brooks HL, et al. Resolution rates of acute pulmonary embolism in man. N Engl J Med 1973; 280:1194–9.
17. Huisman MV, Büller HR, ten Cate JW, et al. Unexpected high prevalence of silent pulmonary embolism in patients with deep venous thrombosis. Chest 1989; 95:498–502.
18. Monreal M, Ruiz J, Olazabal A, et al. Deep venous thrombosis and the risk of pulmonary embolism. A systematic study. Chest 1992; 102:677–81.
19. Stein PD, Terrin ML, Hales CA, et al. Clinical, laboratory, roentgenographic and electrocardiographic findings in patients with pulmonary embolism and no pre-existing cardiac or pulmonary disease. Chest 1991; 100:598–603.
20. Fedullo PF, Auger WR, Moser KM, et al. Hemodynamic response to exercise in patients with chronic, major vessel thromboembolic pulmonary hypertension. Am Rev Resp Dis 1990; 141:A-890.
21. Moser KM, Bloor C, Auger WR, Fedullo PF. Plexogenic and angiomatoid lesions occur in chronic, large vessel thromboembolic pulmonary hypertension. Clin Res 1991; 39:42A.
22. Auger WR, Moser KM. Pulmonary flow murmurs. A distinctive physical sign found in chronic pulmonary thromboembolic disease. Clin Res 1989; 37: 145A.
23. Horn M, Ries A, Neveu C, Moser KM. Restrictive ventilatory pattern in precapillary pulmonary hypertension. Am Rev Respir Dis 1983; 128:163–5.
24. Chow LC, Dittrich HC, Hoit BD, et al. Doppler assessment of changes in right-sided cardiac hemodynamics after pulmonary thromboendarterectomy. Am J Cardiol 1988; 61:1092–7.
25. Fishmann AJ, Moser KM, Fedullo PF. Perfusion lung scan vs. pulmonary angiography in evaluation of suspected primary pulmonary hypertension. Chest 1983; 84:679–83.

26. Ryan KL, Fedullo PF, Davis GB, et al. Perfusion scans understate the severity of angiographic and hemodynamic compromise in chronic thromboembolic pulmonary hypertension. Chest 1988; 93:1180–5.
27. Nicod P, Peterson K, Levine M, et al. Pulmonary angiography in severe chronic pulmonary hypertension. Ann Intern Med 1987; 107:565–8.
28. Auger WR, Fedullo PF, Moser KM, et al. Chronic major-vessel thromboembolic pulmonary hypertension: appearance at angiography. Radiology 1992; 182:393–398.
29. Moser KM, Olson KL, Schlusselberg M, et al. Chronic thromboembolic occlusion in the adult can mimic pulmonary artery agenesis. Chest 1989; 95:503–8.
30. Shure D, Gregoratos G, Moser KM. Fiberoptic angioscopy: role in the diagnosis of chronic pulmonary arterial obstruction. Ann Intern Med 1985; 103:844–50.
31. Winkler MH, Rohrer CH, Ratty SC, et al. Perfusion techniques of profound hypothermia and circulatory arrest for pulmonary thromboendarterectomy. Journal of Extra-Corporeal Technology 1990; 22:57–60.
32. Jamieson SW, Auger WR, Fedullo PF, et al. Experience and results of 150 pulmonary thromboendarterectomy operations over a 29 month period. J Thorac Cardiovasc Surg; in press.
33. Moser KM, Kapitan KS, Channick RW, et al. Bronchial arterial blood flow in chronic thromboembolic pulmonary hypertension. Circulation 1991; 8:II-322.
34. Dittrich HC, Nicod PH, Chow LC, et al. Early changes of right heart geometry after pulmonary thromboendarterectomy. J Am Coll Cardiol 1988; 11:937–43.
35. Levinson RM, Shure D, Moser KM. Reperfusion pulmonary edema after pulmonary artery thromboendarterectomy. Am Rev Respir Dis 1986; 134:1241–5.
36. Olman MA, Auger WR, Fedullo PF, Moser KM. Pulmonary vascular steal in chronic thromboembolic pulmonary hypertension. Chest 1990; 98:1430–4.
37. Moser KM, Auger WR, Fedullo PF, Metersky ML. Resolution of pulmonary vascular "steal" after pulmonary thromboendarterectomy. Clin Res 1993; 41:33A.
38. Glassford DM, Alford WC, Burrus GR, et al. Pulmonary embolectomy. Ann Thorac Surg 1981; 32:28–32.
39. Mattox KL, Feldtman RW, Beall AC, DeBakey ME. Pulmonary embolectomy for acute massive pulmonary embolism. Ann Surg 1982; 195:726–31.
40. Del Campo C. Pulmonary embolectomy: a review. Can J Surg 1985; 28:111–3.
41. Clarke DB, Abrams LD. Pulmonary embolectomy: a 25 year experience. J Thorac Cardiovasc Surg 1986; 92:442–5.
42. McIntyre KM, Sasahara AA. Hemodynamic and ventricular responses to pulmonary embolism. Prog Cardiovasc Dis 1974; 17:175–90.
43. Elliott CG. Pulmonary physiology during pulmonary embolism. Chest 1992; 101(suppl):163S–171S.
44. Hoagland PM. Massive pulmonary embolism. In Goldhaber SZ, ed. Pulmonary Embolism and Deep Venous Thrombosis. Philadelphia: WB Saunders Co, 1985; 179–208.
45. National Cooperative Study. The Urokinase Pulmonary Embolism Trial. Circulation 1973; 47(suppl)1–100.
46. Urokinase-Streptokinase Embolism Trial. Phase 2 results. A cooperative study. JAMA 1974; 229:1606–13.

47. Alpert JS, Smith RE, Ockene IS, et al. Treatment of massive pulmonary embolism: the role of pulmonary embolectomy. Am Heart J 1975; 89:413–8.
48. Miller GAH, Hall RJC, Paneth M. Pulmonary embolectomy, heparin and streptokinase; their place in the treatment of acute massive pulmonary embolism. Am Heart J 1977; 93:568–74.
49. Clarke DB. Pulmonary embolectomy re-evaluated. Ann R Coll Surg 1981; 63:18–24.
50. Coon WW, Coller FA. Clinicopathologic correlation in thromboembolism. Surg Gynecol Obstet 1959; 109:259–69.
51. Sautter RD, Myers WO, Wenzel FJ. Implications of the urokinase study concerning the surgical treatment of pulmonary embolism. J Thorac Cardiovasc Surg 1972; 63:54–9.
52. Goldhaber SZ. Thrombolysis for pulmonary embolism. Prog Cardiovasc Dis 1991; 34:113–34.
53. Trendelenburg F. Ueber die Operative Behandlung der Embolie der Lungenarterie. Arch Klin Chir 1908; 86:686.
54. Sabiston DC. Trendelenburg's classic work on the operative treatment of pulmonary embolism. Ann Thorac Surg 1983; 35:570–4.
55. Greenfield LJ, Bruce TA, Nichols NB. Transvenous pulmonary embolectomy by catheter device. Ann Surg 1971; 62:890–7.
56. Greenfield LJ, Langham MR. Surgical approaches to thromboembolism. Br J Surg 1984; 71:968–70.
57. Timset JF, Reynaud P, Meyer G, Sors H. Pulmonary embolectomy by catheter device in massive pulmonary embolism. Chest 1991; 100:655–8.
58. Brady AJB, Crake T, Oakley CM. Percutaneous catheter fragmentation and distal dispersion of proximal pulmonary embolus. Lancet 1991; 338:1186–9.
59. Stein PD, Sabbah HN, Basha MA, et al. Mechanical disruption of pulmonary emboli in dogs with a flexible rotating-tip catheter (Kensey Catheter). Chest 1990; 98:994–8.

Part Five

PREVENTION

18

Prevention of Fatal Pulmonary Embolism

V. V. KAKKAR

Thrombosis Research Institute
London, England

I. Introduction

Venous thromboembolism is a frequent complication of the primary illness in hospital patients. Apart from the immediate risk to life, the late sequelae of extensive deep vein thrombosis must be considered—swelling of the legs, varicose veins, ulceration, and other trophic changes. It is sometimes asked whether postoperative pulmonary embolism is preventable and, furthermore, whether it is worth preventing, because the mortality caused by this complication is extremely low, and all prophylactic measures require supervision and involve extra work. Data are presented to support the argument that not only should venous thromboembolism be prevented but also that prophylactic measures now available make prevention a practical proposition. The need for prophylaxis is best illustrated by the fact that most cases of major embolism are not diagnosed during life and, thus, are not treated. Two thirds of deaths from pulmonary embolism occur within 30 min after the embolic event—too brief a period for any benefit to be derived from thromboembolic therapy, which has been shown to be highly effective in producing rapid lysis of emboli (1). Furthermore, approximately 80% of pulmonary emboli occur without premonitory signs of peripheral venous thrombosis, and, consequently, treatment with heparin and oral anticoagulants to prevent embolism is often not given. Thus, to adopt a policy of treating massive pulmonary embolism or its precursor, peripheral venous thrombosis, is to expose patients to an unacceptable risk of fatal complications.

The most rational approach, therefore, would seem to be that of developing an effective method of prophylaxis, if the mortality caused by pulmonary embolism and the misery caused by the postphlebitic syndrome are to be significantly reduced. If such a method is to be adopted on a wide scale, it should fulfill the following criteria: It must be simple, safe, and effective; it must be applicable to all types of patients at risk of developing deep vein thrombosis; and it must cover the period of risk, which in surgical patients has been shown to extend from the time of operation through the first 7–10 postoperative days. A number of drugs are now available for preventing fatal pulmonary emboli. These include dextran, oral anticoagulants, low-dose heparin, and low molecular weight heparin.

II. Dextran

A commonly used agent for prevention of venous thromboembolism is dextran, which is a partially hydrolyzed glucose polymer produced from the bacteria *Leuconostoc mesenteriodes*. There are two dextran preparations suitable for clinical use, dextran 70 (average molecular weight 70,000), and dextran 40, or "low molecular weight dextran" (average molecular weight 40,000). The two preparations are not distinct; the lower molecular weight spectrum of one overlaps the upper molecular weight spectrum of the other. A number of studies have demonstrated that dextran infusion started during surgery and continued in the postoperative period is effective in reducing the incidence of deep vein thrombosis (DVT) and pulmonary embolism (PE). In these, the ratio of the incidence of venous thrombosis in treated versus untreated patients was 1:2, and for pulmonary embolism, it was 1:3.8. In a large-scale study, the value of dextran infusion was compared with low-dose heparin against fatal pulmonary embolism after elective operations for general, orthopedic, urological, and gynecological conditions. Out of 3984 patients correctly admitted to the trial, 1993 were allocated to receive dextran 70 and 1991 to receive low-dose heparin. Of 75 patients who died within 30 days of operation, 38 had been given dextran and 37 low-dose heparin. Necropsy was performed in 33 and 32 of these cases, respectively. In six patients in each group, pulmonary embolism was the sole or a contributory cause of death. Of these, five patients in the dextran group and two in the heparin group had received a full course of prophylaxis. Complications of dextran therapy include pulmonary edema in patients with limited cardiac reserve, occasional renal failure, mild allergenic reactions, and rare anaphylactic responses. A survey involving 236 clinics in Sweden showed that approximately 12% of clinicians do not use dextran 70 for prophylaxis because of the risk of serious anaphylactic reactions. It has also been suggested that bleeding complications approach those of oral anticoagulants in frequency. Furthermore, the drug is expensive and must be given intravenously, and its use is restricted to hospitalized patients during the acute phase of their illness.

III. Oral Anticoagulants

Oral anticoagulants, properly employed (started well before operation) are the most effective and proved method of preventing venous thrombosis. In controlled clinical trials the incidence of venous thrombosis was 0–36.0% (average 7.7%) in the treated groups and 1.1%–56.0% (average 20.8%) among controls. Pulmonary embolism occurred in 0%–2.5% (average 0.8%) of the controls (2). The true impact of these data can only be realized by analysis according to patient categories. Encouraging results of oral anticoagulant prophylaxis have been reported in patients undergoing orthopedic surgery, such as reconstructive hip surgery. Among such patients, there has been a reduction of approximately 66% in the incidence of deep vein thrombosis and 80% in the incidence of pulmonary embolism as compared with the randomly allocated controls. Similar results have been reported in patients undergoing thoracic and general abdominal surgery. Embolism is quite frequent in patients with heart disease, particularly in those with congestive cardiac failure. Among such patients, oral anticoagulant therapy was effective in reducing the incidence of deep vein thrombosis by approximately 80%, as compared with untreated controls. A major drawback of oral anticoagulant therapy is the risk of massive hemorrhage during and after operation, despite laboratory control of the dosage given. The incidence of severe hemorrhage in the various reported studies has varied between 2% and 7%, and the mortality rate has been in the range of 0.08%–0.1%. The risk of hemorrhage and the need for strict laboratory control have undoubtedly contributed to the relatively low level of acceptance of this form of prophylaxis among surgeons generally, at least in the United States and the United Kingdom (3).

IV. Low-Dose Heparin

A form of therapy that is both effective and devoid of the drawbacks of oral anticoagulant therapy would meet a real need. Ideally, any agent used for the prophylaxis of deep vein thrombosis should be well tolerated by the patient, have no side effects, require no special monitoring, and produce no bleeding in a clinical situation in which the patient is subjected to major tissue trauma. The promising approach in the past has been the use of low-dose heparin, given subcutaneously, which has been claimed to prevent thrombosis without increasing the risk of hemorrhage. The results of 77 clinical trials of low-dose heparin prophylaxis in a variety of patient populations have now been reported (2). The greatest experience has been acquired in patients undergoing general abdominal, thoracic, and urological operations. Despite variations in the study designs and regimen of low-dose heparin used in these studies, there was evidence of a significant reduction of the incidence of deep vein thrombosis in patients receiving heparin.

In the final analysis, a crucial question concerns the effect of low-dose heparin in the prevention of fatal and nonfatal pulmonary embolism. This end point has been evaluated in several studies. The most important and largest of these was an international multicenter, prospective, randomized, controlled trial that was conducted in 28 centers, each of which had a separate list of allocations to randomize patients into control and heparin groups (5). The heparin-treated patients received calcium heparin 5000 U subcutaneously, 2 h preoperatively and every 8 h for 7 days or until they became ambulant. Patients in the control group did not receive placebo injections. The major end point of the study was fatal pulmonary embolism diagnosed at autopsy. Fatal pulmonary embolism was defined as massive fresh emboli present in the main pulmonary trunk, main pulmonary artery, or in at least two lobar arteries, demonstrated postmortem in patients in whom no other cause of death was found. This study involved 4121 patients over the age of 40 years undergoing a variety of elective major surgical procedures; 2076 of these were in the control group, and 2045 received heparin. The two groups were well matched for age, sex, weight, blood group, and other factors that could predispose to the development of venous thromboembolism. During the postoperative period, 180 patients (4.4%) died, 100 in the control group and 80 in the heparin group. Necropsies were performed on 72% of the patients who died in the control group and 66% of those who died in the heparin group. Sixteen of the control patients and two of the heparin-treated group were found to have died from massive pulmonary embolism ($P < 0.005$). In addition, the emboli found at necropsy in six patients in the control group and in three in the heparin-treated group were considered to have been either only contributory to death or incidental findings, because death in these patients was attributed to other causes. If one takes all pulmonary emboli together, the findings were again significant ($P < 0.005$). A number of parameters were used to assess the frequency of bleeding complications. Wound hematoma developed in 117 controls and 158 patients in the heparin group ($P < 0.01$). However, no significant difference was observed between the two groups in other parameters including perioperative blood loss, mean transfusion requirements for each patient related to their operation, and fall in hemoglobin 1 week after surgery, compared to the preoperative level. These results have been further supported by an overview of 70 randomized trials of low-dose heparin involving nearly

16,000 patients (6). In this meta-analysis, the reduction in deaths attributed to pulmonary embolism was striking, with 19 deaths in patients receiving heparin, as compared with 55 deaths in control patients ($P < 0.001$). However, once again there was clear and consistent evidence for an increased risk of bleeding after administration of subcutaneous heparin (overall, 419 episodes in the heparin group versus 244 in the control group) in nearly 13,500 patients for whom bleeding data were available.

V. Low Molecular Weight Heparins

Low molecular weight heparins represent the most significant recent development in antithrombotic therapy. The impetus for their development came from the pivotal multicenter trial of low-dose prophylaxis, the results of which were published in 1975 and clearly demonstrated the protective effect not only against postoperative deep vein thrombosis but also fatal and nonfatal pulmonary embolism. However, there were two major disadvantages of low-dose heparin that had to be overcome if this form of prophylaxis was to be used on a large scale. Firstly, heparin had to be administered each 8 or 12 h, and second there was a definite increased risk of bleeding, mostly in the form of wound hematoma. Thus, low molecular weight heparins were developed to overcome these two main disadvantages of standard heparin (SH) prophylaxis.

The potential advantages of their use as prophylactic antithrombotic agents are based on their two- to fourfold longer plasma half-life when compared to SH at therapeutic doses and 90%–98% bio-availability following subcutaneous administration, thus enabling them to be administered as a single daily injection. Furthermore, for an equivalent antithrombotic effect, low molecular weight heparins have been shown to cause less hemorrhage in experimental models than SH (7,8) and, therefore, are presumed to be associated with a reduced risk of perioperative bleeding in surgical patients.

Over the past decade, low molecular weight heparins (LMWHs) have been evaluated in a number of double-blind, randomized clinical trials. The first prospective study of the efficacy of low molecular weight heparin in patients was published by Kakkar et al. (9) in 1982. In this study, 150 consecutive patients undergoing major abdominal surgery were investigated. Fifty of these patients received 1250 APTT units of a heparin fraction prepared by gel permeation every 12 h, while the remaining 100 patients received a single injection of 1850 U daily. The units of activity were measured by an APTT assay, and the LMWH had an anti-Xa/APTT ratio of 4. None of the patients died from pulmonary embolism, and three in each group developed deep vein thrombosis detected by the ^{125}I-fibrinogen uptake test. Prophylaxis had to be discontinued in 2 of the 50 patients who received low molecular weight heparin every 12 h. The effect of equal amounts of low molecular weight heparin and unfractionated heparin on the coagulation mechanism was also investigated in this study.

Global clotting assays and platelet function tests indicated that both the low molecular weight heparin and unfractionated heparin produced comparable effects, although intragroup comparisons revealed significant differences in anti-Xa activity, lipoprotein lipase release, and plasma prekallikrein and thromboxane B_2 concentration (9). Thus, this study was first to show that a single daily dose of low molecular weight heparin administered subcutaneously was sufficient to prevent postoperative deep vein thrombosis in 97 out of 100 patients monitored by the ^{125}I-fibrinogen uptake test for at least 10 days. In a follow-up study, Kakkar and Murray (10) assessed the efficacy and safety of the same low molecular weight heparin in the prevention of deep vein thrombosis in a double-blind, randomly allocated trial involving 400 patients, half of whom received low molecular weight heparin and the other half unfractionated heparin. Isotopic deep vein thrombosis was developed by 7.5% of patients receiving unfractionated heparin and 2.5% receiving low molecular weight heparin, the difference in the frequency of deep vein thrombosis in the two groups being statistically significant ($P < 0.05$). No significant difference between the two groups in terms of excessive incisional or total blood loss during surgery was observed. In a further 910 patients included in an "open" study, who again received a single daily injection of low molecular weight heparin every day, 3.4% developed isotopic deep vein thrombosis. Several other randomized, double-blind trials, using almost similar design have subsequently confirmed the original observations reported by Kakkar et al. (9–12).

In a large multicenter Italian trial, Pezzuoli et al. (13) randomized 4498 patients to receive either 7500 anti-Xa IC units of Fraxiparine once daily or placebo (13). Eight (0.36%) deaths occurred to the Fraxiparine group and 18 (0.80%) in the placebo group, the difference being significant ($P < 0.05$). Autopsy was performed in 88.5% of the patients who died, and two deaths were attributed directly to pulmonary embolism in the treated group (0.09%) and four in the placebo group (0.18%). There was also a statistically significant reduction in thromboembolic mortality in favor of low molecular weight heparin (0.36%–0.09%) ($P < 0.05$). Intra- and postoperative bleeding was significantly more frequent in the low molecular weight heparin group ($P < 0.01$), although such bleeding complications did not cause a significant difference in prophylaxis discontinuation. However, in comparison with the placebo group, there was a significantly higher incidence ($P < 0.01$) of wound hematoma.

In a recent meta-analysis study, Nurmohamed et al. (14) analyzed all comparative trials of perioperative prophylaxis against deep vein thrombosis or pulmonary embolism in patients undergoing general surgery (defined as abdominothoracic or gynecological surgery) or orthopedic surgery (defined as elective or traumatic hip surgery), only studies that compared low molecular weight heparin and unfractionated heparin, both agents being given in the currently recommended dose were included in the analysis. A total of 8172 patients were included in this analysis; 6878 patients were in the 17 general surgery trials and 1294 in the 6 orthopedic surgery trials. For the general surgical trials, ^{125}I-fibrinogen leg scanning was used as the end point for the diagnosis of deep vein thrombosis while for orthopedic surgery, only trials in which venography was used in all patients for establishing the presence or absence of deep vein thrombosis were included. For the rate of fatal and nonfatal pulmonary embolism, the diagnosis was accepted if one or more of the following methods or criteria were applied in both study groups: necropsy, perfusion-ventilation scanning, and angiography or clinical diagnosis, total mortality, and major bleeding was defined as clinically overt with one or more of the following criteria: fall in hemoglobin of more than 1.2 g/I, bleeding necessitating reoperation or cessation of prophylaxis, or retroperitoneal or intracranial bleeding.

In the general surgery group, 184 patients out of 3467 patients developed deep vein thrombosis compared to 230 out of 3411 in the unfractionated heparin group. A relative risk of deep vein thrombosis of low molecular weight heparin over standard heparin for all surgical trials was 0.74 (95% CI 0.65–0.86). In contrast, 9 out of 2888 patients in the low molecular weight heparin group and 20 out of 2843 patients in the standard heparin group developed pulmonary emboli. Thus, the relative risk for all pulmonary emboli of low molecular weight heparin over standard was 0.44 (95% CI 0.21–0.95). In the general surgery trials, the absolute mean incidence of major bleeding was 2.6% in each of the two treatment groups. In the general surgery group, 52 out of 1977 patients receiving low molecular weight heparin and 51 out of 1966 receiving standard heparin developed major bleeding—a relative risk of 1.01 (95% CI 0.70–1.48). In the orthopedic group, only 6 out of 672 patients receiving low molecular weight heparin and 8 out of 622 receiving standard heparin developed major bleeding—a relative risk of 0.75 (95% CI 0.26–2.14). The authors concluded that at present, there is no convincing evidence that in general surgery patients, low molecular weight heparin compared with standard heparin generates a clinically important improvement in the benefit to risk ratio. However, low molecular weight heparins may be preferable for orthopedic surgery patients, in view of the large risk reduction for venous thrombosis.

VI. The Definitive Trial

There is no doubt that several studies have clearly shown that low molecular weight heparins represent the most significant development in antithrombotic therapy. As already stated, they have been evaluated in a number of randomized clinical trials and have been shown to be particularly effective in preventing postoperative venous thromboembolism in patients undergoing major abdominal and orthopedic surgery. However, to date, in all the randomized clinical trials designed to compare the safety and efficacy of low molecular weight heparin and standard heparin, limited numbers of patients have been included, and, thus, it has not been possible to answer the following critical questions that need to be resolved before recommending their use on a large scale: Is the risk of perioperative bleeding significantly reduced when low molecular weight heparin is compared to standard heparin for prophylaxis? Does the bleeding induced by heparin prophylaxis, particularly low molecular weight heparin, significantly alter the outcome of surgery? What factors, in addition to heparin prophylaxis, constitute an increased risk of bleeding? How long should prophylaxis be continued, because a recent large study (15) has claimed that the risk of postoperative deep vein thrombosis/pulmonary embolism persists for a considerable time following discharge from hospital? A multicenter randomized, double-blind, comparative trial of low molecular weight heparin (Fragmin) and standard heparin for the prevention of postoperative venous thromboembolism in patients undergoing major abdominal surgery has been recently completed (16). Surgeons in 19 hospitals took part in this study; 3938 patients were entered into this trial. This sample size was calculated on an assumption based on the previous multicenter trial (International Multicentre Trial 1975), which showed an incidence of bleeding events of 10%. Given that a 30% reduction in these events would be clinically significant, it was estimated that at least 3600 evaluable patients would be required with equal numbers in each group, to give a 90% probability of detecting the difference at the 5% level of confidence. The sample size was increased by 10% to allow protocol violations. Eligible patients were randomly allocated to receive subcutaneously either 2500 U of low molecular weight heparin (Fragmin) once daily plus a placebo injection or 5000 U of standard heparin twice daily. Of 3938 patients entered in the trial, 129 were excluded from the analysis because in the vast majority, the scheduled operation was cancelled. Of the remaining 3809 patients, 1894 received low molecular weight heparin and 1915 standard heparin. The two groups were well matched with respect to age, sex, weight, height and body mass index, and other risk factors that could predispose to a higher incidence of postoperative deep vein thrombosis/pulmonary embolism. Over 60% of patients had more than two risk factors known to predispose to a higher frequency of thromboembolism, and 37.6% of patients were operated for malignant disease. Of 3809 patients included in this study, perioperative deaths occurred in 110 patients (2.8%): 63 in the low molecular weight heparin group and 47 (2.5%) in the standard heparin group. This difference is not statistically significant (PR 1.36, C 10.93–1.97, $P = 0.13$). Ninety-two (84%) deaths occurred in patients who were operated for malignant disease. Autopsy was performed in 58% of patients, but in those suspected of sudden death caused by cardiovascular or respiratory disease, autopsy was performed in all cases. Pulmonary emboli were detected in 27 patients (0.7%): 13 (0.7%) of the low molecular weight heparin group and 14 (0.7%) in the standard heparin group. Sudden death occurred in eight of these patients, and autopsy was performed in each case. Five (0.26%) patients in the low molecular weight heparin group and three (0.16%) in the standard heparin group were found to have died from acute massive pulmonary embolism. The diagnosis of deep vein thrombosis was made in 11 (0.6%) patients in each group.

The safety of the heparins was assessed by using objective criteria, and the bleeding was classified as major and minor. Ninety-three indices of major bleeding events were observed in 69 (3.6%) patients in the low molecular weight heparin group and 141 indices in 91 (4.8%) patients in the standard heparin group. Nonparametric testing revealed that the difference in the indices had a statistical significance of $P = 0.058$. To assess the severity of bleeding in the two groups, the patients were scored according to various indices of major bleeding with 1 point being allocated for each event. Severe bleeding (scoring 2 or more) occurred less frequently in the low molecular weight heparin group with 18 (1.0%) versus 36 (1.9%) patients in the standard heparin group (RR 0.51, CI 0.29–0.89, $P = 0.02$). Similarly, wound hematoma were less commonly seen in the low molecular weight heparin group; 27 (1.4%) versus 52 (2.7%) (RR 0.52, CI 0.33–0.83, $P = 0.007$). Furthermore, 20 bleeding episodes in 18 (0.95%) patients in the low molecular weight heparin group and 38 episodes in 33 (1.72%) patients in the standard heparin group required further surgery, either for the evacuation of hematoma or reoperation to control bleeding (RR 0.55, CI 0.31–0.98, $P = 0.05$). Injection site bruising was also less common in the low molecular weight heparin group; 74 (3.9%) versus 120 (6.3%) (RR 0.62, CI 0.47–0.83, $P = 0.001$).

The follow-up assessment was performed on 3358 (91%) of 3699 evaluable patients. Nineteen patients (0.57%) died: 10 (0.60%) in the low molecular weight heparin group and 9 (0.53%) in the standard heparin group. Twenty-five (0.74%) patients developed thromboembolic complications, 15 in the low molecular weight heparin group and 10 in the standard heparin group (RR 1.53, CI 0.69–3.40, $P = 0.39$). Pulmonary embolism occurred in nine (0.5%) patients in the low molecular weight heparin group and five (0.3%) in the standard heparin group. Of the three patients who had fatal pulmonary emboli (confirmed at autopsy), two received low molecular weight heparin, and one received standard heparin. All patients who survived received anticoagulant therapy.

In summary, this prospective, randomized, double-blind trial designed essentially to compare the safety of two drugs, and involving 3809 patients, has demonstrated that low molecular weight heparin has greater safety as compared with standard heparin, with a significant difference in the objective indices of major bleeding during the postoperative period. Severe bleeding occurred less frequently in the low molecular weight heparin group; significantly fewer wound fewer wound hematomas developed, and a lesser number of patients required further surgery for the evacuation of hematoma or reoperation to control bleeding. Evidence has also been provided that both antithrombotic agents appear to be of equal efficacy in preventing postoperative venous thromboembolic complications. Furthermore, for the first time, a high-risk profile of patients who are likely to bleed has been established, and the data have also been presented on the prospective follow up of the majority (91%) of patients following discharge from hospital to assess the incidence of postdischarge venous thromboembolic complications.

VII. A Reduction in Both Fatal Pulmonary Embolism Detected at Necropsy and Postoperative Deep Vein Thrombosis over 15 Years

Following the publication of the International Multicentre Trial (1975), low-dose heparin prophylaxis was adopted on a large scale. However, it is not known whether such a wide use of prophylaxis in fact has resulted in a reduction in the frequency of fatal pulmonary embolism. In fact, a recent study from Sweden examined necropsy findings from medical and surgical departments in one hospital by performing four annual reviews over a 30-year time period (17). This study concluded that the "overall incidence of venous thromboembolism has not changed over 30 years." On the other hand, it has also been claimed that there has been a reduction in the incidence of pulmonary embolism in surgical patients (17). However, no information has been provided whether the frequency

Table 1 Total and Postoperative (PO) Fatal Pulmonary Emboli (FPE)[a]

	No.			
Years	All necropsies	Total FPE	PO FPE	% FPE PO
1976–1980	2660	4.5 (120)	1.2 (33)	27.5
1981–1985	2354	2.3 (54)[b]	0.6 (13)[c]	24.1
1986–1990	2963	2.1 (62)	0.4 (12)	19.4

Chi-square tests for linear trend with time for total and postoperative FPE and the percentage of FPE that were postoperative: All chi squares were >50, P = 0.00001.

[a]At necropsy as a percentage of all necropsies, and the percentage of FPE that are PO (% FPE PO) over 25 years.

[b]When compared with the previous 5-year period: $P < 0.0001$.

[c]When compared with the previous 5-year period: $P = 0.02$. The other comparisons were nonsignificant by conventional levels of statistical significance ($P > 0.05$).

of spontaneous deep vein thrombosis has also changed or remained constant during this period. These issues have been addressed in a recent retrospective analysis, in which all necropsy reports between 1976 and 1990 were analyzed, and those that reported the cause of death as fatal pulmonary embolism were checked to ascertain whether they occurred postoperatively (18). In order to assess the frequency of spontaneous venous thrombosis, all diagnostic venograms, totaling 6436, performed in our hospital from 1976 to 1990 were also reviewed. Those showing evidence of fresh thrombus were subclassified into two groups: "spontaneous," occurring in patients referred from the local primary care physicians within the King's Health District, and "postoperative," occurring in patients following surgery performed in our hospital. The statistical significance tests for the comparison of two proportions was with the appropriate methods using both the chi-square test with Yates correction and the "Z" test, which was referred to the tables of the normal distribution. The test for the comparison of two rates was also the "Z" test. The chi-square test for trend was analyzed by computer using the "EPI-INFO" package.

During 1976–1990, 7977 autopsies were performed. When compared with the previous 5-year period (1976–1980), there was a highly significant reduction in the frequency of total fatal pulmonary embolism from 4.5 to 2.3 per 100 necropsies ($P = 0.0001$) as well as postoperative fatal pulmonary embolism from 1.2 to 0.6 per 100 necropsies ($P = 0.0001$). However, in the subsequent 5 years (the period between 1986 and 1990), the differences in both total fatal pulmonary embolism and postoperative fatal pulmonary embolism were not significant.

The King's District Health Authority was formed in 1974, and, hence, the data on the population characteristics were available from 1975 onwards. As shown in Table 2, the number of patients discharged from hospital per year has remained constant during this period of observation. There was a marked reduction in the annual rate of postoperative deep vein thromboses per 100,000 population diagnosed by venography. A significant fall in the rate occurred between 1976 and 1980 and 1981 and 1985; however, the rate of spontaneous deep vein thrombosis per 100,000 population remains almost constant (Table 3). The greatest fall in the rate of venographically diagnosed deep vein thromboses

Table 2 Characteristics of the District Health Authority

Year	Patient discharges	District population	% Over 65
1975	35,000	242,000	13.7
1980	36,000	220,000	15.0
1985	37,500	215,000	14.4
1990	36,800	211,000	13.7

Table 3 Hospital Diagnosis Rate of Spontaneous and Postoperative Deep Venous Thrombosis (DVT) by Venography per 100,000 Residents in the District per Year

Years	Spontaneous DVTs	Postoperative DVTs
1976–1980	26.6	49.9
1981–1985	29.5	24.7[a]
1986–1990	27.3	21.7

[a]When compared with the previous 5-year period: $P <$ 0.0001. The other comparisons were nonsignificant by conventional levels of statistical significance ($P > 0.05$).

was concurrent with the maximal decline in the finding of fatal pulmonary embolism at necropsy.

During the period of this study, several significant changes occurred at our hospital. In the early 1970s heparin was gradually introduced in surgical clinical trials, and many surveillance studies were undertaken. In the late 1970s, several studies were performed that compared groups receiving thromboprophylaxis with placebo control groups. Subsequently, in the 1980s, control groups received standard low-dose heparin and comparative studies with differing, but progressively more efficacious, regimens of heparin prophylaxis (including a combination of heparin and dihydroergotamine-DHE, or low molecular weight heparin) were undertaken. It is more than likely that the wider adoption of prophylaxis in all surgical patients during the time period 1980–1985 compared with 1976–1980 was responsible for the observed significant reduction in the frequency of postoperative fatal pulmonary embolism. However, these conclusions must be considered in the light of inherent limitations of necropsy data that essentially represents a highly selected population and may not represent true hospital or community disease rates (19).

VIII. Adoption of Low Molecular Weight Heparin Prophylaxis

The evidence that low molecular weight heparin and standard heparin can prevent venous thromboembolism in most postoperative patients is irrefutable. Furthermore, as already stated, a number of studies have also demonstrated that a fixed dose of low molecular weight heparin administered as a single daily subcutaneous injection is at least as effective a prophylactic agent as standard heparin given every 8 or 12 h. Therefore, low molecular weight heparin prophylaxis has a potential advantage of better acceptance by the patients, and its adoption on a large scale should save considerable nursing time. However, one of the main unresolved questions in the past related to the presumed greater safety of low molecular weight heparin. This critical question was answered by the results of a large multicenter, randomized, double-blind comparative trial involving approximately 4000 patients. As already stated ($P = 0.058$), serious bleeding during the perioperative period was significantly reduced with the low molecular weight heparin, which was primarily due to a reduction in the frequency of postoperative bleeding complications. Furthermore, there were significantly less wound hematomas in the low molecular weight heparin group, as well as fewer patients requiring evaluation of hematoma or reoperation to control bleeding.

Another concern about the adoption of heparin prophylaxis in the past has been whether the bleeding induced significantly alters the outcome of surgery, particularly anastomic failure in patients having colinic or gastroesophageal anastomosis, wound infection, and wound dehiscence. In a recent report of the National Confidential Enquiry into Peri-Operative Deaths (NCEPOD, 1990), the frequency of such complications in 1109 patients who died was analyzed. When the complication rate calculated in each of the NCEPOD surgical groups was applied to the multicenter trial data (20), the following number of events would be aspected: anastomic failure in five, wound dehiscence in four, and wound infection in seven. In fact in the 110 patients who died during the peri-operative period in the multicenter trial, anastomic failure occurred in 8 (7.3%), wound dehiscence in 1 (0.26%), and wound infection in 12 (11.0%). Although an accurate comparison can only be made in a double-blind, randomized trial having a control group, the comparison with the NCEPOD data does appear to suggest that the use of heparin prophylaxis does not significantly alter the outcome of surgery.

The other unresolved issue for a wider adoption of low molecular weight heparin prophylaxis in the past has related to the duration for which heparin prophylaxis had to be administered. It had been claimed by some studies that the risk of postoperative deep vein thrombosis and pulmonary embolism persists for a considerable time following discharge from hospital. In the multicenter trial (as already stated), 3358 patients were followed up at a minimum of 4 weeks after discharge; 19 patients died, 10 in the low molecular weight heparin group and 9 in the standard heparin group. Fifteen (79%) of these had malignant disease. Of three patients (0.09%) who died because of fatal pulmonary embolism, one was suffering from disseminated malignant disease; another had an operation for carcinoma of the rectum and had been readmitted with a recent cerebrovascular accident, and the third was a Parkinsonian patient who had an operation for fibroid uterus and had been diagnosed and subsequently treated for active tuberculosis. Therefore, it can be argued that long-term prophylaxis would not have made a significant difference to the final prognosis in these three cases.

Recently, discussion has also focussed on the cost-effectiveness of thromboprophylaxis in surgery, particularly because the decision-making process is lately, to a considerable extent, based on economic implications. A number of studies have evaluated the cost-effectiveness of various strategies for routine use of thromboprophylaxis (21–26). The results in general indicate that thromboprophylaxis is cost-effective and, besides saving lives by preventing fatal pulmonary embolism, also saves money.

The results of the International Multicentre Trial published in 1975 laid the foundation for the worldwide adoption of low-dose heparin prophylaxis. The first postoperative study of the efficacy of low molecular weight heparin in patients was published in 1982 (27). This pivotal study paved the way for many studies that have followed, confirming the original observation that a single daily fixed dose of low molecular weight heparin prevented most postoperative deep vein thrombosis and was likely to be more acceptable to patients and save nursing time. The results of the multicenter trial indicate that both low molecular weight heparin and standard heparin are equally effective in preventing postoperative venous thromboembolism, but a specific preparation of low molecular weight heparin (Fragmin™ is safer than standard heparin and, therefore, is less likely to cause serious bleeding complications (20).

IX. Current Practices of Prevention

In a recent survey (28), a random sample of 1920 surgeons in the United States and Western Europe were asked to complete a questionnaire concerning their practices and beliefs about the prevention of venous thromboembolism. Seventy percent of the respondents were general, vascular, or orthopedic surgeons. A total of 886 surgeons responded. The questionnaire asked the following questions: whether they use prophylaxis, what methods they use, when did they start and stop prophylaxis, which patients receive prophylaxis, and what risk factors did they consider important.

X. Reasons for Not Using Prophylaxis

Of the 886 respondents, 113 (13%) replied that they did not use prophylaxis. Reasons stated by the nonusers were that DVT is not a problem in my practice (62 respondents), prophylaxis is too expensive (20 respondents, United States only), prophylaxis is not effective (13 respondents), and organizational problems (5 respondents, United States and United Kingdom only). Thus, the most surprising finding was a perception that DVT is not a problem in their clinical practice. Expense was a reason for not using prophylaxis stated by more than half of the U.S. respondents, and this may be related to the private health care schemes in the United States. Expense was not a major concern in Western Europe.

XI. Methods of Prophylaxis Used

More than 90% of respondents in the United Kingdom and Switzerland, 100% in Germany, and 65% in the United States claimed to use subcutaneous heparins (Fig. 1). Warfarin was used by 35% of respondents in the United States, partly reflecting the inclusion of orthopedic surgeons in the U.S. sample. A similar rate of warfarin use has been reported for British orthopedic surgeons. Fewer vascular and general surgeons in the European countries used warfarin. Dextrans and

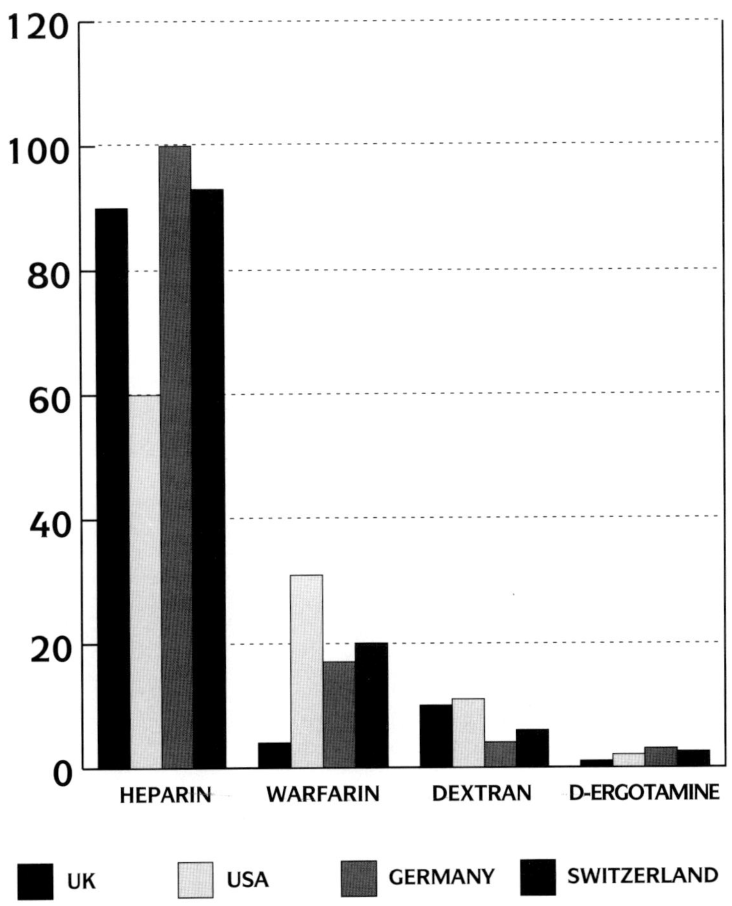

Figure 1 The proportion of respondents using pharmacological methods of prophylaxis.

dihydroergotamine are not commonly used in any of the countries included in the survey.

Elastic stockings—the simplest form of mechanical prophylaxis—are used by more than half of U.S. and Swiss surgeons and 75% of U.K. surgeons, and are used almost universally in Germany (Fig. 2). Intermittent calf compression is unpopular in Germany and Switzerland but more favored in the United States (59%) and the United Kingdom (32.6%). Few surgeons choose electrical calf stimulation.

Less than 30% of respondents from the United Kingdom, United States,

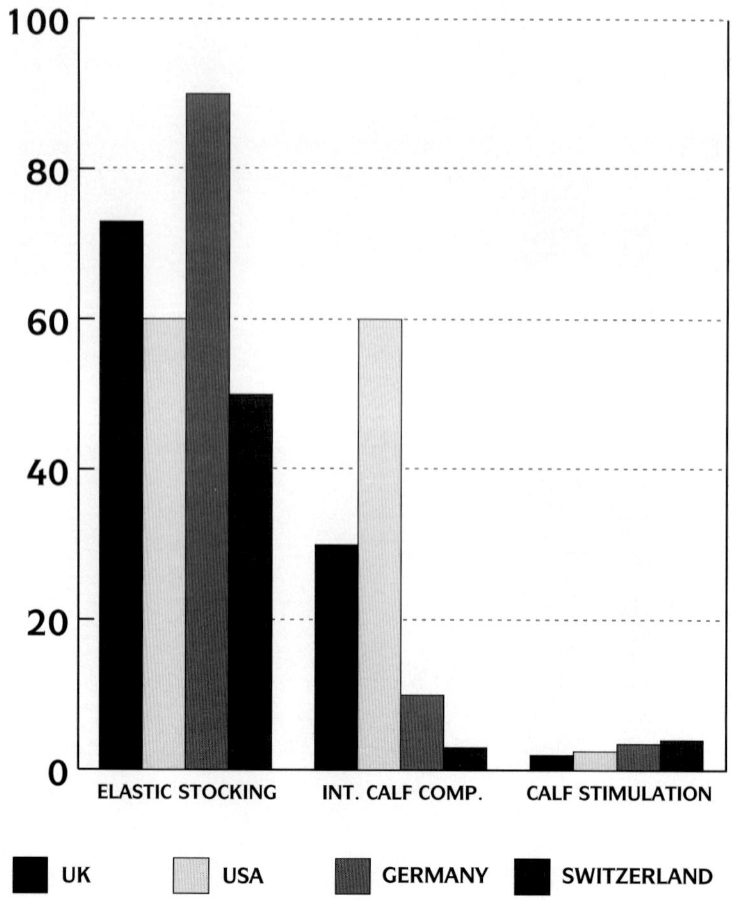

Figure 2 The proportion of respondents using mechanical methods.

and Switzerland and less than 10% in Western Germany take the option of combining pharmacological and mechanical methods. Nevertheless, some surgeons do combine methods, and nearly as many use elastic stockings as use heparin, which indicates that many surgeons are tailoring prophylaxis to the perceived needs of their patients.

XII. When Was Prophylaxis Stopped?

The majority initiated prophylaxis before surgery, and a few began during surgery. Between 20% and 30%, however, had a variable or unspecified schedule, presumably responding to the perceived clinical situation. Prophylaxis beginning after surgery was mainly confined to U.S. orthopedic surgeons administering warfarin, although about 20% of German respondents (who might include some heparin users) also started postoperatively. Most surgeons ended prophylaxis when the patient was mobilized rather than setting up a standard regimen (Fig. 3).

XIII. What Risk Factors Are Important?

Surgeons in the United Kingdom considered age, previous DVT, type of surgery, carcinoma, obesity, and immobility as important in evaluating the risk of DVT. The perceived risk factors varied between countries, and few of the Swiss respondents rated old age as a major risk factor, although they ranked obesity highest.

XIV. Use of Prophylaxis Is Increasing

Comparing the results of this survey with a similar survey of U.K. surgeons conducted in 1980 demonstrates a substantial increase in the use of subcutaneous heparin (approximately 25% in 1980 versus 90% in 1991 in the United Kingdom) and elastic stockings (about 15% in 1980 and nearly 80% in 1991 in the United Kingdom). This trend is an encouraging indication that the message concerning the efficacy and cost-effectiveness of the measures for preventing PE is getting through. Furthermore, a survey of the pharmaceutical industry involved in manufacturing heparin and low molecular weight heparin fractions and fragments has indicated that over the past 10 years, there has been nearly 300% increase in heparins produced, and clinical use of heparin continues to grow. Based on the data of the current increasing use of heparin prophylaxis in various countries throughout the Western hemisphere, the increase in heparin production that continues to grow, and proven efficacy of heparin prophylaxis in reducing the

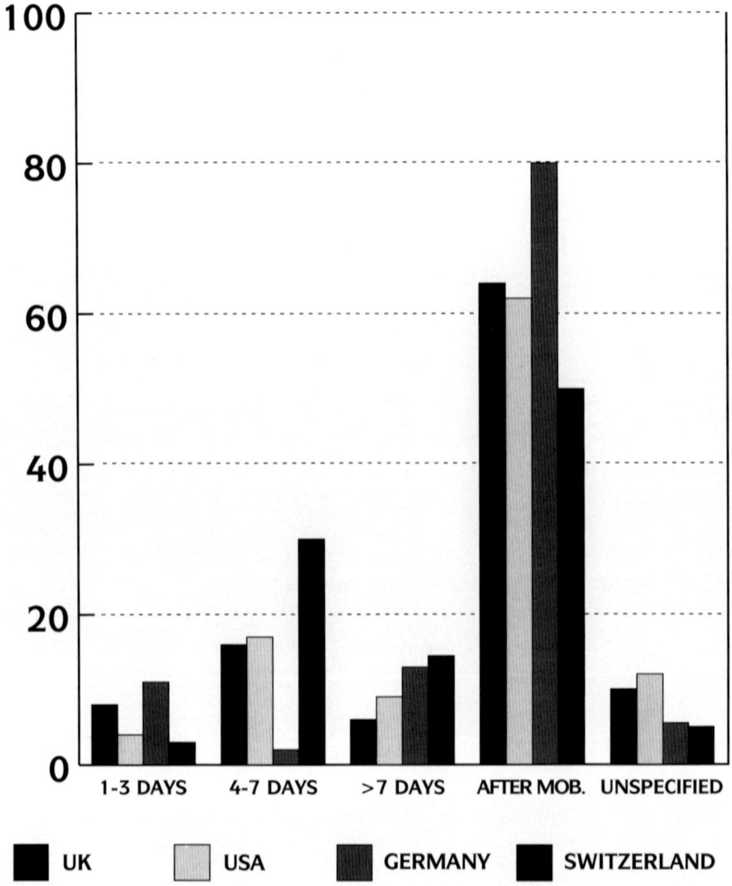

Figure 3 Most surgeons discontinue prophylaxis when the patient is mobilized.

mortality caused by fatal pulmonary embolism in all high-risk hospitalized patients, a very conservative estimate indicates that approximately 200,000 lives are being saved each year. However, still many high-risk patients are not protected in a number of countries. This is partly because individual surgeons, no matter how extensive their personal practices are, will never recognize the success of their prophylactic actions, yet will invariably be reminded of their failures in terms of bleeding complications. However, in view of such circumstances, what should be the role of a practicing clinician now that we have a safe, effective prophylactic therapy that is acceptable to patients and simple for nursing staff to use? It is believed that the emphasis is now on the clinicians who must protect all high-risk patients using low molecular weight heparin prophylaxis.

References

1. Donaldson GA, Williams C, Schnnez JG, Sharo RS. A re-appraisal of the application of the Trendelenburg operation to massive fatal pulmonary embolism. N Engl J Med 1963; 268:171–4.
2. Kakkar VV. Prevention of venous thromboembolism. In: Bloom A, Thomas D, eds. Thrombosis and Haemostasis. Edinburgh: Churchill Livingstone, 1990:803–19.
3. Gruber UF, Saldeen T, Brolcop T, et al. Incidence of fatal postoperative pulmonary embolism after prophylaxis with dextran 70 and low dose heparin: an International Multicentre Study. B Med J 1980; 280:69–72.
4. Bergqvist D. Prevention of postoperative thrombosis in Sweden. World J Surg 1981; 4:489–95.
5. Prevention of Fatal Postoperative Pulmonary Embolism by Low Doses of Heparin. An International Multicentre Trial. Lancet 1975; ii:45–51.
6. Collins R, Scrimgeour A, Yusef S, Peto R. Reduction in fatal pulmonary embolism and venous thrombosis by perioperative administration of subcutaneous heparin. Overview of results of randomized trials of general, or orthopaedic and urological surgery. New Engl J Med 1988; 318:1162–73.
7. Carter CJ, Kelton JG, Hirsh J, Cerskus AL, Santros AV, Gent M. The relationship between the haemorrhagic and antithrombotic properties of low molecular weight heparins and heparin. Blood 1982; 59:1239–42.
8. Holmer E, Matsson C, Nilsson S. Anticoagulant and antithrombotic effects of low molecular weight heparin fragments in rabbits. Thromb Res 1982; 25:475–9.
9. Kakkar VV, Djazaeri B, Fok J, Fletcher M, Scully MF, Westwick J. Low molecular weight heparin in the prophylaxis of venous thrombosis. B Med J 1982; 284:375–9.
10. Kakkar VV, Murray WJG. Efficacy and safety of low-molecular-weight heparin (CY 216) in preventing postoperative venous thromboembolism: a co-operative study. Br J Surg 1985: 71:786–91.
11. Clinical studies in prophylaxis of thrombosis. In: Barrowcliffe TW, Johnson EA, Thomas DP, eds. Low Molecular Weight Heparin. Chichester, UK: John Witerg & Sons, 1992:153–81.
12. Hirsh J, Levine MM: Low molecular weight heparin. Blood 1992; 79:1–17.
13. Pezzuoli G, Neriserneri GG, Settembrini P, Coggi G, Olivari H, Buzzetti G, Chierichetti S, Scotti A, Scatigoa M, Carnovali M. Prophylaxis of fatal pulmonary embolism in general surgery using low molecular weight heparin (CY216): a multicentre, double blind, randomized controlled trial versus placebo (STEP). Int. Surg 1989; 74:205–10.
14. Nurmohamed MT, Rosendaal FR, Buller HR, Dekker E, Hommes DW, Vandenbronche Jan P, Briet E. The efficacy and safety of low molecular weight

heparin versus standard heparin in general and orthopaedic surgery: a meta-analysis. Lancet 1992; 340:152–6.
15. Huber O, Bounameaux H, Borst F, Rohner A. Postoperative pulmonary embolism after hospital discharge—an underestimated risk. Arch Surg 1992; 127:310–3.
16. Kakkar VV, Cohen AT, Edmondson RA, et al. A multicentre, randomized, double blind, comparative trial of low molecular weight heparin and standard heparin for the prevention of postoperative venous thromboembolism in major abdominal surgery. Lancet 1992; in press.
17. Lindblad B, Eriksson A, Bergqvist D. Autopsy-verified pulmonary embolism in a surgical department: analysis of the period from 1951 to 1988. Br J Surg 1988; 78:849–52.
18. Edmondson RA, Cohen AT, Ward VP, Kakkar VV. A reduction in both fatal pulmonary embolism and venous thrombosis over 15 years. Submitted for publication.
19. Horowitz RE, Tatter D. Lethal pulmonary embolism. In: Sherry S, Brinkhaus KM, Genton E, Stengl J, eds. Thrombosis. Washington: National Academy of Science, 1969:19.
20. Kakkar VV, Cohen AT, Edmonson RA, Phillips MJ, Cooper DJ, Das SK, Maher KT, Sanderson RM, Ward VP, Kakkar S. Low molecular weight versus standard heparin for prevention of venous thromboembolism after major abdominal surgery. Lancet 1993; 341:259–65.
21. Salzmann EW, Davies GC. Prophylaxis of venous thromboembolism. Analysis of cost effectiveness. Ann Surg 1980; 191:207–16.
22. Hull RD, Hirsh J, Sackett DL, Stoddart GL. Cost effectiveness of primary and secondary prevention of fatal pulmonary embolism in high risk surgical patients. Can Med Assoc J 1982; 127:900–5.
23. Oster G, Tuden RL, Colditz GA. A cost-effectiveness analysis of prophylaxis against deep vein thrombosis in major orthopaedic surgery. JAMA 1987; 257:203–8.
24. Paiement GD, Bell D, Wessinger SJ, Harris WH. New advances in the prevention, diagnosis and cost effectiveness of venous thromboembolic disease in patients with total hip replacement. In: Paiement D, Braod RA, eds. The Hip. St Louis: Mosby, 1987; 94–119.
25. Hillson SD, Rich EC. Two strategies for prophylaxis of fatal postoperative pulmonary embolism. Cost effectiveness analysis. Int J Tech Assess Health Care 1990; 6:470–9.
26. Bergqvist D, Jendteg S, Lindgren B, Mätzsch T, Persson U. The economics of general thromboembolic prophylaxis. World J Surg 1988; 12:349–55.
27. Kakkar VV, Djazaeri B, Fok J, Fletcher M, Scully MF, Westwick J. Low molecular weight heparin and prevention of postoperative deep vein thrombosis. Nr Med J 1982; 284:375–9.
28. Current practices of prevention. Cooke ED. Venous Thromboembolism—A Continuing Challenge. Jersey: Symposium, 1992.

19

Prevention of Pulmonary Embolism: The Nonpharmacological Approach

SAMUEL Z. GOLDHABER

Harvard Medical School
and Brigham and Women's Hospital
Boston, Massachusetts

I. Introduction

Pulmonary embolism (PE) is easier and less expensive to prevent than it is to diagnose and to treat. Virtually all hospitalized patients should receive prophylactic measures against venous thromboembolism. The method of PE prevention that is utilized should be based on an assessment of the patient's level of risk for PE and on whether a patient is most likely to benefit from nonpharmacological, pharmacological, or combined modalities. Because the risk of PE continues after discharge from the hospital, prophylaxis should be continued at home among those patients at moderate or high risk for venous thromboembolism.

The most commonly used nonpharmacological measures are graduated compression stockings (GCSs) and intermittent pneumatic compression (IPC) boots. Overall, there are five nonpharmacological approaches to PE prophylaxis, including several strategies that combine various preventive modalities (Table 1).

Vascular compression with GCSs or IPC boots is effective among surgical patients because it counters the otherwise unopposed perioperative venodilatation that appears causally related to postoperative venous thrombosis. Comerota et al. (1) monitored the contralateral cephalic vein of 21 patients undergoing total hip replacement. They used a continuous on-line recorder that graphed the

Table 1 Nonpharmacological Approaches to Pulmonary Embolism (PE) Prophylaxis

Modality	Mechanism of action
Graduated compression stockings (GCS)	Prevent venous stasis
Intermittent pneumatic compression (IPC) boots	Prevent venous stasis Increase endogenous fibrinolytic activity
Inferior vena caval (IVC) interruption	Prevents PE by mechanical blocking effect but does not prevent deep venous thrombosis
Combined nonpharmacological methods (e.g., GCS + IPC)	Additive or synergistic effect
Combined nonpharmacological plus pharmacological approach (e.g., IPC + low-dose heparin)	Additive or synergistic effect

ultrasonographically imaged venous diameter. In this study, excessive operative venodilation correlated with postoperative deep venous thrombosis.

II. Types of Nonpharmacological Prophylaxis

A. Graduated Compression Stockings

Graduated compression stockings produce a higher femoral vein flow than uniform compression (2). For example, the commonly used GCSs that have compression of 18 mm Hg at the ankle, 14 mm Hg at the calf, 8 mm Hg popliteal, 10 mm Hg at lower thigh, and 8 mm Hg at midthigh produce a 36% increase in femoral vein blood flow velocity compared with a 10% increase among subjects who receive 11 mm Hg of uniform compression. Among low-risk, general-surgery patients, GCSs can reduce the frequency of venous thrombosis by more than half compared with no prophylaxis (3,4). Graduated compression stockings should be considered as first-line prophylaxis against PE among all hospitalized patients, except for those with peripheral vascular disease whose condition may be worsened by vascular compression.

B. Intermittent Pneumatic Compression (IPC) Boots

Intermittent pneumatic compression boots (Fig. 1) are devices that provide intermittent inflation of air-filled cuffs that prevent venous stasis in the legs and appear to stimulate the endogenous fibrinolytic system. To test the latter hypothesis, patients undergoing general surgery were randomized either to specially designed IPC devices applied to the *arms* or to no prophylaxis (5). Postoperatively, the development of deep venous thrombosis of the *legs* was assessed in both groups. Venous thrombosis developed in 32% of the controls compared with 14% of the group that received IPC. Therefore, the reduction of

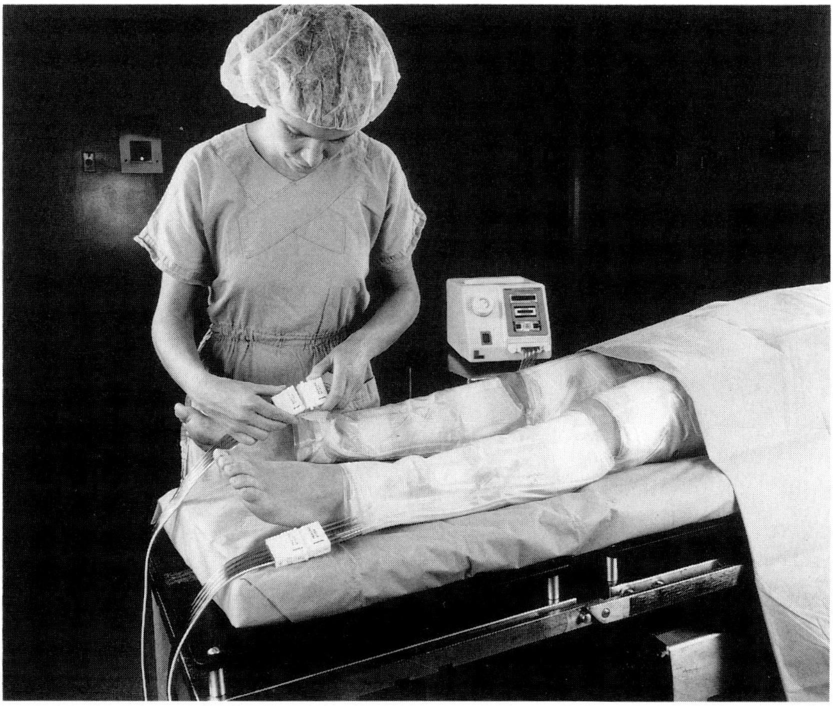

Figure 1 The Kendall Sequential Compression device expels blood from the legs, and its mechanical force may enhance fibrinolytic activity. The three compartments produce graded sequential compression of the ankle, calf, and thigh, with pressures of 35, 30, and 20 mm Hg, respectively, causing a 240% increase in peak blood flow velocity.

thrombosis in the legs with an IPC device for the arms suggests that IPC causes an increase in endogenous fibrinolytic activity.

Sequential gradient compression (e.g., pressures of 35, 30, and 20 mm Hg at the ankle, calf, and thigh, respectively, applied sequentially for 12 s) produces a 240% increase in peak blood flow velocity (6). By comparison, a one-chamber IPC boot inflated with 35 mm Hg of pressure over the calf for 12 s produces a 180% increase in blood flow velocity. Not surprisingly, thigh high sequential gradient leg compression cleared venographic dye from the cusps of venous valves in the thighs eight times more quickly than single-chamber calf IPC (7).

C. Inferior Vena Caval (IVC) Interruption

Inferior vena caval interruption is usually accomplished with a filter device (Fig. 2) that mechanically blocks thrombus in the IVC and, thus, prevents PE (see

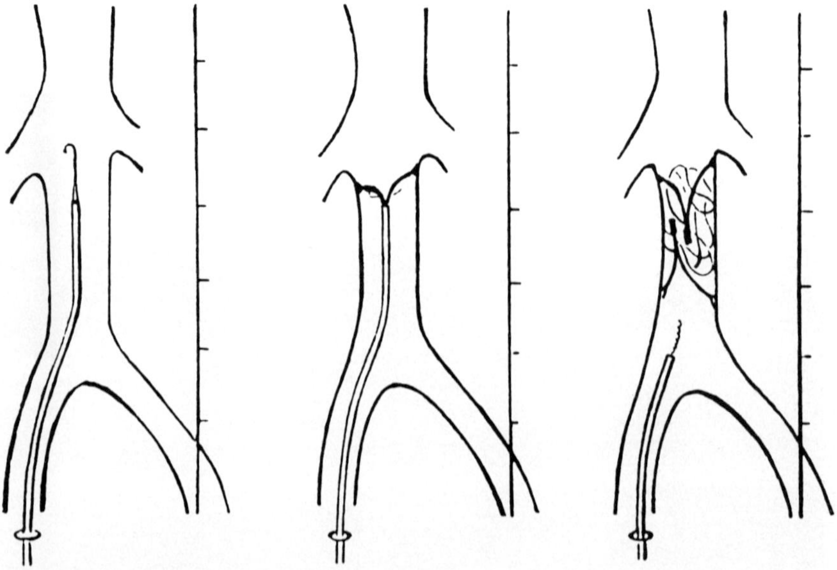

Figure 2 *Left panel*: The Bird's Nest filter is positioned in the IVC. *Middle panel*: fixation to the wall of the IVC is accomplished with wire hooks. *Right panel*: the mesh of the filter resembles a bird's nest and becomes evident as the introducer is withdrawn.

Chap. 20). These devices have no effect on the thrombotic process and do not prevent venous thrombosis of the upper extremities, pelvis, or deep leg veins. Inferior vena cava interruption should be used prophylactically only when patients are at extremely high risk for PE. One typical setting would be in a patient who had suffered a recent PE but required urgent, high-risk (e.g., orthopedic) surgery. Occasionally, a patient will have contraindications to GSCs and IPC because of recent DVT, as well as contraindications to pharmacological prophylaxis because of conditions such as active internal bleeding or recent neurosurgery. Such a patient, if at high risk for PE, would also benefit from IVC interruption.

Percutaneous IVC filter placement should be utilized, rather than a surgical cutdown technique, in almost all patients who require IVC interruption (8). The three exceptions are (a) a hypocoagulable state (e.g., thrombocytopenia) that requires direct surgical control of the vessel, (b) anticipated noncompliance with rest orders in the postprocedure period, and (c) obstructing thrombus along the routes of insertion (e.g., both femoral veins and the right internal jugular vein) (9,10). For percutaneous insertion, the femoral vein is punctured with a single-wall puncture technique. A 5 or 6 French pigtail catheter is positioned in the IVC; an inferior vena cavagram is then obtained to assess vena caval patency, size, and anatomy.

A new generation of filters has been developed with emphasis on smaller diameter sizes that are suitable for percutaneous insertion. For example, the Bird's Nest filter has the advantage of a small sheath size, 12 French, with an 11 French preloaded filter catheter, thus avoiding the necessity of handling the filter (10).

D. Combined Nonpharmacological Methods

The two nonpharmacological methods of GCSs and IPC may work through complementary mechanisms. Graduated compression stockings provide continuous stimulation of linear blood flow velocity and prevent dilation of the venous system in the legs. Intermittent pneumatic compression devices compress the veins more forcefully than GCSs but for a relatively brief period. In a randomized trial of patients undergoing general surgery, GCSs, plus IPC was more effective than IPC alone in preventing venous thrombosis (11).

E. Combined Nonpharmacological Plus Pharmacological Approach

Vascular compression to prevent venous stasis and low-dose heparin to prevent hypercoagulability are prophylaxis strategies that require a combined nonpharmacological plus pharmacological approach. Among patients undergoing general surgery, several studies have demonstrated that GCSs plus low-dose heparin is more effective than low-dose heparin alone in reducing the frequency of venous thrombosis (12,13).

III. Special High-Risk Groups (Table 2)

A. Orthopedic Surgery

Patients undergoing lower extremity orthopedic surgery are at very high risk of PE. These patients should ordinarily receive combined nonpharmacological and pharmacological prophylaxis (e.g., IPC plus adjusted low-dose warfarin) while hospitalized, followed by some form of prophylaxis for approximately 1 month

Table 2 Recommendations for Pulmonary Embolism (PE) Prophylaxis Among Special High-Risk Groups

High-risk group	Recommended PE prophylaxis
Orthopedic surgery in lower extremity	IPC plus pharmacological prophylaxis, followed by some prophylaxis after hospital discharge
Gynecological cancer surgery	IPC or intensive pharmacological prophylaxis
General surgery	Combined nonpharmacological or combined nonpharmacological plus pharmacological modalities
Immobilized medical patients	Nonpharmacological or pharmacological prophylaxis

after hospital discharge. Patients undergoing total knee replacement are at as high a risk of developing PE as patients undergoing total hip replacement (14).

Foley et al. (14) studied 403 patients undergoing total knee or hip replacement; their protocol required PE prophylaxis with adjusted low-dose warfarin (target prothrombin time 1.2–1.4 times the control value, corresponding to an International Normalized Ratio [INR] of approximately 1.5–2.0). In addition, patients were studied with pre and postoperative lung scans so that the rate of perioperative PE could be calculated. Patients with changes in their scans postoperatively underwent pulmonary angiography. The rate of postoperative PE was 4% overall: 3% asymptomatic PE and 1% symptomatic PE, without any difference in frequency between hip and knee surgery.

Most trials of PE prophylaxis utilize the development of deep venous thrombosis (DVT) of the legs as a surrogate end point for PE. In a randomized controlled trial (15) of sequential gradient IPC versus no prophylaxis among patients undergoing total hip replacement, the end point was DVT assessed by leg phlebography. There was a very significant reduction in DVT among patients who received IPC prophylaxis begun postoperatively in the recovery room. The DVT rates were 52% in the no-prophylaxis control group compared with 25% in the IPC group. The rate of proximal vein thrombosis was 27% in the no-prophylaxis group compared with 14% in the IPC group.

In a randomized controlled trial (16) of sequential gradient IPC versus adjusted low-dose warfarin (target INR approximately 2.0) among patients undergoing total hip replacement, the nonpharmacological and pharmacological prophylaxis modalities had similar efficacy. The end point was venographically confirmed DVT of the legs, and the frequency of DVT was 17% in each group.

B. Gynecological Cancer Surgery

Patients who develop proximal leg DVT and PE after gynecological cancer surgery often have no evidence of calf vein thrombosis. The thrombi appear to arise de novo in the pelvic or proximal deep veins of the leg (17). Therefore, non-pharmacological prophylaxis among these patients should, if feasible, ordinarily consist of thigh length sequential gradient IPC. However, even isolated calf IPC in one randomized trial was effective in reducing the rate of venous thrombosis from 35% in the no-prophylaxis group to 13% in the IPC group (18). If pharmacological prophylaxis is employed, it should be more intensive than fixed low-dose heparin (5000 U twice daily), which appears to be ineffective (19).

C. General Surgery

In a meta-analysis of 45 randomized controlled trials of DVT prophylaxis among general surgery patients without cancer, combined modalities were found to be more effective than any single prophylaxis method (20). Based on a very small number of studies, IPC plus GCSs resulted in the lowest rate of postoperative DVT, only 4.5% (95% CI 1.1%, 8.0%). Graduated compression stockings plus low-dose heparin had a DVT rate of 6.3% (95% CI 0%, 17.6%).

D. Immobilized Medical Patients

Among bedridden patients in a respiratory intensive care unit, one study found that PE occurred in 27% who were autopsied (21). Half of these PEs were not diagnosed before death. In another study, among immobilized patients who are not critically ill, fibrinogen leg scanning identified DVT in 13% (22). Therefore, immobilized medical patients should routinely receive nonpharmacological or pharmacological prophylaxis.

IV. Prevention of Pulmonary Embolism After Hospital Discharge

The danger of postoperative PE continues for more than 1 month after surgery. In an analysis of autopsied surgical patients in Malmo, Sweden, where the autopsy rate remained high throughout the study, PE that was considered the cause or a major contributor to death occurred in 25% of PE patients between postoperative days 15 and 30, and in 15% after postoperative day 30 (Fig. 3) (23).

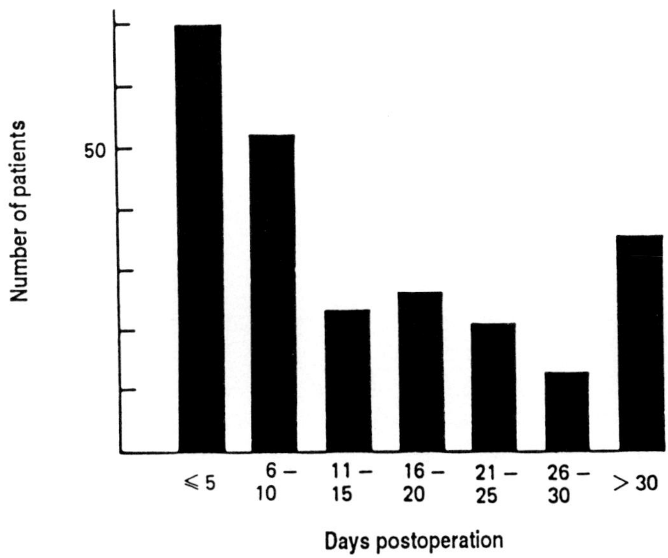

Figure 3 The interval between operation and death in patients with autopsy proven fatal PE or PE contributing to the cause of death. (From Bergqvist D, Lindblad B, 1985.)

In a recently completed study of general surgical patients in Geneva, Switzerland, delayed PEs occurred a median of 6 days after discharge and 18 days after surgery (24). The authors calculated that the rate of postoperative PE increases by 30% when PEs that occur within 30 days of hospital discharge are not overlooked.

Among 51 general surgery patients in London who had not developed DVT 2 days before hospital discharge, 13 did develop DVT during the first 6 weeks at home: one during the first 3 days, seven between 4 and 6 days, three between 7 and 10 days, and two after more than 10 days (25). These studies of "late" PE and DVT indicate that venous thromboembolism continues to be an important risk after hospital discharge. Indeed, many patients may be less mobile at home than in the hospital. Therefore, patients at moderate or high risk for venous thrombosis should continue to receive prophylaxis against PE after hospital discharge.

V. Cost-Effectiveness of Pulmonary Embolism Prevention

Prophylaxis not only saves lives but is also cost-effective. In an analysis of patients undergoing major orthopedic surgery, all prophylaxis methods saved health care dollars (26). In a separate analysis of general surgery patients, GCSs were the most cost-effective approach (27).

VI. Summary

Prophylaxis against PE continues to be underutilized, despite its endorsement by an NIH Consensus Development Conference (28). Effective pharmacological and nonpharmacological methods exist to prevent the majority of PEs. The World Health Organization should endorse the intensification of PE prophylaxis efforts, with particular attention to special high-risk patients during hospitalization and for the first month after hospital discharge.

References

1. Comerota AJ, Stewart GJ, Alburger PD, Smalley K, White JV. Operative venodilation: a previously unsuspected factor in the cause of postoperative deep vein thrombosis. Surgery 1989; 106:301–9.
2. Sigel B, Edelstein AL, Savitch L, Hasty JH, Felix WR. Type of compression for reducing venous stasis. A study of lower extremities during inactive recumbency. Arch Surg 1975; 110:171–5.
3. Jeffery PC, Nicolaides AN. Graduated compression stockings in the prevention of postoperative deep vein thrombosis. Br J Surg 1990; 77:380–3.
4. Allan A, Williams JT, Bolton JP, Le Quesne LP. The use of graduated compression

stockings in the prevention of postoperative deep vein thrombosis. Br J Surg 1983; 70:172–4.
5. Knight MTN, Dawson R. Effect of intermittent compression of the arms on deep venous thrombosis in the legs. Lancet 1976; ii:1265–7.
6. Nicolaides AN, Fernandes JF, Pollock AV. Intermittent sequential pneumatic compression of the legs in the prevention of venous stasis and postoperative deep venous thrombosis. Surgery 1980; 87:69–76.
7. Mittelman JS, Edwards WS, McDonald JB. Effectiveness of leg compression in preventing venous stasis. Am J Surg 1982; 144:611–3.
8. Dorfman GS. Percutaneous inferior vena caval filters. Radiology 1990; 174:987–92.
9. Grassi CJ, Goldhaber SZ. Interruption of the inferior vena cava for prevention of pulmonary embolism: transvenous filter devices. Herz 1989; 14:182–91.
10. Goldhaber SZ, Grassi CJ. Management of pulmonary embolism. In: Sabiston DC, Jr, ed.. Textbook of Surgery—Update 8. Philadelphia: WB Saunders Co, 1990: 115–27.
11. Scurr JH, Coleridge-Smith PD, Hasty JH. Regimen for improved effectiveness of intermittent pneumatic compression in deep venous thrombosis prophylaxis. Surgery 1987; 102:816–20.
12. Törngren S. Low dose heparin and compression stockings in the prevention of postoperative deep venous thrombosis. Br J Surg 1980; 67:482–4.
13. Wille-Jorgensen P, Thorup J, Fischer A, Holst-Christensen J, Flamsholt R. Heparin with and without graded compression stockings in the prevention of thromboembolic complications of major abdominal surgery: a randomized trial. Br J Surg 1985; 72:579–81.
14. Foley M, Maslack MM, Rothman RH, Casey MP, Lugano EM, Parry CE, Balderston RA, Booth RE Jr. Pulmonary embolism after hip or knee replacement: postoperative changes on pulmonary scintigrams in asymptomatic patients. Radiology 1989; 172:481–5.
15. Hull RD, Raskob GE, Gent M, McLoughlin D, Julian D, Smith FC, Dale NI, Reed-Davis R, Lofthouse RN, Anderson C. Effectiveness of intermittent pneumatic leg compression for preventing deep vein thrombosis after total hip replacement. JAMA 1990; 263:2313–7.
16. Paiement G, Wessinger SJ, Waltman AC, Harris WH. Low-dose warfarin versus external pneumatic compression for prophylaxis against venous thromboembolism following total hip replacement. J Arthroplasty 1987; 2:23–6.
17. Clarke-Pearson DL, Synan IS, Colemen RE, Hinshaw W, Creasman WT. The natural history of postoperative venous thromboemboli in gynecologic oncology: a prospective study of 382 patients. Am J Obstet Gynecol 1984; 148:1051–4.
18. Clarke-Pearson DL, Synan IS, Hinshaw WM, Coleman RE, Creasman WT. Prevention of postoperative venous thromboembolism by external pneumatic calf compression in patients with gynecologic malignancy. Obstet Gynecol 1984; 63:92–8.
19. Clarke-Pearson DL, Coleman RE, Synan IS, Hinshaw W, Creasman WT. Venous thromboembolism prophylaxis in gynecologic oncology: a prospective, controlled trial of low-dose heparin. Am J Obstet Gynecol 1983; 145:606–13.

20. Colditz GA, Tuden RL, Oster G. Rates of venous thrombosis after general surgery: combined results of randomised clinical trials. Lancet 1982; ii:143–6.
21. Neuhaus A, Bentz RR, Weg JG. Pulmonary embolism in respiratory failure. Chest 1978; 73:460–5.
22. Kierkegaard A, Norgren L, Olsson C-G, Castenfors J, Persson G, Persson S. Incidence of deep vein thrombosis in bedridden non-surgical patients. Acta Med Scand 1987; 222:409–14.
23. Bergqvist D, Lindblad B. A 30-year survey of pulmonary embolism verified at autopsy: an analysis of 1274 surgical patients. Br J Surg 1985; 72:105–8.
24. Huber O, Bounameaux H, Borst F, Rohner A. Postoperative pulmonary embolism after hospital discharge: an underestimated risk. Arch Surg 1992; 127:310–3.
25. Scurr JH, Coleridge-Smith PD, Hasty JH. Deep venous thrombosis: a continuing problem. Br Med J 1988; 297:28.
26. Oster G, Tuden RL, Colditz GA. A cost-effectiveness analysis of prophylaxis against deep-vein thrombosis in major orthopedic surgery. JAMA 1987; 257:203–8.
27. Oster G, Tuden RL, Colditz GA. Prevention of venous thromboembolism after general surgery. Cost-effectiveness analysis of alternative approaches to prophylaxis. Am J Med 1987; 82:889–9.
28. NIH Consensus Development Statement: Prevention of venous thrombosis and pulmonary embolism. JAMA 1986; 256:744–9.

20

Surgical Prevention of Pulmonary Embolism

MAKIS J. TSAPOGAS

State University of New York at Stony Brook
Stony Brook
Albany Medical College
Albany, New York
Royal College of Surgeons of England
King's College School of Medicine
and University of London
London, England
and Academy of Athens
Athens, Greece

I. Introduction

Significant progress has been made over the last 20 years in the prevention, early detection, and management of deep vein thrombosis (DVT) and pulmonary embolism (PE) (1–6). Morbidity and mortality, however, still remain high. (7,8). Mechanical and pharmacological prophylactic measures, when appropriately applied, substantially decrease their incidence (9,10).

In spite of these advances in prophylaxis, earlier detection, and management, in about 10% of patients the established therapy is ineffective or leads to high risk for bleeding (11). In such instances, several techniques for interruption of the inferior vena cava (IVC) have been employed over the years, with varying degrees of success. More recently this is usually accomplished with a filter device. These are so designed as to retain sizable thrombi originating from the veins of the lower extremities. Thus, pulmonary embolism is prevented, while, in general, patency of the IVC is maintained.

II. Indications for Interruption of the IVC

The main indications are (a) contraindication to anticoagulants, e.g., in patients following recent surgery or trauma and those sensitive to heparin or with bleeding diathesis; and (b) recurrent episodes of thromboembolism, despite anticoagulation and adequately elevated clotting factors.

Special indications for IVC interruption may be considered for (a) patients with a history of severe cardiopulmonary disease who develop even small emboli, (b) candidates for embolectomy (12), (c) patients with propagating iliofemoral thrombosis who will undergo major surgery, and (d) persistent septic PE.

Indications for prophylaxis are limited. Consideration is given to a small number of particularly vulnerable patients. The benefit/risk ratio for them is carefully assessed before a decision is reached.

III. Older Techniques of IVC Interruption

Review of techniques extensively used in the past is useful. It demonstrates the various stages of the developmental process in this area. An additional reason is that some of them are still in use in certain parts of the world.

A. Ligation

John Hunter (13) ligated the femoral vein in 1784 to prevent PE. Trousseau (14) in 1868 considered the use of a barrier between a thrombosed femoral and the larger veins. Bottini suggested ligation of the IVC in 1893, and this was popularized by Alton Ochsner (15). For this procedure, a transverse right upper quadrant incision is made that is extended to the flank for the retroperitoneal approach. A suture is placed just below the level of the renal veins to prevent formation of thrombi in the cul-de-sac. Each gonadal vein is individually ligated. The reported incidence of operative mortality, recurrent emboli, and postphlebitic syndrome is significant. In addition, cardiac output is compromised because of inadequate venous return.

B. Filtration

De Weese and others (12,16) recognized the advantages of this technique over complete occlusion of the IVC by ligation and proposed a suture grid. Stapler plication was later advocated by Ravitch et al. (17). A problem caused by these techniques is the intimal disruption, which may lead to thrombosis.

C. External Clips

A variety of external clips were designed to compress the IVC either within a narrow slot between parallel orifices or within a series of channels (18). These allow blood flow while preventing passage of large thrombi. Operative mortality was reduced, but the incidence of cava occlusion was significant (19).

There are no major differences among the various types of available clips.

Most of them do not produce measurable pressure differential but cause significant wave dumping of the pulsatile flow. Complete occlusion of the IVC at the clip site occurs fairly frequently. In most instances, however, patency is subsequently reestablished. Sudden occlusion sometimes produces treatable functional hypovolemic hypotension, which could mimic recurrent thromboembolism. Inferior vena cava plication may not be feasible in seriously ill patients who cannot withstand surgery.

IV. Older Filters

Intraluminal techniques for temporary caval filtration were developed by Eichelter and Schenk (20). However, the danger of embolism from trapped thrombi during the removal of the device was significant. This led to the development of detachable types that are so designed as to retain sizable emboli, while IVC patency is maintained (21). Their placement is relatively easy, and they were proven to be the safest method for IVC interruption.

The selection of the appropriate filter is crucial. Factors for consideration include: high filtering efficiency, preservation of blood flow, stability after positioning, and low incidence of complications. None of the available devices fulfills all these requirements at different clinical settings.

A. Mobin-Uddin Umbrella (MUU)

This device was extensively used in the past but is no longer available in the United States. It resembles an inverted umbrella with six flat stainless steel spokes and is covered with a thin silastic membrane. The 28-mm size was preferred because filter migration was low (22). Recurrent PE was only 0.5%, although there was a very high incidence (60%–70%) of IVC occlusion and significant venous stasis in the legs.

B. Kimray-Greenfield Stainless Steel Filter (KGF)

This filter (Fig. 1A) (23) was first described in 1973 and is designed to provide maximal entrapment area. Emboli larger than 3 mm are retained while blood flow is maintained. It consists of six stainless steel wires forming a conical device, with a maximum diameter of 30 mm. Its geometry permits filling by thrombi to 80% of its depth, before the effective cross-sectional area is reduced to 64%. This represents the amount required to produce a pressure gradient across it (24). This filter was initially placed surgically and later percutaneously, via the femoral or jugular vein, usually below the renals (Fig. 2) (25). Its insertion is achieved by a 26 French sheath.

Studies were carried out to compare the degree of effectiveness of KGF

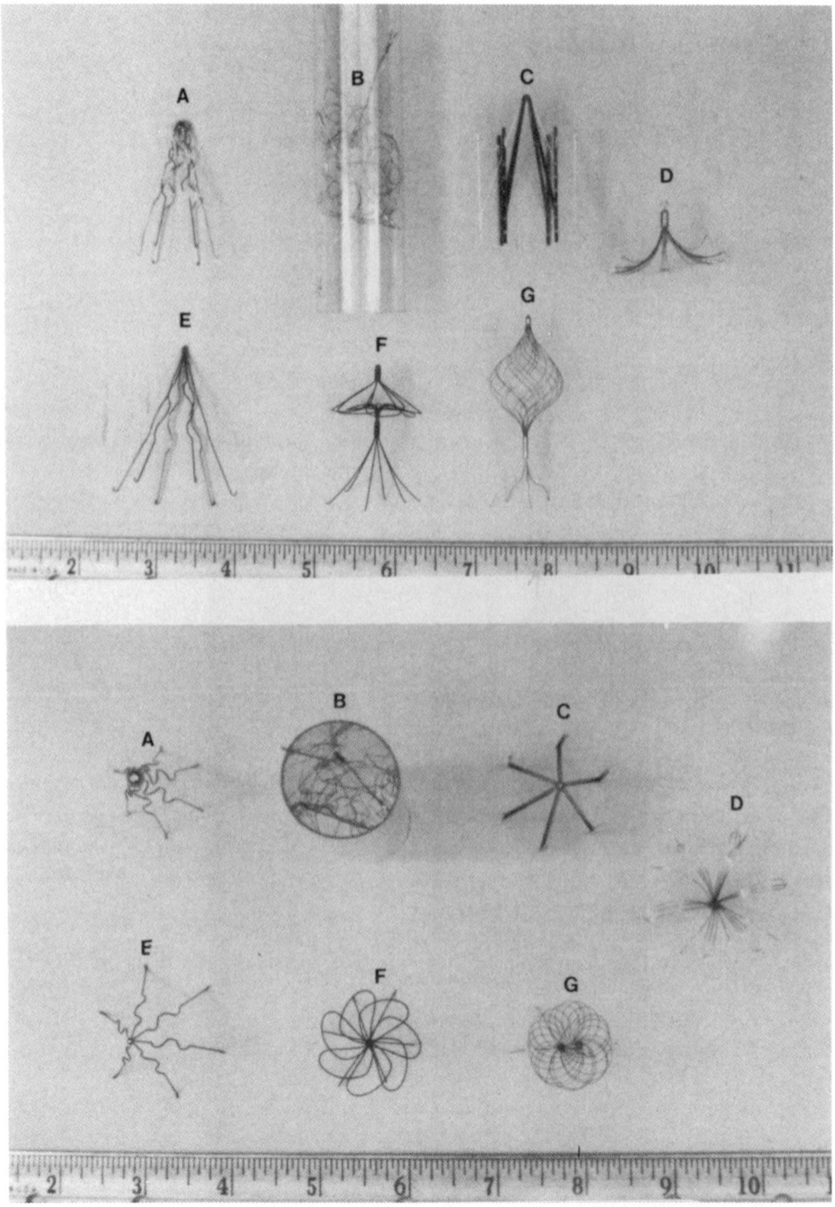

Figure 1 Lateral (top) and axial (bottom) views of vena cava filters: (A) Stainless Steel Greenfield, (B) Bird's Nest, (C) Vena Tech (LGM), (D) Amplatz, (E) Titanium Greenfield, (F) Nitinol, (G) Gunther. (From Ref. 23.)

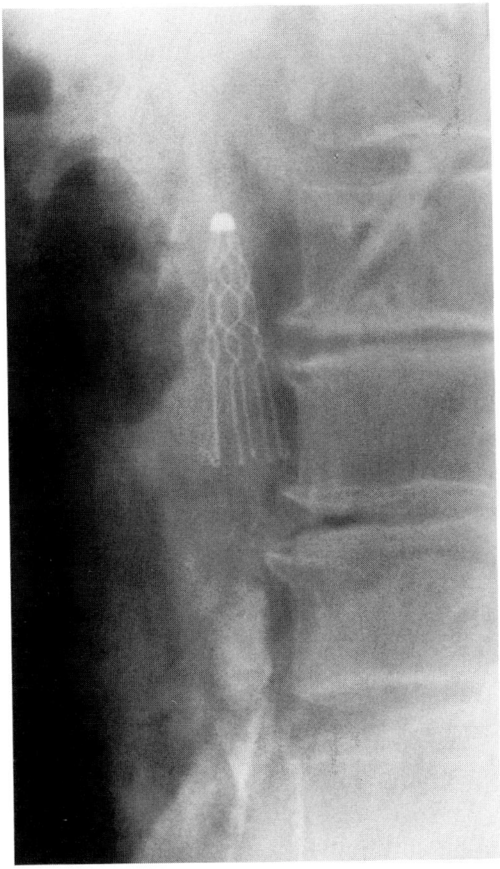

Figure 2 Radiograph showing Stainless Steel Greenfield Filter in place. (From Ref. 25.)

and its complications by employing the percutaneous versus the surgical approach. The percutaneous route was considered the technique of choice because of the safety, relatively easy insertion, and lower cost, 58% that of the surgical (26). When the source of recurrent emboli is above the renal veins, the filter is positioned suprarenally. At that level, it has an advantage over other devices because it maintains high caval patency.

In certain patients, such as those with Megacava, the filter is placed in the iliac veins percutaneously (27). This approach is also indicated in the presence of technical difficulty in reaching the IVC, because of marked iliac vein tortuosity.

The advantages of the KGF are (a) low recurrent embolization (5%)

(28,29), (b) IVC patency rate of 95%–97% (30,31), and (c) low incidence of misplacement and migration (32). The procedure is carried out under local anesthesia.

Following the filter's insertion, anticoagulants can be given when there are definitive indications and meticulous laboratory control is assured. It has not yet been fully determined whether with this regimen, extension of DVT can be prevented. Its early detection and appropriate management may diminish the incidence of postphlebitic syndrome (33), although some reports claim otherwise (34).

The KGF was proven over the last 15 years to be reliable in minimizing the incidence of PE. Based on in vitro studies, tilting of the device, which sometimes occurs, was initially considered a major disadvantage (35). Subsequent experimental and clinical studies have shown that it is not of major significance (36). The main disadvantage of this device is its large sheath (26 French), designed to accept standard size stainless-steel filter. This resulted in high incidence of DVT at the insertion site. A variable range of thrombosis was reported, from 10%–24% (37), to 30%–41% (38). In such cases, noninvasive testing is a useful diagnostic tool (39). Because of this problem, a modified version of the filter was developed.

V. Newer Filters and Other Devices

A. Titanium Greenfield Filter (TGF)

In this new version (Fig. 1E) (23), the carrier system was reduced to size 12 French, resulting in only 3% femoral vein thrombosis (40). Distal migration, angulation, and, in some cases, penetration of the IVC were reported (41). For this reason, the limb and hook design was additionally modified. The new device was initially tested in sheep (42). Its length was increased to 4.7 cm, as opposed to 4.4 cm of the stainless-steel filter. The base was made broader, from the previous 30 mm to a diameter of 38 mm. The recurved hook is set at an angle of 80 degrees, and the measured force of fixation on the IVC wall is more than 22 mm (38).

For the placement of the filter, a guide wire is inserted percutaneously under local anesthesia, through the femoral or jugular vein. The dilator system, which has an attached 14 French sheath, is advanced into the IVC to the desired level through another small incision adjacent to that for the guide wire or before its insertion. Once the aimed level is reached, the dilator and wire are retracted, leaving the sheath behind. The carrier component is then inserted through it. A new handle system allows one-handed removal of the carrier for the discharge of the filter. Therefore, the other hand is free to stabilize the sheath. The carrier and sheath are then withdrawn, while gentle pressure is applied on the insertion site. The entire procedure is performed under fluoroscopy. This device has the additional advantage that the titanium aloe is not ferromagnetic, and, therefore, the potential concern when this is exposed to magnetic resonance imaging (MRI) is avoided.

A multicenter study on the use of this modified filter was undertaken on 186 patients (38). In 75% of them, contraindication to anticoagulation was the reason for inserting the filter. Thirty-five patients died during the 30-day postinsertion period. Recurrent embolism was suspected in six of them (3%), and in two this was confirmed at autopsy. Venous thrombosis at the insertion site was observed in 8.7% of patients. The reported incidence of migration and caval penetration were significantly low.

B. Bird's Nest Filter (BNF) and Its Modification

This filter (Fig. 1B) (23) was first clinically tested in 1982. It was designed to overcome some of the disadvantages of the KGF, such as malposition, premature filter release, IVC perforation, and femoral vein thrombosis at the insertion site (43). It consists of wires shaped by the operator appropriately in a cluster like a bird's nest (Fig. 3) (25). Migration observed with the original model was corrected by using firmer securing struts, 0.46 mm in diameter. The BNF delivery system consists of a 12 French sheath. It was designed to be inserted over a 0.038-in. guide wire and an 11 French filter-carrying catheter. This filter is for percutaneous use only and is claimed to have potential advantages over the KGF. In preliminary studies based on 440 patients (44), this was found to be effective. The incidence of clinically suspected recurrent PE was 2.7%. Inferior vena cava occlusion was reported as 2.9% after a 6-month follow-up period. The patients received a first- or second-generation device. Because the filter consists of a cluster of wires, meticulous alignment with the IVC is not necessary. Filter migration was rarely reported when the modified BNF was used.

C. Vena Tech Filter (LGM)

This Food and Drug Administration (FDA-USA)-approved version (Fig. 1C) (23) of the LGM-France device is made of Phynox, has a 10 French carrier, a 12 French sheath, and is for percutaneous use. The IVC diameter is known to be affected by respiration movements and cardiac pulsation. Stabilizing side rails welded to the limbs of the filter cone remain parallel to the caval wall and, thus, are relatively unaffected by diameter changes (Fig. 4) (25,45).

In the first 100 patients of a multicenter European trial, the reported complications were tilting, 8%; malposition, 16%; and incomplete opening of the filter, 3% (46). The incidence of malposition was observed to decrease as the operator's experience increased. After a 1-year follow-up, there was a 13%

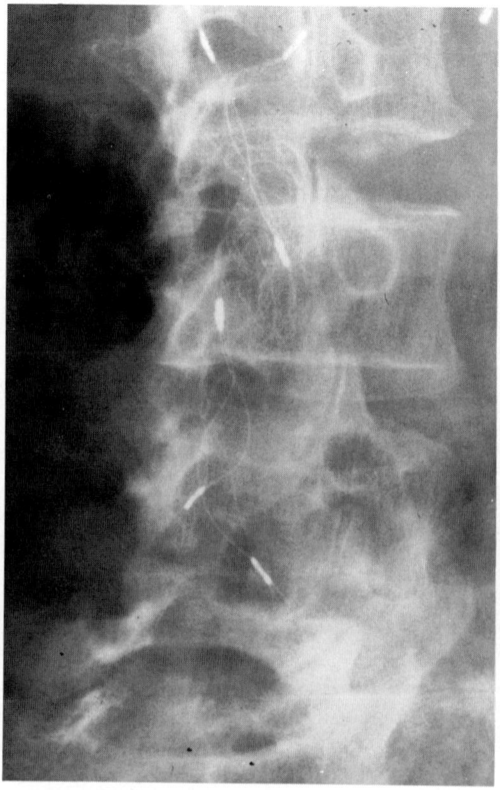

Figure 3 Bird's Nest Filter in place. (From Ref. 25.)

displacement, recurrent PE was 2%, and IVC occlusion was 8%. Several thousand of this filter have already been placed to the present date.

D. Simon-Nitinol Filter (SNF)

This device (Fig. 1F) (23) was approved by the FDA in 1980. It has the shape of an umbrella dome with seven petal loops and six legs for fixation to the caval wall. It is made of thermal aloe, consisting of nickel and titanium. The wires, which are straight in cool environment, reform at body temperature into a predetermined shape (Fig. 5) (25). It is easily inserted through the femoral or jugular route with a 7 French carrier and a 9 French sheath. Initial results of a multicenter trial showed an incidence of 1.8% recurrent PE and 9.7% IVC occlusion (47).

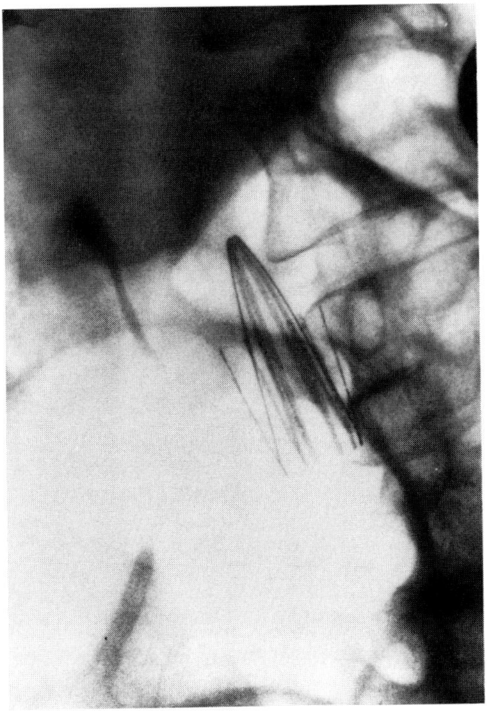

Figure 4 Inserted Vena Tech Filter. (From Ref. 25.)

E. Gunther Basket Filter (GBF)

This relatively new device (Fig. 1G) (23) is fairly easy to place percutaneously and can be removed within 24–48 h. It presents an advantage especially in patients with renal cancer that extends into the vein. Perioperative protection, therefore, is needed because the intraluminal part of the tumor and thrombus may dislodge and occlude the pulmonary circulation (48,49).

F. Amplatz Filter

This cone-shaped stainless steel filter (Fig. 1D) (23) is designed in such a way as to lie in the IVC in an inverted position, and it is retrievable. Although the latter can be considered an advantage, in actual practice there would be very few indications for it. This device is not generally available (11).

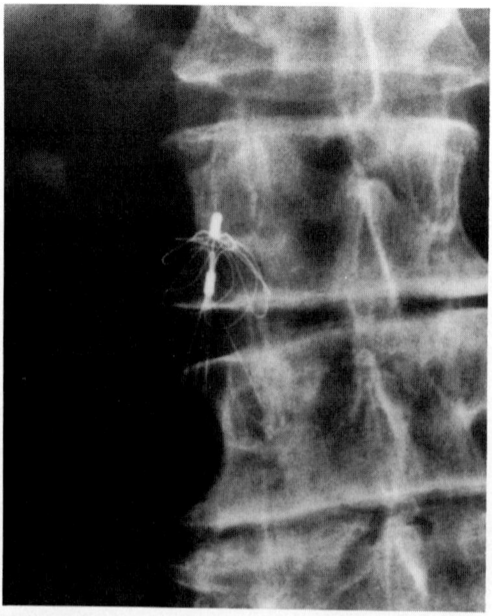

Figure 5 Postinsertion Nitinol Filter. (From Ref. 25.)

G. Hunter-Sessions Balloon (HSB)

This device is not a filter, but it is an inflatable sphere that is inserted transvenously to occlude completely the IVC. It can be used in anticoagulated patients. It prevents major recurrent thromboembolism, although it is associated with a fairly high incidence of postphlebitic syndrome. However, recurrent emboli may occur after the balloon placement through collateral circulation, which may be significant (50).

H. General Technical Principles

A good-quality venacavogram is necessary before the insertion of a device, to obtain information on (a) the IVC anatomy and the location of the renal veins; (b) possible presence of thrombus and its extent; (c) the caval diameter, which is essential for the selection of appropriate size and type device; and (d) presence of IVC anomalies and the degree of collateral circulation (51).

Careful percutaneous insertion is achieved with an open-ended, single-wall cut needle with an attached syringe to detect inadvertent arterial entry. The right transfemoral route is preferred because it is technically easier and better tolerated by the patient. The left femoral vein approach presents certain difficulties. The reasons are that the left iliac vein is compressed by its corresponding artery and the degree of its angulation into the IVC (52).

VI. Discussion—Future Research

There has been considerable difference of opinion as to the specialist best qualified to perform the procedures for IVC interruption. Comprehensive training of the physician is the most important parameter. Therefore, he or she may be a vascular surgeon, interventional radiologist, cardiologist, or vascular medicine specialist. A well-coordinated team that includes several specialists working in harmony is the most effective approach that benefits the patient. It also provides optimum learning exposure for the trainees.

Clear definition of the indications for IVC interruption is of obvious importance. There is general consensus on their use in patients on whom anticoagulants are contraindicated or have been ineffective. Many also agree that such an indication exists in iliofemoral thrombosis, especially when there is free-floating thrombus.

In a series of 84 patients, Magnant et al. (53) reported that filters were inserted because of contraindication to anticoagulants in 64%, anticoagulation failure in 25%, and preoperative prophylaxis in 11%. The underlying disease was lower extremity DVT in 50% and PE in 45%. Filters without documented thromboembolism were inserted in 5% of their patients. However, debate continues on the prophylactic role of these devices.

There has been a tendency during the last few years for more liberal application of filters, e.g., in patients with chronic neurological problems or following spine and hip surgery. Filters were also inserted in patients with disseminated cancer or multisystem organ failure. Their clinical value in such instances has been questioned (53). Careful assessment of the benefit/risk ratio is essential, and filters should only be inserted very selectively. The small size and easier placement of some devices, although advantageous, should not encourage a more liberal use beyond the otherwise well defined clinical indications.

None of the available devices fulfils all the criteria of "the ideal" filter. Highly desirable characteristics include easy percutaneous insertion, small and simple caliber release mechanism that is well-controlled, effective filtering without significant changes of flow, low cost, easy repositioning, biocompatible durable material, and nonferromagnetic properties for MRI compatibility. Assessment of each available device has to be based on these criteria. They could also contribute toward improving those already existing or in developing new ones.

In the present-day practice, selection of the appropriate filter requires consideration of a number of factors. Balance is to be maintained between their effectiveness in clot trapping and high IVC patency. Objective assessment of the relative merits and complication rate among the various devices is needed. There is at times discrepancy between in vitro and in vivo studies, e.g., on the significance of the KGF tilting tendency. Although in vitro studies showed major deficiencies when this becomes tilted, in vivo work in sheep did not confirm these findings (35,36).

Definitive conclusions from different clinical studies on the comparative merits of the available devices cannot be drawn accurately for several reasons. Indications for intervention are variable, e.g., in some recent series prophylaxis was the main reason for insertion of the filter. Another reason is that the follow-up is often based on different parameters and at times limited to clinical examination and/or telephone contacts. Appropriate follow-up investigations are necessary, as in patients suspected of having PE (54).

A device is selected according to the individual requirements of the patient. When full life expectancy is anticipated, a filter such as the GF, tested over a long period of time for durability and high IVC patency, is suitable. Because of the latter property, this is also indicated for suprarenal placement.

Retrievability is in principle a desirable quality, although in actual practice there are limited indications for it. Moreover, a filter with a satisfactory fixation is not easily retrievable. Even if this property is initially present, it is not maintained for long because the device becomes embedded within the residual organized thrombus and the neighboring tissues. Therefore, retrieval may damage the IVC intima. This filter is of course valuable for certain patients for whom it is only needed for a limited period of time, such as those with renal carcinoma that protrudes inside the IVC.

When the IVC is larger than 30 mm in diameter, there are two possible types of management. The BNF is suitable because it fits effectively in larger vena cavas up to 40 mm. Alternatively, a device can be placed in each of the two common iliac veins.

It is apparent that the SNF, because of its small (7 French) carrier and its 3-cm length, is particularly suitable for small femoral veins or when the distance between the renal and iliac veins is short.

When MRI is required to evaluate the status of the IVC and/or other neighboring structures, a device other than one made of stainless steel is used to avoid artifacts and poor imaging.

No device, even when carefully selected and correctly placed, can entirely eliminate the risk of recurrent embolization, which at times may originate from unconventional sites. Awareness of this possibility leads to appropriate investigations and results in better management. Sources of emboli may include the collateral circulation through the ovarian, spermatic, or epigastric veins. Superficial collaterals can develop through the wide-caliber gonadal veins that drain into the right renal vein and IVC. Emboli so formed cannot be controlled by most caval interruption procedures. They can also pass through an IVC interruption or develop at that site. In complete occlusion, collateral flow commonly takes place through central channels, the ascending lumbar and vertebral veins. Complex collaterals in the lumbar and pelvic plexuses do not allow passage of clinically significant emboli.

Duplication of the IVC can be a pathway for recurrent embolism following interruption. Emboli may also originate from the right heart, hepatic, renal, or upper extremity veins. Management depends on the source and extent of the thromboembolus as well as the general condition of the patient.

VII. Summary—Conclusions

Despite major advances in the prevention, detection, and management of DVT and PE, the morbidity and mortality still remain high. Inferior vena cava interruption is a valuable modality. The main indications are contraindication to anticoagulants, failure of anticoagulation, and extensive iliofemoral thrombosis with free-floating thrombus. For prophylaxis alone, their role is very limited.

The knowledge of older techniques of interruption, such as ligation, external clips, and the original filters, are not only of historical value but also because some of them are still in use in certain parts of the world.

Criteria for "the ideal" filter have been established. Although none of the available devices fulfills all of them, they are still valuable. Among the better known are the Kimray-Greenfield, Titanium Greenfield, Bird's Nest, LGM/Vena Tech, Simon-Nitinol, Gunther Basket, and the Hunter-Sessions Balloon device.

Selection of the appropriate filter is crucial and is based on the individual needs of each patient. The important parameters include the ability to retain major clots and high IVC patency as well as infrequent and minimal complications.

A well-coordinated team preferably consisting of a vascular surgeon, interventional radiologist, cardiologist, and vascular medicine specialist, all having been comprehensively and specifically trained in this area, is the most effective way to secure the best possible results for the patient. In addition, a team provides excellent learning experience for the trainees.

New randomized prospective studies are warranted to define exactly the role of the existing devices. They would also contribute toward the development of newer filters, even more effective and with fewer complications.

References

1. Tsapogas MJ, Flute PT, Cotton LT, et al. Lysis of experimental thrombi by streptokinase. Br J Surg 1962; 50:334–7.

2. Tsapogas MJ, Flute PT. Experimental thrombolysis with streptokinase and urokinase. Br Med Bull 1964; 20:223–6.
3. Tsapogas MJ. Effects of fibrinolytic agents on experimental and clinical thrombosis. J Clin Pathol 1964; 17:360–1.
4. Tsapogas MJ, Peabody RA, Wu KT, et al. Controlled study of thrombolytic therapy and deep vein thrombosis. Surgery 1973; 74:973–84.
5. Peabody RA, Halse T, Tsapogas MJ. Rapid method for preparation of human fibrinogen labeled with I^{125}. J Nucl Med 1973; 15:195–7.
6. Wu KT, Tsapogas MJ, Jordan FR. Prophylaxis of deep venous thrombosis by hydroxychloroquine sulfate and heparin. Surg Gynecol Obstet 1977; 145:714–7.
7. Benotti JR, Dalen ED. The natural history of pulmonary embolism. Clin Chest Med 1984; 5:403–10.
8. Consensus Conference: Prevention of venous thrombosis and pulmonary embolism. JAMA 1986; 256:744–9.
9. Tsapogas MJ, Miller R, Peabody RA, et al. Detection of post-operative venous thrombosis and effectiveness of prophylactic measures. Studies with fibrinogen I^{125} technique. Arch Surg 1970; 101:149–54.
10. Tsapogas MJ, Goussous H, Peabody RA, et al. Post-operative venous thrombosis and the effectiveness of prophylactic measures. Arch Surg 1971; 103:561–7.
11. Greenfield LJ, DeLucia A III. Endovascular therapy of venous thromboembolic disease. Surg Clin North Am 1992; 72:969–89.
12. Spencer FC. Experimental evaluation of partitioning of the inferior vena cava to prevent pulmonary embolism. Surg Forum 1960; 10:680–9.
13. Hunter J. Observation on inflammation of internal coat of veins. Trans Soc Improvement Med Chir Knowledge (London) 1793; 1:18.
14. Hoagland PM. Massive pulmonary embolus. In Goldhaber SZ, ed. Pulmonary Embolism and Deep venous Thrombosis. Philadelphia: WB Saunders Co, 1985:179.
15. Ochsner A, Ochsner JK, Saunders HS. Prevention of pulmonary embolism by caval ligation. Ann Surg 1970; 171:923.
16. De Weese MS, Hunter DC. A vena cava filter for the prevention of pulmonary emboli. Arch Surg 1963; 86:852–68.
17. Ravitch MM, Snodgrass E, McEnamy T, et al. Compartmentation of the vena cava with the mechanical stapler. Surg Gynecol Obstet 1966; 122:561.
18. Moretz WH, Rhode CM, Shepherd MH. Prevention of pulmonary emboli by partial occlusion of the inferior vena cava. Am Surg 1959; 25:617–26.
19. Greenfield LJ. Vena caval interruption and pulmonary embolism. Clin Chest Med 1984; 5:495–504.
20. Eichelter P, Schenk WG Jr. Prophylaxis of pulmonary embolism: A new experimental approach with initial results. Arch Surg 1968; 97:348.
21. Mansour M, Chang AE, Sindlar WF. Interruption of the inferior vena cava for the prevention of recurrent pulmonary embolism. Am Surg 1985; 51:375–9.
22. Mensoian JO, LoGerfo FW, Weitzman AF, et al. Clinical experience with the Mobin-Uddin vena cava umbrella filter. Arch Surg 1980; 115:1179–81.
23. Bergan JJ, Yao JST. Venous Disorders. Philadelphia: WB Saunders Co, 1991:556.
24. Messmer JM, Greenfield LJ. Greenfield caval filters: long term radiographic follow up study. Radiology 1985; 9:613–8.

25. Athanassoulis CA. Vena Cava filters. Personal collection. Harvard University, Cambridge, MA 1993.
26. Hye RJ, Mitchell AT, Dory CE, et al. Analysis of the transition to percutaneous placement of Greenfield filters. Arch Surg 1990; 125:1550–3.
27. Ramchandani P. Bilateral iliac vein filtration. An effective alternative to caval filtration in patients with Megacava. Arch Surg 1991; 126:390–3.
28. Greenfield LJ, Michna BA. Twelve-year clinical experience with the Greenfield vena cava filter. Surgery 1988; 104:706–12.
29. Geisinger MA, Zelch MG, Risius B. Recurrent pulmonary emboli after Greenfield filter placement. Radiology 1987; 165:383–4.
30. Gomez GA, Cutler BS, Wheeler HB. Transvenous interruption of the inferior vena cava. Surgery 1983; 93:612–9.
31. Cimochowski GE, Evans RG, Zarins CK, et al. Greenfield filter versus Mobin-Uddin umbrella. J Thorac Cardiovasc Surg 1980; 79:358–65.
32. Pais SO, Tobin KD. Percutaneous insertion of the Greenfield filter. AJR 1989; 152:933–8.
33. Tsapogas MJ. Venous thrombosis; Part II. Management. Ala J Med Sci 1987; 24:301–5.
34. Jones B, Fink JA, Donovan DL, et al. Analysis of benefit of anticoagulation after placement of Kimray-Greenfield filter. Surg Gynecol Obstet 1989; 169:400–2.
35. Katsamouris AA, Waltman AC, Delichatsios MA, et al. Inferior vena cava filters; in vitro comparison of clot-trapping and flow dynamics. Radiology 1988; 166:361–6.
36. Thompson BH, Cragg AH, Smith TP, et al. Thrombus-trapping efficiency of the Greenfield filter in vivo. Radiology 1989; 172:979–81.
37. Mewissen MW, Erickson SJ, Foley WD, et al. Thrombosis at venous insertion sites after inferior vena cava filter placement. Radiology 1989; 173:155–7.
38. Greenfield LJ, Cho KJ, Proctor M, et al. Results of a multicenter study of the modified hook-titanium Greenfield filter. J Vasc Surg 1991; 14:253–7.
39. Tsapogas MJ. Venous thrombosis Part I. Etiology, diagnosis and prevention. Ala J Med Sci 1987; 24:176–82.
40. Greenfield LJ, Savin MA. Comparison of titanium and stainless steel Greenfield vena cava filters. Surgery 1989; 106:820–8.
41. Greenfield LJ, Cho KJ, Pais SO, et al. Preliminary clinical experience with the titanium Greenfield vena caval filter. Arch Surg 1989; 124:657–9.
42. Greenfield LJ, Cho KJ, Tauscher JR. Evolution of hook design for fixation of the titanium Greenfield filter. J Vasc Surg 1990; 9:345–53.
43. Roehm JOF. The Bird's nest filter: a new percutaneous transcatheter inferior vena cava filter. J Vasc Surg 1984; 1:498–501.
44. Roehm JOF, Johnsrude IS, Barth MH, et al. The Bird's nest inferior vena cava filter; progress report. Radiology 1988; 168:745–9.
45. Awh MH, Taylor FC, Lu CT. Spontaneous fracture of a Vena-Tech inferior vena cava filter. AJR 1991; 157:177–8.
46. Ricco JB, Crochet D, Sebilotte P, et al. Percutaneous transvenous caval interruption with the LGM filter; early results of a multicenter trial. Ann Vasc Surg 1988; 3:242–7.

47. Grassi CJ. Inferior vena caval filters: analysis of five currently available devices. AJR 1991; 156:813–21.
48. Gunther RW, Schild H. Basket filter for prevention of pulmonary embolism. Semin Intervent Radiol 1986; 3:220–6.
49. Fobbe F, Dietzel M, Korth R, et al. Gunther vena cava filter; results and long term follow up. AJR 1988; 151:1031–4.
50. Hunter JA, DeLaria GA, Goldin MD, et al. Inferior vena cava interruption with the Hunter-Sessions balloon; 18 years' experience in 191 cases. J Vasc Surg 1989; 10:450–6.
51. Grassi CJ, Goldhaber SZ. Interruption of the inferior vena cava for prevention of pulmonary embolism. Herz 1989; 14:182–91.
52. Rose BS, Simon DC, Hess ML, et al. Percutaneous transfemoral placement of the Kimray-Greenfield filter. Radiology 1987; 165:373–6.
53. Magnant JG, Walsh DB, Juravsky LI, Cronenwett JL. Current use of inferior vena cava filters. J Vasc Surg 1992; 16:701–6.
54. Tsapogas MJ. Pulmonary Embolism Part I: incidence, pathophysiology and diagnosis. Ala J Med Sci 1987; 165:373–6.

21

Summary and Remarks

HENRI DENOLIN

Hôpital Universitaire Saint-Pierre
Brussels, Belgium

I. Introduction

Pulmonary embolism (PE) usually results from a venous thrombus coming loose at its point of origin and reaching the pulmonary arterial circulation through the venous system. Other materials may cause embolism, such as fat, gases, parasites, and foreign bodies, but those are rare occurrences, and so they are not discussed in this book.

Pulmonary embolism (PE) continues to confront the clinician and pathophysiologist with complex problems, and it was in the hope of throwing some light on such issues that a meeting was held late in Geneva in 1991 to debate the several aspects of the disease. The reports presented at that meeting constitute the subject matter of this volume.

Numerous reports emphasize the frequent occurrence of PE and the sizable mortality deriving from it. Yet, available figures are far from clear-cut or at all dependable. For one thing, PE usually represents a *complication* of a background disease that predisposes to venous thrombosis (major surgery, malignancy, overweight, contraceptive medication, prolonged immobilization, etc.), sometimes themselves being responsible for the patient's death. For another, most cases of PE are diagnosed only clinically—and we know how little value that approach can have. Accordingly, there is a very great need for extensive, diversified, and well-structured epidemiological studies in view of developing more effective strategies for PE prevention. In that respect, we must gratefully acknowledge the fact that in very recent times some important epidemiological information has been contributed from unexpected quarters such as China and the Republic of Cameroun (see pertinent chapters in this book).

The anatomical data reported by Wagenvoort illustrate the great variability of embolus size and evolution, in turn accounting for the variability of clinical pictures and signs over time. At the same time, such considerations emphasize the need for detecting any permanent pulmonary hypertension. In some patients surviving a PE, indeed, embolus material fails to dissolve in time and progresses to create a state of chronic thromboembolic pulmonary hypertension that may be amenable to surgical correction (endarterectomy of endothelialized thrombi), with reported mortality rates of 13% and falling, and definitely brilliant long-term results.

The *clinical diagnosis* of PE is most unreliable. The more common symptoms of acute pulmonary embolization are dyspnea and pleural pain—both being anything but specific. Yet these two symptoms must raise the suspicion of PE, especially in situations that may invite thrombosis like orthopedic, gynecological, or major abdominal surgery, or any of the favoring conditions mentioned earlier.

Because in the great majority of cases, embolus material originates in the veins of the lower limbs, a careful study of leg veins is mandatory. In that respect, we now have noninvasive diagnostic tools that are both sensitive and specific, as explained in an article by Goldhaber and Morpurgo (1) of the WHO/ISFC Task Force. The methods include compression ultrasonography, impedance plethysmography, and Doppler imaging. While a positive diagnosis of proximal venous thrombosis of the legs does not necessarily mean or prove that the patient has PE, the therapeutical implications of the two diseases are the same, and a contributory diagnosis may sometimes obviate the need for more invasive studies. Conversely, PE cannot be excluded when a negative noninvasive or even venographic leg examination is elicited.

Because the clinical diagnosis of PE is unreliable, several tests have been proposed for validating it; none of these are perfect, and all offer various degrees of sensitivity and specificity.

Such tests include the following:

The pulmonary ventilation-perfusion scan. As clearly explained in Dalen's text, a "nondiagnostic" scan does not rule out PE. Palla and Giuntini stress the interest of a plain chest X-ray picture, both in association with scanning and as a sole, time-honored procedure.

Echocardiography may reveal the degree of dilatation of the right heart and tricuspid valve regurgitation; in some cases it may even reveal a thrombus lodged in the right atrium or ventricle—more rarely in the inferior vena cava. The value of transesophageal echocardiography in the diagnosis of PE remains undecided.

Electrocardiography has been explored in numerous studies for many years, but the method is now considered to be poorly sensitive and far from specific in the diagnosis of PE. Only a massive pulmonary embolization may produce some characteristic evidence expressing severe right ventricle overload. Other than that, electrocardiography remains of value in the differential diagnosis between PE and acute myocardial infarction.

Arterial blood gas analysis is of limited diagnostic value because it lacks specificity; it may, however, prove useful in the follow-up of PE patients.

Much effort has been expended to find a blood test at once easy to perform and diagnostically serviceable, such as we have available for myocardial infarction. Elevated D-dimer assays may be found in PE but also in other disorders; a normal D-dimer assay, on the other hand, does not disprove PE. Ideally, the diagnosis of PE should be based on one or two sufficiently sensitive and specific tests, but none of those just named satisfies both requirements. In fact, the only method capable of yielding objective evidence of PE is angiography—lamentably an invasive procedure and one that calls for adequate equipment and expert handling. In a very recent article, Oudkerk et al. (2) have explored the cost:benefit ratios of different strategies used for diagnosing PE. They estimate that the best single method is pulmonary angiography, but lung perfusion-ventilation scintigraphy and Doppler sonography for the detection of deep vein thrombosis of the legs may cut down the proportion of patients needing pulmonary angiography by as much as 40% or 50%. On the other hand, in a recent article published in *Cardiologia*, Morpurgo (3) argued that it made no sense to look for a rigid algorithm whereby to assess patients suspected to have PE because of the protean character of the disorder, and more so because most of the tests proposed may not be available and/or feasible at all times.

Other diagnostic methods are currently being investigated, one being nuclear magnetic resonance, but they stand in need of validation as well as standardization.

II. The Prevention and Treatment of Pulmonary Embolism

It is often easier and less expensive to prevent complications than to diagnose and treat them when they occur—a rule most apposite in the case of venous thrombosis and PE.

Several factors may influence the choice of preventive and therapeutic methods: thus, the nature of underlying disease, the degree and duration of immobilization, the patient's age and tolerance of anticoagulants; and in the case of PE, severity of the pulmonary accident in the individual case.

The prevention of venous thrombosis, in turn, comprises the gentle touch in surgery, the use of elastic stockings, and treatment with low molecular weight heparin. In the presence of massive PE, one should consider recourse to thrombolytic drugs or even to surgical embolectomy.

Current therapeutic resources are indeed manifold—but here, too, there is no way to propose just one and the same approach for all cases because of the capricious evolution of venous thrombosis and its complications. All we can do is formulate a few general recommendations. First of all, we must suspect PE or consider its likelihood in a number of disease conditions, particularly when suddenly compounded by new symptoms. Next, once a PE is suspected, no stone should be left unturned to confirm or disprove the diagnosis—lest the patient be needlessly exposed to prolonged, potentially dangerous anticoagulant, or fibrinolytic treatment, or conversely be deprived of the same, direly needed treatment.

If the patient's hemodynamic status is not too worrisome, it will be wise to wait for diagnostic confirmation before starting anticoagulant or thrombolytic therapy. As Duroux (4) puts it tersely in his preface to the book of Simonneau and Huet, *Embolie pulmonaire et thrombose veineuse profonde* "thromboembolic disease is underestimated, underdiagnosed, and undertreated."

New diagnostic methods should be developed and evaluated. Physicians should be better informed in matters of prevention and actual treatment. And patients should be grouped whenever possible into hospital centers specializing in this area of medicine, so as to afford maximal accumulation of data where they will do the most good.

References

1. Goldhaber SZ, Morpurgo M. Diagnosis, treatment and prevention of pulmonary embolism. JAMA 1992; 268:1721–33.
2. Oudkerk M, Van Beek, EJR, Van Dutton WLJ, Büller HR. Cost-effective analysis of various strategies in the diagnostic management of pulmonary embolism. Arch Intern Med 1993; 153:947–54.
3. Morpurgo M. Do we really need an algorithm for the diagnostic work-up of a patient with suspected pulmonary embolism? Cardiologia 1992; 37:383–4.
4. Duroux P. Preface. In: Simonneau G. and Huet. Embolie pulmonaire et thrombose veineuse profonde. Paris: Masson, 1990.

AUTHOR INDEX

Italic numbers give the page on which the complete reference is listed.

C

E

F

G

H

I

J

K

L

M

N

O

P

S

X

Y

Z

SUBJECT INDEX

D

F

G

J

K

L

M

N

O

P

R

S

T